Optical Imaging
for Biomedical and
Clinical Applications

T0221416

Optical Imaging for Biomedical and Clinical Applications

Edited by
Ahmad Fadzil Mohamad Hani and Dileep Kumar

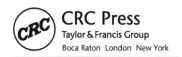

CRC Press
Taylor & Francis Group
Boca Raton London New York

CRC Press is an imprint of the
Taylor & Francis Group, an **informa** business

MATLAB® is a trademark of The MathWorks, Inc. and is used with permission. The MathWorks does not warrant the accuracy of the text or exercises in this book. This book's use or discussion of MATLAB® software or related products does not constitute endorsement or sponsorship by The MathWorks of a particular pedagogical approach or particular use of the MATLAB® software.

CRC Press
Taylor & Francis Group
6000 Broken Sound Parkway NW, Suite 300
Boca Raton, FL 33487-2742

First issued in paperback 2019

© 2018 by Taylor & Francis Group, LLC
CRC Press is an imprint of Taylor & Francis Group, an Informa business

No claim to original U.S. Government works

ISBN-13: 978-0-4987-5037-0 (hbk)
ISBN-13: 978-0-367-87571-8 (pbk)

This book contains information obtained from authentic and highly regarded sources. Reasonable efforts have been made to publish reliable data and information, but the author and publisher cannot assume responsibility for the validity of all materials or the consequences of their use. The authors and publishers have attempted to trace the copyright holders of all material reproduced in this publication and apologize to copyright holders if permission to publish in this form has not been obtained. If any copyright material has not been acknowledged please write and let us know so we may rectify in any future reprint.

Except as permitted under U.S. Copyright Law, no part of this book may be reprinted, reproduced, transmitted, or utilized in any form by any electronic, mechanical, or other means, now known or hereafter invented, including photocopying, microfilming, and recording, or in any information storage or retrieval system, without written permission from the publishers.

For permission to photocopy or use material electronically from this work, please access www.copyright.com (http://www.copyright.com/) or contact the Copyright Clearance Center, Inc. (CCC), 222 Rosewood Drive, Danvers, MA 01923, 978-750-8400. CCC is a not-for-profit organization that provides licenses and registration for a variety of users. For organizations that have been granted a photocopy license by the CCC, a separate system of payment has been arranged.

Trademark Notice: Product or corporate names may be trademarks or registered trademarks, and are used only for identification and explanation without intent to infringe.

Library of Congress Cataloging–in–Publication Data

Names: Kumar, Dileep, 1985- author. | Hani, Ahmad Fadzil Mohamad, author.
Title: Optical imaging for biomedical and clinical applications / Dileep Kumar & Ahmad Fadzil Mohamad Hani
Description: Boca Raton : Taylor & Francis / CRC Press, 2018. | Includes bibliographical references.
Identifiers: LCCN 2017028543| ISBN 9781498750370 (hardback : alk. paper) | ISBN 9781315368351 (ebook)
Subjects: | MESH: Optical Imaging--methods | Image Enhancement | Skin Diseases--diagnostic imaging | Eye Diseases--diagnostic imaging
Classification: LCC R857.O6 | NLM WN 195 | DDC 616.07/54--dc23
LC record available at https://lccn.loc.gov/2017028543

Visit the Taylor & Francis Web site at
http://www.taylorandfrancis.com

and the CRC Press Web site at
http://www.crcpress.com

Dedication

This book was made possible with the unwavering support of all authors of the book chapters; former students—Leena, Dr. Hermawan, Dr. Lila, Dr. Hanung, Toufique, Aamir Shahzad; colleagues—Dr. Naufal, Dr. Norashikin, Dr. Nidal, Dr. Aamir, Dr. Ibrahima, Professor Fabrice; and collaborators—Dr. Norashikin, Dr. Suraiya, Dr. Adawiyah, Dr. Felix Yap, Dr. Nor Fariza. Their dedication, perseverance and undying search for answers during the course of the research work and clinical studies have led to this piece of work. This book is dedicated to them.

Contents

Preface

We are motivated to compile the findings of several research and pre-clinical observational studies at Hospital Kuala Lumpur and Hospital Selayang that investigated the use of optical imaging techniques in dermatology for monitoring of skin pigmentation diseases such as vitiligo and in ophthalmology to enhance colour fundus images system in diagnosing retina-related eye sicknesses, such as diabetic retinopathy.

Optical imaging is an effective medical imaging technique for in vitro and in vivo applications. It is yet a vast field, from the understanding of effectiveness of the technique to the analysis of the images. It involves biomedical optics, photon propagation in tissues, bioluminescence and fluorescence as well as hardware components that are required such as light sources, filters and detectors. The discussion also includes various optical microscopic imaging techniques along with the whole animal body imaging technique specially used to image small animals.

Investigating the optical characteristics of ulcer tissues based on their histology and cellular composition to detect their corresponding content in ulcer colour images is central in developing algorithm that is able to identify granulation tissue regions on the exterior of ulcers to provide an objective assessment of the healing condition of chronic ulcers. This is very significant in detecting early stages of ulcer healing especially where granulation tissue is spreading slowly over the ulcer surface and cannot be detected visually. This work essentially utilises the optical imaging technique to characterise haemoglobin pigments and determining its content within and below the visible surface of ulcers. Identified regions of haemoglobin distribution can then be utilised as image markers to identify areas of granulation tissue indicating the ulcer healing progression and reflects on the efficacy of the ulcer management and treatment.

The physician's global assessment of skin pigmentary skin disorders such as vitiligo, requires visual inspection but pigmentation changes due to treatment and takes 3 to 6 months to discern visually by the dermatologist. Therapeutic responses of vitiligo treatments can be different from patient to patient and are typically very slow and time consuming. Segmentation of vitiligo lesion areas can be performed after the separation process that produces skin images due to melanin and haemoglobin only. The repigmentation progression due to treatment of the lesion areas is measured objectively. Measurements generate equivalent PGA scores that are useful to physicians in evaluating the efficacy of the treatment in a shorter time period for example in 6 weeks.

In colour fundus images, the low contrast between the blood vessels and the varying contrast of its surrounding background makes it visually difficult to determine the retinal vasculature accurately. In addition, fundus images are found to have both multiplicative and additive noise, and can contain artefacts. This contrast problem can be overcome by using fundus fluorescein angiography (FFA) that creates fundus images of high contrast; however, because of its invasive nature, injecting contrast agent is not a preferred method. RETICA, a non-invasive image improvement scheme is developed and addresses the issue of low and varying contrast image, through RETINEX for contrast normalisation and ICA for contrast enhancement.

With TDCE-RETICA, the presence of noise in the fundus image is also addressed. The novelty of this technique is that the noise level has been effectively reduced by TDCE. RETICA with TDCE provides a mechanism to reduce noise and resolve low and varied contrast in colour fundus images and provides an efficient and non-invasive manner for retinal fundus image analysis and interpretation. It is a practical non-invasive alternative to the invasive fluorescein angiogram for retinal imaging and further analysis and interpretation for diagnosis and monitoring of vision threatening complications.

It is a difficult task to localise suitable veins in patients having certain physiological characteristics such as dark skin tone, deep veins and the presence of scars, tattoos or hair on the skin. To overcome the problem of difficult venous access, several techniques can be used. As NIR imaging is considered to be the most suitable among the techniques in terms of usability, cost and efficiency, the optimisation of NIR illumination in order to overcome the difficulty of veins localisation for different skin tone subjects is presented. Hyperspectral venous image data acquired from 252 subjects, arrived at an optimised range of illumination wavelengths. It was concluded that the wavelength range of 800–850 nm is the optimum range for illumination in NIR imaging for all skin tone subjects.

We hope the book addresses problems from the medical sciences to engineering principles transcending disciplines and professions.

Ahmad Fadzil Mohamad Hani, FASc, FIEM, PEng, PhD
Dileep Kumar, PhD
Centre for Intelligent Signal and Imaging Research (CISIR)
Universiti Teknologi PETRONAS
Bandar Seri Iskandar, Perak.

MATLAB® is a registered trademark of The MathWorks, Inc. For product information, please contact:

The MathWorks, Inc.
3 Apple Hill Drive
Natick, MA 01760-2098 USA Tel: 508 647 7000
Fax: 508-647-7001
E-mail: info@mathworks.com
Web: www.mathworks.com

Acknowledgements

We would like to acknowledge Universiti Teknologi PETRONAS for the financial, laboratory and programming support at CISIR (Centre for Intelligent Signal and Imaging Research). We also acknowledge the various university internal funds and external grants received from the Malaysian Ministry of Science, Technology and Innovation, and the Ministry of Higher Education for the research work. We would like to thank our collaborators; dermatologists from the Department of Dermatology, Hospital Kuala Lumpur and ophthalmologists from the Department of Ophthalmology, Hospital Selayang.

Acknowledgements

Editors

Professor Ahmad Fadzil Mohamad Hani is an expert in the area of image processing and computer vision. He graduated with a BSc (1st Class Honours) in electronic engineering in 1983, earned his MSc in telematics in 1984 and PhD in image processing in 1991 from the University of Essex, UK. He has been actively involved in machine vision and medical imaging research since the early 1990s. His research activities range from fundamental signal and image processing to pattern recognition to developing vision and image analysis applications in the biomedical imaging area such as in retinal vasculature imaging for grading severity of diabetic retinopathy and digital analysis leading to objective assessment for treatment efficacy of ulcer wounds and psoriasis lesions, and bio-optics for skin pigmentation analysis. His current research challenges are developing new analysis techniques for early osteoarthritis and drug addiction using MRI (magnetic resonance imaging)/MRS (magnetic resonance spectroscopy), and neuroergonomics using fNIRS (functional near-infrared spectroscopy). He has authored over 200 research articles in journals and conference proceedings, granted several patents and won several awards for his work. He is a senior professor and heads the Centre for Intelligent Signal & Imaging Research (CISIR), a Ministry of Higher Education Higher Institution Centre of Excellence at Universiti Teknologi PETRONAS.

Professor Fadzil is a Fellow of the Academy of Sciences, Malaysia and a Fellow of Institution of Engineers Malaysia. He is a registered professional engineer with Board of Engineers, Malaysia and a senior member of the Institution of Electrical & Electronic Engineers Inc. He is a member of the Governing Board of the International Neuroinformatics Coordinating Facility (INCF). In industry, he is a member of the Board of Directors of ViTrox Corporation Bhd., an R&D and public-listed company that develops and manufactures automated vision inspection systems. He is also a member of the Board of Directors of Prince Court Medical Centre, Kuala Lumpur.

Dr. Dileep Kumar is an expert in the area of biomedical imaging, focusing on the development of image processing/analysis methods that are incorporated into decision support systems/tools. He graduated with a

Bachelor of Technology (BTech) in information technology from Uttar Pradesh Technical University (UPTU), Lucknow, India, in 2006, earned his master of technology (MTech) from Indian Institute of Information Technology, Allahabad, India in 2008 and PhD in electrical engineering from the Universiti Teknologi PETRONAS, Malaysia in 2014. His current research interests include medical image analysis, image processing, pattern recognition, medical imaging, medical physics, bioengineering and biomedical systems. In particular, quantitative analysis of biomedical image/signal data, technological development for the acquisition of biomedical images and development of new algorithm/techniques have been a focusing point of his research. He is currently working as research scientist/manager at the Centre for Intelligent Signal & Imaging Research (CISIR), a Ministry of Higher Education Higher Institution Centre of Excellence at Universiti Teknologi PETRONAS. Dr. Dileep has published more than 25 scientific articles; obtained 2 IPR's, filed 6 patents and one of his patents was granted in 2015. He has received 'Best Researcher Award' (1 award/year) at Universiti Teknologi PETRONAS in 2015, 'Need Based Award' by Osteoarthritis Research Society International (OARSI) in 2013, 'Young Investigator Collaborative Research Award' in the year 2015 by OARSI (one of the six recipients from all over the world and the first from SEA) and 'Young Engineers Award', given by the Institution of Engineers, India in 2010 (one of the three recipients). He has been actively involved in the peer-review process of several high-ranked journals, serving as an associate editor for the *SM Journal of Orthopedics*, served in the Technical Program Committee in various international conferences and occupies in the executive committee board of professional organisations.

Contributors

Leena Arshad
Centre for Intelligent Signal and
  Imaging Research
Department of Electrical and
  Electronic Engineering
Universiti Teknologi PETRONAS
Malaysia

Ibrahima Faye
Centre for Intelligent Signal and
  Imaging Research
Department of Fundamental Studies
Universiti Teknologi PETRONAS
Malaysia

Ahmad Fadzil Mohamad Hani
Centre for Intelligent Signal and
  Imaging Research
Department of Electrical and
  Electronic Engineering
Universiti Teknologi PETRONAS
Malaysia

and

SIRIM Tech Venture Sdn Bhd
Selangor
Malaysia

Suraiya H. Hussein
Damansara Specialist Hospital
Damansara Utama
Petaling Jaya
Malaysia

Lila Iznita Izhar
Centre for Intelligent Signal and
  Imaging Research
Department of Electrical and
  Electronic Engineering
Universiti Teknologi
  PETRONAS
Malaysia

Nidal Kamel
Centre for Intelligent Signal and
  Imaging Research
Department of Electrical and
  Electronic Engineering
Universiti Teknologi
  PETRONAS
Malaysia

Dileep Kumar
Centre for Intelligent Signal and
  Imaging Research
Department of Electrical and
  Electronic Engineering
Universiti Teknologi
  PETRONAS
Malaysia

and

Department of Psychology
University of Otago
Dunedin
New Zealand

Aamir Saeed Malik
Centre for Intelligent Signal and
    Imaging Research
Department of Electrical and
    Electronic Engineering
Universiti Teknologi PETRONAS
Malaysia

Fabrice Meriaudeau
Centre for Intelligent Signal and
    Imaging Research
Department of Electrical and
    Electronic Engineering
Universiti Teknologi PETRONAS
Malaysia

Nor Fariza Ngah
Department of Opthalmology
Selayang Hospital
Selangor
Malaysia

Hanung Nugroho
Department of Information
    Technology and Electrical
    Engineering
Gadjah Mada University
Yogyakarta
DIY
Indonesia

Hermawan Nugroho
Faculty of Engineering
Computing and Science
Swinburne University of
    Technology Sarawak
Malaysia

Mohamad Naufal Mohamad Saad
Centre for Intelligent Signal and
    Imaging Research
Department of Electrical and
    Electronic Engineering
Universiti Teknologi PETRONAS
Malaysia

Aamir Shahzad
Centre for Intelligent Signal and
    Imaging Research
Department of Electrical and
    Electronic Engineering
Universiti Teknologi
    PETRONAS
Malaysia

and

Department of Electrical and
    Electronic Engineering
COMSATS Institute of Information
    Technology
Islamabad
Pakistan

Norashikin Shamsudin
Department of Medicine
Faculty of Medicine and Health
    Science
Universiti Putra Malaysia
Serdang
Malaysia

Toufique Ahmed Soomro
Centre for Intelligent Signal and
    Imaging Research
Department of Electrical and
    Electronic Engineering
Universiti Teknologi
    PETRONAS
Malaysia

Norashikin Yahya
Centre for Intelligent Signal and
    Imaging Research
Department of Electrical and
    Electronic Engineering
Universiti Teknologi PETRONAS
Malaysia

chapter one

Introduction to optical imaging

Dileep Kumar and Ahmad Fadzil Mohamad Hani

Contents

1.1 Introduction

Medical imaging has brought revolutionary changes to the medical diagnostic field. In medical radiology, various imaging modalities are being used to study the biological view of different anatomical and molecular structures of human and animals for diagnostics [1]. Various imaging

1

modalities, such as x-ray, ultrasound and computed tomography (CT) that work based on radiography for structural tissue visualisation are widely used for imaging internal tissue organs, whereas magnetic resonance imaging (MRI), positron emission tomography (PET), single-photon emission computed tomography (SPECT) and optical imaging that work based on radiology are used for structural and molecular change measurements. The mechanisms in these modalities, for example, x-rays and CT involve radiation of x-rays to see through soft tissues [2]. In the case of ultrasound, being an anatomical modality, it involves sound waves to measure different anatomical structures of internal organs [3]. MRI involves interaction of RF (radio frequency) energy with underlying tissues to obtain structural and physiological features [4]. PET and SPECT falls under nuclear imaging and these modalities are being used to measure chemical changes in tissue using radioactive tracers [5]. Optical imaging uses the visible light spectrum of electromagnetic radiation and its interaction with internal tissues to evaluate molecular changes [6]. Each of the above modality has its own advantages and limitations. A comparison of different imaging modalities is given in Table 1.1.

Although most imaging modalities are able to visualise internal tissues not all modalities are able to measure molecular changes associated with internal organs in humans and animals. Molecular changes in underlying internal tissues can be visualised using MRI, PET, SPECT and optical imaging techniques. However, imaging modalities such as

Table 1.1 Comparison between different medical imaging techniques

Modality	Soft tissue contrast	Resolution	Penetration level	Nonionizing radiation	Data acquisition	Cost
X-ray imaging	Poor	Excellent	Organ-tissue	No	Fast	Low
Ultrasound (US) imaging	Good	Good	Organ-tissue	Yes	Fast	Low
X-ray CT	Good	Excellent	Organ-tissue	No	Slow	Moderate
MRI and its derivatives	Excellent	Excellent	Organ-tissue	Yes	Slow	High and very high
PET	Excellent	Low	Tissue-cellular-molecular	No	Slow	Very high
SPECT	Excellent	Low	Tissue-cellular	No	Slow	Very high
Optical imaging	Excellent	Moderate	Tissue-cellular-molecular	Yes	Fast	Low

PET and SPECT involve the use of contrast agent or radioactive tracers that make these modalities invasive. Nuclear imaging modalities are widely used for animal imaging in preclinical environment [7]. MRI has the potential to visualise internal tissues as well as measure molecular changes corresponding to the internal tissues in the body. However, MRI for the measurement of chemical changes requires contrast enhance agents that is injected prior to MR (magnetic resonance) scanning in subjects [8]. So far, optical imaging modalities using visible, ultraviolet (UV) and infrared light and the special properties of photons are noninvasive and have proven to be effective in visualising details of internal tissues and organs as small as cells and molecules level. It also takes advantage of various colors of light to visualise and measure several properties of tissue at the same time while other modalities are unable to do so [6].

Optical imaging techniques can be broadly classified as bioluminescence imaging and fluorescence imaging [9]. Bioluminescence imaging is used for imaging molecules in small animals where the light is emitted into living organisms. The discovery of fluorescence and fluorescence microscopy has been instrumental in imaging the single-cell structures at the microscopic levels with the help of microscopic lenses. Fluorescent images are obtained using a light source of specific wavelength to excite the targeted molecule, which in turn emits light of longer wavelength than absorbed. This emitted light is used to generate fluorescent optical images. Optical imaging techniques being investigated meet the challenges and improvement in molecular imaging in preclinical examination and patient concern. Combination of targeted molecules in vivo and optical contrast agents imaging sensitivity are driven in parts for molecular imaging in order to emphasise an optical imaging systems [10]. By combining optical imaging techniques such as bioluminescence imaging and fluorescence with near-infrared (NIR) spectrum, the signal-to-background ratio for detecting specific molecular signals can be increased and similarly can be achieved with other molecular imaging modalities. In advanced cases, a fundamentally simplified gene expression imaging is produced using bioluminescent and fluorescent proteins that act as synthesised optical active biomarkers. It is also noted that optical imaging with its advancements can now be used in clinical practices for some applications and it is widely investigated for future research directions toward its application in clinics.

In this chapter, biomedical optics, photon propagation in tissues, bioluminescence and fluorescence are discussed followed by the parameters and components required for optical imaging such as light sources, filters, and detectors. In addition, microscopic imaging techniques for whole animal body imaging using optical imaging are discussed.

1.2 Biomedical optics

1.2.1 Background on photon propagation

In optical imaging, electromagnetic radiation ranging from 400 to 700 nm, referred to as the visible light spectrum, is used to produce images through microscopy, endoscopy and colonoscopy for biomedical applications [11]. The range of spectrum can be extended to the soft UV (short wavelengths) and NIR (long wavelengths) ranges in order to perform advanced optical imaging such as fluorescence and multispectral imaging. Unlike x-rays with wavelengths ranging from 0.01 to 10 nm, which are able to penetrate deep through tissues, visible light spectrum used in optical imaging interacts with tissues to a certain depth. Light interaction is defined in terms of reflection, refraction, diffusion, interference propagations, etc. Parameterisation of optical photon propagation is in terms of total emission or reflection within a solid angle.

Whenever a photon beam is incident on biological tissue, scattering or absorption phenomenon is observed and can be measured in terms of scattering coefficient, μ_s and absorption coefficient, μ_a. This is referred to as the transport coefficient (also termed as extinction coefficient or total interaction coefficient) and is given by

$$\mu_t = \mu_s + \mu_a \tag{1.1}$$

For biological tissues (also considered as turbid medium), the absorption coefficient is insignificant compared to scattering coefficient, that is, $\mu_a \ll \mu_s$; thus, the transport coefficient, $\mu_t = \mu_s$. If the photons undergo several scattering events, then the scattering coefficient is reduced as expressed by

$$\mu_s' = \mu_s(1 - g) \tag{1.2}$$

Here, g is the scattering anisotropic coefficient, which is typically in the range of 0.8–1.

Absorption coefficient is defined as the probability of photon absorption in a medium per unit path length. The reciprocal of absorption coefficient is called the mean absorption length. Optical parameters for the biological tissues are wavelength-dependent. For example, different layers of skin have different absorption coefficients with respect to the wavelength of optical photon beam, as shown in Figure 1.1.

The scattering coefficient, μ_s, is defined as the probability of photon scattering in a medium per unit path length. Biological tissues typically have a scattering coefficient of 100 cm^{-1}. The inverse of μ_s is the scattering mean free path (MFP). Biological structure interaction with light leads

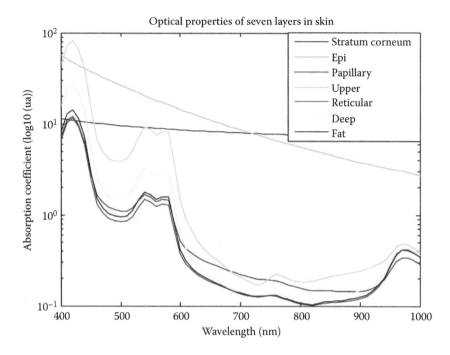

Figure 1.1 Wavelength vs. absorption coefficient for seven layers of skin. (Adapted from A. P. Dhawan, B. D'Alessandro, and X. Fu, *Biomedical Engineering, IEEE Reviews* in, vol. 3, pp. 69–92, 2010.)

to optical scattering ranging between whole cells and membrane [11]. Scattering of light is inversely proportional to the wavelengths but more precisely it remains comparatively stable in the visible range spectrum. The MFP is given in terms of scattering and absorption coefficients as reciprocal of transport coefficient as expressed by

$$MFP = \frac{1}{\mu_t} \tag{1.3}$$

With, $\mu_t = \mu_s + \mu_a$ and $\mu_a \ll \mu_s$,

$$MFP = \frac{1}{\mu_s} \tag{1.4}$$

Transport TMFP in terms of μ_s' for which the beam has undergone several scattering is expressed by

$$TMFP = \frac{1}{\mu_s'} \tag{1.5}$$

This generally holds for most tissues assuming that scattering is dominant over absorption, that is, $\mu_a \ll \mu_s'$. Therefore, the relationship between two parameters is given as $MFP = TMFP\,(1 - g)$; higher values of g increases forward scattering of light with longer duration to diffuse, leading to in-depth penetration using microscopic technique [12].

1.2.2 Fluorescence and bioluminescence phenomenon

Fluorescence is a phenomenon in which a molecule emits light when it returns to the ground state after being excited by an external light source [13]. Light produced by the molecule while relaxing to the ground state is of a longer wavelength relative to the wavelength of the excitation light. The duration of time for which the molecule is in excitation state is considered as the lifetime of the molecule. The material's ability of absorbing light photons of a particular wavelength and entering into excitation state and emitting the light of longer wavelength while returning to ground state is called the fluorescence property of the material. The fluorescence process can be divided into three steps: (1) excitation of molecule to new state by an external light source of specific wavelength within certain femtoseconds, (2) vibrational relaxation state in the excited mode for certain picoseconds and (3) molecule emitting light photons at a longer wavelength while returning to the ground state, which requires some nanoseconds [13]. The entire molecular fluorescence lifetime from excitation to relaxing to ground state is measured in billionths of a second. Such phenomenon is used by many of the fluorescent microscopic imaging devices for optical imaging of the biological tissues.

Bioluminescence is the phenomenon of bio-organisms producing light by the enzymatic reaction of a luciferase enzyme with its substrate luciferin. This luciferase enzyme is obtained from a firefly, which is a natural source of luciferase and is widely used in bioluminescence process to measure molecular changes in tissues of small animals. Luciferin is injected into a small animal and passes through blood tissues including the brain and placenta causing emissions of light from the molecules of small animals. The emitted light reaches its peak after 10–12 min and loses its intensity slowly over 60 min [10]. This time frame taken to lose emitted light intensity is sufficient to capture microscopic images of these molecular tissues in small animals. There are many natural sources of luciferase enzyme from other organisms that produce light of different wavelengths possibly leading to different colors such as red, green, blue, etc. [10].

1.3 Optical imaging hardware

An optical imaging system consists of three main components: (1) light source that is being emitted into tissues and reflected in the form of images, (2) filters form an integral part of optical imaging system that generally removes any artefacts produced during acquisition, and (3) optical detectors or photon detectors as the source component required to detect the optical beams that is being reflected from light source after filtration. The following subsections describe the three components of an optical imaging system.

1.3.1 Light sources

Light sources for an optical imaging technique can be of any form but the choice of a light source depends on the type of application. For biological applications, the light source for optical imaging should be predictable, stable, measurable and reliable [14]. It should also be adjustable to appropriate wavelengths, beam size and intensity for specific applications. The most commonly used light sources for optical imaging in biomedical applications are lasers (gas and solid state), broadband lamps that are capable of providing UV to NIR range of wavelengths and light-emitting diodes (LEDs) [15].

1.3.1.1 Broadband lamps

Most commonly available broadband light sources are high-pressure arc lamps and incandescent lamps. UV to NIR (200–1000 nm) intense broadband emission can be obtained from high-pressure arc lamps. These lamps typically use xenon, mercury or mercury–xenon gases. These lamps are to be handled with utmost care because of their explosive nature. Xenon lamp has strong UV output while incandescent lamps cover the visible range to NIR range. Xenon and incandescent lamps are the simplest light sources and commonly used in quartz tungsten halogen lamp. The latest available broadband light sources are supercontinuum light sources, which generate light through propagation of high-power pulse via a nonlinear media. Most supercontinuum light sources can generate huge wattages of optical power in a broad wavelength range from visible to NIR [15].

1.3.1.2 Light emitting diodes

LEDs are solid-state light sources based on semiconductors of p- and n-type in a p–n junction, which emit light when both the terminals are kept under different voltages [16]. Depending on the band gap of the p–n junction, LEDs can cover full range of wavelengths from UV to NIR. LEDs can generate different colours of light for various applications. LEDs offer better SNR (signal-to-noise ratio) for vascular imaging applications since haemoglobin has higher absorption in the visible range of wavelengths below 650 nm [17]. Quantitative analysis of biomedical imaging involves repeatable measurements and requires consistency; here, LEDs' controllable intensity stability plays a vital role in such applications [18].

1.3.1.3 Gas or solid-state lasers

Lasers are light sources that can emit coherent and polarised light, which exhibit monochromatic (peaked) spectrum. Optical imaging techniques such as fluorescence and Raman spectroscopy most often use lasers. Lasers can couple effectively with the optical fibres because of their sharp and intense monochromatic type. Most commonly available lasers are gas or solid-state lasers obtained using He–Ne (helium–neon), CO_2 (carbon dioxide), Ar^+ (argon), nitrogen sapphire, Nd:YLF (neodymium–yttrium lithium fluoride) and Nd: YVO_4 (neodymium–yttrium orthovanadate) solid states. The choice of lasers is made depending on the requirement of wavelength, size, power and cost [15]. Lasers are the prime source of light in the imaging techniques such as fluorescence imaging, optical tomography, etc. Lasers are used to excite the fluorescence signals in biological tissues in order to observe the abnormalities in the tissue through fluorescence imaging [13].

1.3.2 Filters used in optical imaging

Optical filters are the most common requirement of an optical imaging system. Filters that are often used in optical imaging are notch filters (NF), neutral density (ND), band-pass (BP), short-pass (SP) and long-pass (LP) filters [19]. ND filters provide full band attenuation in applications with very strong intensity for detectors. SP filter allows signals with smaller wavelengths and attenuates longer wavelength light while LP filter allows only longer wavelengths and attenuate shorter wavelengths. BP filters allow the particular band (range) of wavelengths to pass and blocks the rest but NF does the opposite. These filters can be narrowband or broadband depending on the size of the pass band.

Filters are mostly dependent on dispersion, interference or absorption. Absorbing filters work on the principle of either transmitting or absorbing the light. Interference filters work on the principle of either transmitting or reflecting the light; none of the light is absorbed. Dispersive filters work on the principle where the light incident on it is dispersed into different wavelengths according to the application [19]. Optical filters are critical in order to obtain sharp and high contrast images by blocking the scattered light from reaching the detector. The scattered light received from the unwanted tissues is blocked by optical filters in order to image the specific tissue [20]. In biomedical optical imaging, optical filters are chosen based on the requirements of the application and the type of light source used.

1.3.3 Photon detectors

Photon detectors are light sensors that sense light incident on it. There are several types of detectors available for biomedical optical imaging and are generally classified into two groups namely, single- and multichannel detectors. Depending on the application, the choice of detector is made by considering several factors such as wavelength range, signal level, physical size and the data acquisition speed.

1.3.3.1 Single-channel photon detectors

The most commonly available single-channel photon detectors are PIN diode, avalanche photo diode (APD) and photomultiplier tube (PMT) [15]. PIN diodes are made up of silicon or In GaAs (indium gallium arsenide). Silicon photodiode operates in the range of 200–1100 nm and has a peak response at 900 nm, whereas In GaAs operates in the range of 800–1700 nm and has a peak response at 1500 nm. Signal is linearly dependent on the input light and there is no requirement of any high voltage. Because of very low sensitivity and small photoactive area, PIN photodiodes are often used in monitoring the excitation of intensity in fluorescence spectroscopy. However, the APD has a higher sensitivity compared to PIN photodiode due to the avalanche multiplication that results in the first stage of gain. A suitable APD is selected based on the range of wavelengths, size of detection area and electrical bandwidth [15]. In applications like fluorescence microscopy with very low signal detection level, APDs are used because of its higher sensitivity and faster response time. The PMT is made up of electron collector (anode), photon electron converter (cathode) and electron multiplier. With higher bandwidth and gain, PMTs are capable of photon counting in very low or short pulses of light. PMTs are selected based on wavelength, beam size and intensity requirements. Most common photodetectors in PET scanners are PMTs, which are used for small animal imaging [21].

1.3.3.2 Multichannel photon detectors

Multichannel detectors are preferred over single-channel detectors because of its high quantum yield, multichannel capability and low dark signal. Silicon-based charge coupled device (CCD) is the most preferred detectors among multichannel photon detectors. There are three different types of CCDs that are commonly used for optical imaging namely, CCD with back illumination, CCD with front illumination and back-illuminated CCD with deep depletion, as depicted in Figure 1.2. The wavelength operability range of these types are as follows: (1) front-illuminated operates well in the range 400–1000 nm with maximum quantum peaked at 700 nm, (2) back-illuminated operates in the range 250–1000 nm with maximum quantum peak at 500 nm, (3) back-illuminated deep depletion operates in the range 300–1000 nm with maximum quantum peak at 800 nm [15].

CCD with front illumination is useful for strong light detection while CCD with back illumination is useful for the low-intensity light signals.

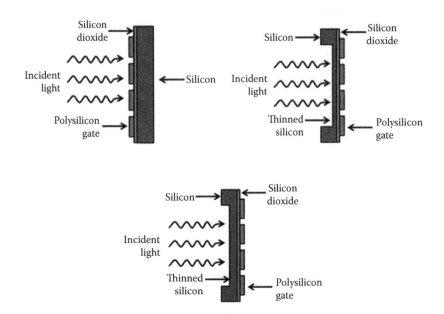

Figure 1.2 CCD sensor array types. (a) CCD with front illumination, (b) CCD with back illumination and (c) back illuminated with deep depletion CCD.

Back-illuminated CCD with deep depletion is used for very low-intensity light signals. In order to increase the speed of the sensors, the CCD multisensors are combined with the light amplifiers often called as intensified CCD (ICCD). The amplifier works as a shutter to intensify the light for the speed gating. Thus, ICCDs are very fast operating detectors.

1.3.4 Optical imaging modalities

At present, various imaging modalities are available that use principles of biomedical optics. The most commonly used biomedical optical imaging techniques are optical coherence tomography (OCT), endoscopy, multispectral endoscopy photoacoustic imaging, diffuse optical tomography (DOT), diffuse reflectance imaging and microscopic techniques such as fluorescence microscopy, stimulated emission depletion (STED), confocal microscopy and multiphoton microscopy. These modalities are portable, cost-effective, and are being used for in vivo and noninvasive imaging of tissues, spanning from molecular and cellular levels. Example images of these optical imaging techniques are shown in Figure 1.3a–d. A brief discussion of each modality is given below and in the following section. The detailed discussion on microscopic optical imaging modalities is given in Section 1.4.

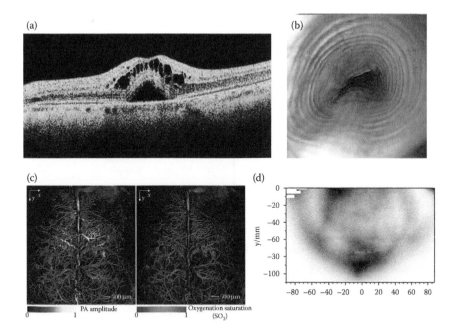

Figure 1.3 Example of images taken from optical imaging modalities. (a) OCT view of cross section of the layers below the eye surface, (b) feline oesophagus: endoscopic view, (c) photo acoustic image of mouse brain, and (d) breast mammography result using diffuse optical imaging.

OCT employs similar principle of back-reflection and backscattering of sounds in ultrasound imaging; instead OCT uses infrared light. OCT enables tissue microstructures to be visualised in real time which makes it to be used as an alternative to the traditional biopsy and histopathology methods [14].

OCT works on the principle of backscattering of the incident light called as low-coherence interferometry [22]. The images are produced from the scattering of light caused by the objects with the incident light resulting in high-resolution cross-sectional and internal biological tissue imaging [23]. It is an in vivo and in situ imaging technology that has the capability of imaging the tissue pathology with the resolution of 1–15 μm. OCT is considered as an "optical biopsy" method because of its capability of imaging the tissue microstructures without the necessity of removing the specimens [22]. A general schematic representation of OCT is shown in Figure 1.4.

OCT is very useful in the following clinical situations [23]:

1. In situations where standard excisional biopsy is hazardous or impossible. This includes tissues such as eye, arteries or nervous tissues.

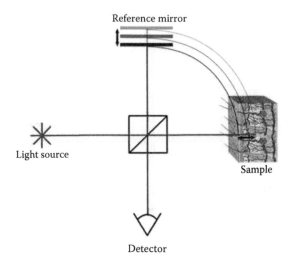

Figure 1.4 OCT set-up schematic representation. (Adapted from A. Z. Freitas et al., Optical coherence tomography: Development and applications, 2014 under CC BY-NC-SA 3.0 license. Copyright 2010. Available from http://dx.doi.org/10.5772/12899.)

2. In cases where standard excisional biopsy has sampling error. OCT has the capability to improve sensitivity by minimising the sampling errors.
3. It can be used to provide assistance in interventional procedures like the microsurgical procedures related to vessels and nerves, in order to visualise under the tissue surface.

Recently, OCT has been used in a wide range of applicability in the field of ophthalmology, dermatology, odontology, brain investigations for traumatic brain injury investigation of stroke, etc. Examples of using OCT in various biomedical applications are as follows.

OCT was first applied in ophthalmology to obtain retinal tomographies [22]. OCT is capable of imaging the eye tissues in a similar way as that of histology but in noninvasive and in situ manner and in real time. In order to increase the depth and resolution, OCT is operated in the NIR region that has very less attenuation [24]. This made ophthalmologists to image not only retina but also the anterior segments and cornea making OCT as the most preferred imaging technique to assess eye pathologies in the most convenient way. The retinal OCT image in Figure 1.5 shows different layers of the retina [24].

Brain investigations using OCT was first used in neurosurgery to differentiate between the tumoral and normal cortex tissues in the brain by using optical backscattering [25]. OCT can depict the data on micron scale by providing information on spatial relations between the adjacent tissues.

An HD-OCT scan of a healthy eye

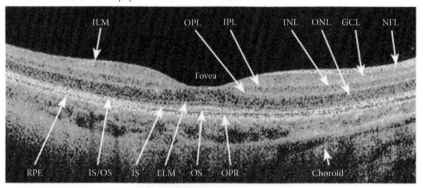

NFL: Nerve fiber layer	OPL: Outer plexiform layer	IS/OS: Interface between IS and OS
ILM: Inner limiting membrane	ONL: Outer nuclear layer	RPE: Retinal pigment epithelium
GCL: Ganglion cell layer	ELM: External limiting membrane	OPR: Outer photoreceptor/
IPL: Inner plexiform layer	IS: Photoreceptor inner segment	RPE compplex
INL: Inner nuclear layer	OS: Photoreceptor outer segment	

Figure 1.5 Retinal OCT image with different layers. (Image taken from http://www.healthpartners.com.au/portals/1/Images.)

Functional brain activity can also be investigated using OCT imaging technology such as evaluating the response of microvascularisation in establishing neuronal activity through metabolic and hemodynamic responses to brain activation [25]. It has been reported that effects of stroke on structural and hemodynamic changes of the brain of rodent models can also be evaluated using the OCT, such as in Reference 26. Brain tissue characterisation for stroke or traumatic brain injuries in rats have been obtained using OCT-imaging technologies, as shown in Figure 1.6 [25].

Endoscopy is a procedure that allows doctors to view and operate internal organs and vessels of the body by using specialised instruments; for example, flexible tube with attached camera is inserted through small cut or opening in the body. It allows surgeons to view inside the body without making large incisions [27].

Photoacoustic imaging works on the principle of conversion of absorbed optical energy into acoustic energy, as acoustic waves scatter less than the optical waves in tissue, resulting in sharp and precise molecular imaging. Photoacoustic imaging generates images with higher resolution in diffusive regimes and optical ballistic [28].

DOT is an imaging technique that uses NIR light source in the form of array in order to illuminate tissue to be imaged. The illuminated tissue causes scattering of light in multiple ways that is detected using the array of detectors, and the localised optical properties of the tissues illuminated are inferred using the model propagation of physics. Detecting tumors in brain and breast is the important application of DOT [29].

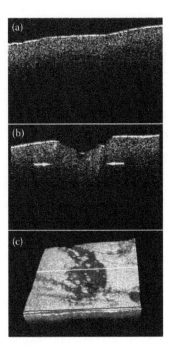

Figure 1.6 OCT images of a rat brain, 12 h after stab injury. (a) Normal brain tissue, (b) affected by traumatic lesion, (c) three-dimensional reconstruction—normal tissue (red line) and injured tissue (yellow line). (Image taken from E. Osiac et al., *Romanian Journal of Morphology and Embryology*, vol. 55, pp. 507–512, 2014.)

1.4 *Optical imaging techniques based on microscopy*

Microscopic imaging techniques involve passing of visible light on the object to be imaged to obtain minute details through single or multiple lenses based on the resolution (magnification) required. The microscopic image is viewed and digitally formed using photodetectors. Usually, Abbe's diffraction limit is used to limit the resolution as denoted by

$$d = \frac{\lambda}{2na} \tag{1.6}$$

Here, d is the shortest distance between two discrete objects that can be separated, na the numerical aperture of the lens, and λ the wavelength of the light source used to obtain microscopic image [9].

1.4.1 Fluorescence microscopy

Fluorescence microscopy set-up, as shown in Figure 1.7, consists of a light source (mainly mercury arc lamp), detector, emission and excitation filters and dichroic mirror. The photon beam is radiated from the mercury arc lamp out of which a particular wavelength light beam is filtered with the help of the excitation filter. This filtered beam is used to excite the electrons in the sample specimen to the excitation state, waits for its lifetime, and returns to the ground state by emitting light of larger wavelengths but at a reduced energy level. These beams are again filtered with the help of an emission filter, which filters out unwanted wavelengths of light beam and passes the required wavelengths of light beam for the photodetectors. The photodetectors then convert these light beams into a visible image for viewing the fluorescent biological tissue. The function of dichroic mirror is to reflect the smaller wavelength beams and pass the beams with larger wavelengths; these are used to guide the light beam from the source to the sample specimen. Xenon or mercury arc tubes are usually used for fluorescence microscopy technique [13].

1.4.2 Confocal microscopy

Confocal microscopy is a technique in which both the object and the corresponding image generated are in focus, as depicted by the schematic representation of confocal microscopy set-up in Figure 1.8. The out-focal data that are generated in the case of normal microscopy is eliminated by the use of confocal pinholes. These confocal pinholes act as spatial filters, which

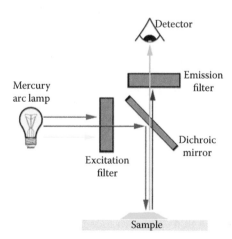

Figure 1.7 Fluorescence microscopy.

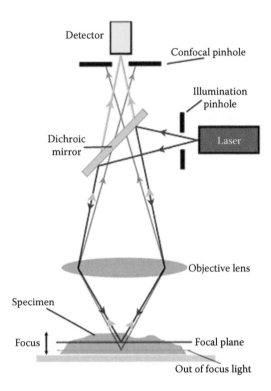

Figure 1.8 Confocal microscopy.

filter out the out-focal beams. Only in-focal light beams are used to create the images, whereas above-focal and below-focal light beams are filtered out using the pinholes. Lasers are used as the light source instead of arc lamps as in the case of general fluorescence imaging because lasers form very bright and sharp wavelength light sources. Thus, confocal images are the sharper but of lesser brightness as compared to fluorescence images. Highly sensitive PMTs are used as photon detectors in order to pick up very low-intensity signals due to filtered out-focal data by the pinhole filters.

1.4.3 *Multiphoton imaging*

In multiphoton imaging two or three photons are excited. A pulsed laser light source is used where the pulse gap produced is very small between two consecutive pulses. Most commonly used multiphoton technique is a two-photon excitation that was introduced in 1990. Using this technique, two photons are excited simultaneously with very short pulse gap, but the fluorescence emission is same for both these pulses, that is, both the photons come to ground state after the same duration of time by emitting

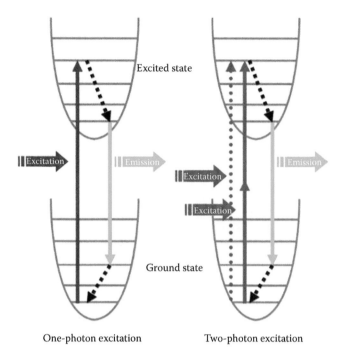

One-photon excitation   Two-photon excitation

Figure 1.9 Single photon and two-photon excitation and relaxation. (Reproduced from V. E. Centonze and J. G. White, *Biophysical Journal*, vol. 75, pp. 2015–2024, 1998.)

light of higher wavelength, which is shown in Figure 1.9 while a single-photon and multiphoton images are shown in Figure 1.10.

As seen from Figure 1.6, a significantly narrower spread of pixel intensities is observed in the confocal image whereas wider spread is obtained using multiphoton imaging. Confocal imaging also has a lower signal-to-background ratio. High contrast images can be obtained using multiphoton even at significant depths for a light-scattering sample [30].

1.4.4 Stimulated emission depletion

STED [30] is one of the most widely used microscopic techniques used to obtain high-resolution microscopic images called as super resolution microscopy. Super resolution microscopy uses STED in order to create sub-diffraction limit features that are obtained by altering the effective point spread function of the excitation pulse using a second laser suppressing fluorescence emission through fluorophores placed at a distant location from the center of excitation. Before the spontaneous emission occurs, the molecule is sent back to ground state by the stimulated emission. This stimulated emission is obtained with the use of a two overlapping synchronised

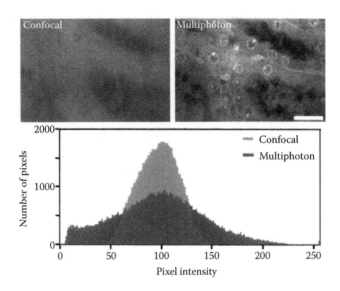

Figure 1.10 Confocal-multiphoton comparison. (Reproduced from V. E. Centonze and J. G. White, *Biophysical Journal*, vol. 75, pp. 2015–2024, 1998.)

laser beams, which arrive one after the other with the time gap of less than the lifetime of molecule excited. The second pulse is of doughnut shape in order to reduce the spreading of the pulse and make the scanning of sample sharper. The pulses are shown in Figure 1.11. STED produces sharper and high-resolution images than that of confocal microscopy.

1.4.5 Other techniques

Apart from the techniques discussed above, there are many more microscopic imaging techniques available in the literature. Some of them are multipoint excitation for far-field microscopy, 4Pi confocal microscopy, near-field microscopy, Raman scattering microscopy with coherent anti-Stokes

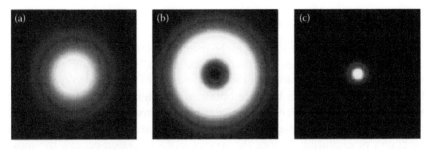

Figure 1.11 (a) Excitation spot, (b) doughnut shaped de-excitation and (c) remaining area allowing fluorescence.

[31], far-field sum frequency generation imaging, near-field sum frequency generation imaging, etc. A microscopic technique for specific application is chosen based on the requirements such as light source, cost and resolution.

1.5 Optical imaging techniques for whole body animal imaging

Whole animal imaging techniques has a vital role in the study of the effectiveness of diagnosis on small animals such as tumors growing or regressing and response to medication. Whole animal imaging can be performed in various noninvasive techniques such as optical imaging, x-ray CT, ultrasound imaging, MRI and radio-nuclei imaging (such as PET and SPECT). As discussed earlier, optical imaging is relatively simple and minimally invasive among the techniques with no ionising radiation required for acquiring images.

Fimaging and bioluminescence imaging are used to obtain whole body imaging. Fluorescence imaging is the technique in which molecules of the tissue are excited with external light source and because of the fluorescence material the molecule gets excited and releases longer wavelength

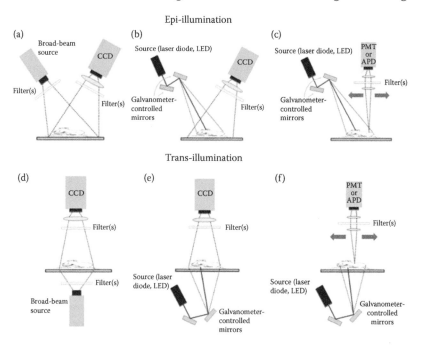

Figure 1.12 Schematic rendering of different methods that can be used for whole-body fluorescence imaging. (Image taken from F. Leblond et al., *Journal of Photochemistry and Photobiology B: Biology,* vol. 98, pp. 77–94, 2010.)

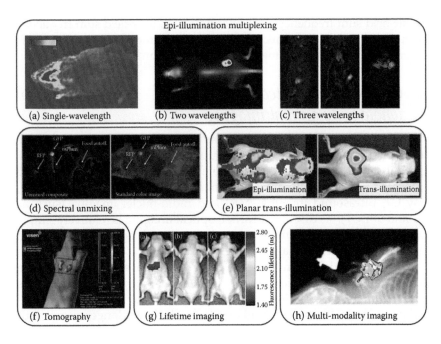

Figure 1.13 Whole animal body imaging techniques. (Image taken from F. Leblond et al., *Journal of Photochemistry and Photobiology B: Biology*, vol. 98, pp. 77–94, 2010.)

light ranging in between UV to NIR range when settling down to ground state. Similarly, the bioluminescence is the natural property of certain living tissues that emit light when it meets certain substrate.

The response of the treatment on small animals is studied using the whole body imaging technique in order to view the inner biological structures of animals. As discussed in the previous sections, it requires suitable light source such as arc lamps, LEDs or lasers depending on the application for which imaging is done. It requires the detectors such as CCDs, PMTs, etc. and proper probes in order to obtain efficient images through proper incident of lights onto the objects along with proper filters and polarisers to filter out the unwanted lights that are being emitted by the object being imaged. In obtaining whole body images two types of illumination are used: Epi-illumination and Trans-illumination. Epi-illumination is the technique that works on reflectance mode, that is, the source as well as detector are on same side of the imaging object. Trans-Illumination is the technique that works on transmission mode, that is, light is injected from one side of the object, and light is detected from the other side using detectors. This can be seen in Figure 1.12. Some typical optical images captured using various whole animal body imaging techniques are shown in Figure 1.13. These images of a mouse are taken using different techniques and modalities of whole animal body imaging techniques.

1.6 Summary

Optical imaging is one of the best medical imaging techniques for in vitro and in vivo applications. Molecular imaging is one of the specialities of optical imaging. Optical imaging is yet a vast field, from the understanding of the effectiveness of the technique to analysis of the images. This chapter has presented various optical microscopic imaging techniques along with the whole animal body imaging technique specially used to image small animals. The reader is referred to the articles in the references for detailed information about optical imaging.

References

1. V. E. Centonze and J. G. White, Multiphoton excitation provides optical sections from deeper within scattering specimens than confocal imaging, *Biophysical Journal*, vol. 75, pp. 2015–2024, 1998.
2. R. Fitzgerald, Phase-sensitive x-ray imaging, *Physics Today*, vol. 53, pp. 23–26, 2000.
3. H. D. Liang and M. J. K. Blomley, The role of ultrasound in molecular imaging, *The British Journal of Radiology*, vol. 76, pp. S140–50, 2003
4. E. Terreno, D. D. Castelli, A. Viale, and S. Aime, Challenges for molecular magnetic resonance imaging, *Chemical Reviews*, vol. 110, pp. 3019–3042, 2010.
5. T. F. Massoud and S. S. Gambhir, Molecular imaging in living subjects: Seeing fundamental biological processes in a new light, *Genes and Development*, vol. 17, pp. 545–580, 2003.
6. A. P. Dhawan, B. D'Alessandro, and X. Fu, Optical imaging modalities for biomedical applications, *Biomedical Engineering, IEEE Reviews in*, vol. 3, pp. 69–92, 2010.
7. F. Leblond, S. C. Davis, P. A. Valdés, and B. W. Pogue, Pre-clinical whole-body fluorescence imaging: Review of instruments, methods and applications, *Journal of Photochemistry and Photobiology B: Biology*, vol. 98, pp. 77–94, 2010.
8. A. Martinez-Möller, M. Souvatzoglou, G. Delso, R. A. Bundschuh, C. Chefd'hotel, S. I. Ziegler, N. Navab, M. Schwaiger, and S. G. Nekolla, Tissue classification as a potential approach for attenuation correction in whole-body PET/MRI: Evaluation with PET/CT data, *Journal of Nuclear Medicine*, vol. 50, pp. 520–526, 2009.
9. R. B. Schulz and W. Semmler, Fundamentals of optical imaging, in *Molecular Imaging I*. W. Semmler and M. Schwaiger (Eds.), Berlin Heidelberg: Springer-Verlag, 2008, pp. 3–22.
10. G. D. Luker and K. E. Luker, Optical imaging: Current applications and future directions, *Journal of Nuclear Medicine*, vol. 49, pp. 1–4, 2008.
11. L. V. Wang and H.-i. Wu, *Biomedical Optics: Principles and Imaging*. Hoboken, NJ: John Wiley & Sons, 2012.
12. V. Ntziachristos, Going deeper than microscopy: The optical imaging frontier in biology, *Nature Methods*, vol. 7, pp. 603–614, 2010.
13. V. Ntziachristos, Fluorescence molecular imaging, *Annual Review of Biomedical Engineering*, vol. 8, pp. 1–33, 2006.
14. J. G. Fujimoto and D. Farkas, *Biomedical Optical Imaging*. New York: Oxford University Press, 2009.

15. J. Zhao and H. Zeng, Advanced spectroscopy technique for biomedicine, in *Biomedical Optical Imaging Technologies*. R. Liang (Ed.), Berlin Heidelberg: Springer-Verlag, 2013, pp. 1–54.
16. N. G. Yeh, C.-H. Wu, and T. C. Cheng, Light-emitting diodes—Their potential in biomedical applications, *Renewable and Sustainable Energy Reviews*, vol. 14, pp. 2161–2166, 2010.
17. T. J. Allen and P. C. Beard, High power visible light emitting diodes as pulsed excitation sources for biomedical photoacoustics, *Biomedical Optics Express*, vol. 7, pp. 1260–1270, 2016.
18. R. Liang, *Biomedical Optical Imaging Technologies: Design and Applications*. Heidelberg, New York and London: Springer Science & Business Media, 2012.
19. O. Aharon, A. Safrani, R. Moses, and I. Abdulhalim, Liquid crystal tunable filters and polarization controllers for biomedical optical imaging, in *Photonic Devices+Applications*. I. C. Khoo (Ed.), CA: San Diego, 2008, pp. 70500P–70500P-15.
20. C. Hodgson and T. Erdogan, Optical filters for multiphoton microscopy, *Biophotonics International*, vol. 13, p. 32, 2006.
21. J. Tian, *Molecular Imaging: Fundamentals and Applications*. Germany: Springer Science & Business Media, 2013.
22. D. Huang, E. A. Swanson, C. P. Lin, J. S. Schuman, W. G. Stinson, W. Chang, M. R. Hee, T. Flotte, K. Gregory, and C. A. Puliafito, Optical coherence tomography, *Science (New York, NY)*, vol. 254, p. 1178, 1991.
23. W. Drexler and J. G. Fujimoto, *Optical Coherence Tomography: Technology and Applications*. Berlin Heidelberg: Springer-Verlag, 2008.
24. A. Freitas, M. Amaral, and M. Raele, Optical coherence tomography: Development and applications, in *Laser Pulse Phenomena and Applications*, Dr. F. J. Duarte (Ed.), InTech, 2010. DOI: 10.5772/12899. Available from: https://www.intechopen.com/books/laser-pulse-phenomena-and-applications/optical-coherence-tomography-development-and-applications.
25. E. Osiac, T.-A. Bălşeanu, B. Cătălin, L. Mogoantă, C. Gheonea, S. N. Dinescu, C. V. Albu, B. V. Cotoi, O.-S. Tica, and V. Sfredel, Optical coherence tomography as a promising imaging tool for brain investigations, *Romanian Journal of Morphology and Embryology*, vol. 55, pp. 507–512, 2014.
26. E. Osiac, T.-A. Bălşeanu, L. Mogoantă, D. I. Gheonea, I. Pirici, M. Iancău, S. I. Mitran, C. V. Albu, B. Cătălin, and V. Sfredel, Optical coherence tomography investigation of ischemic stroke inside a rodent model, *Romanian Journal of Morphology and Embryology*, vol. 55, pp. 767–772, 2014.
27. M. Uram, *Endoscopic Surgery in Ophthalmology*. Philadelphia: Lippincott Williams & Wilkins, 2003.
28. J. Xia, J. Yao, and L. V. Wang, Photoacoustic tomography: Principles and advances, *Electromagnetic waves (Cambridge, MA)*, vol. 147, p. 1, 2014.
29. D. A. Boas, D. H. Brooks, E. L. Miller, C. A. DiMarzio, M. Kilmer, R. J. Gaudette, and Q. Zhang, Imaging the body with diffuse optical tomography, *Signal Processing Magazine, IEEE*, vol. 18, pp. 57–75, 2001.
30. Y. Peng and A. Hua, Mechanism of STED microscopy and analysis of the factors affecting resolution, SPIE 7544, Sixth International Symposium on Precision Engineering Measurements and Instrumentation, 75440F (28 December 2010), 2010, pp. 75440F-75440F-9, doi.org/10.1117/12.885681.
31. F. L. Labarthet and Y. R. Shen, Nonlinear optical microscopy, in *Optical Imaging and Microscopy: Techniques and Advanced Systems*, P. Török and F.-J. Kao, Eds. Berlin: Springer, 2003, pp. 169–196.

chapter two

Skin image analysis granulation tissue for healing assessment of chronic ulcers

Ahmad Fadzil Mohamad Hani and Leena Arshad

Contents

2.1 Chronic ulcers and healing assessment

2.1.1 Ulcers healing progression

In pathology, a wound refers to an injury that causes discontinuity of the anatomical structure and function of skin tissues [1,2]. When the skin is injured due to a certain trauma, it goes through a series of overlapping procedures to repair the damaged tissues. Chronic wounds or ulcers occur when the injured tissues do not follow a normal course of healing within an expected period of time due to untreated underlying aetiologies or improper wound management [3,4]. Non-healing ulcers could reside for years, exposing the patients to the risk of infection and limb amputation, further leading to pain and discomfort.

According to recent studies, more than 3.0% of the adult population has the potential to develop chronic wounds during their lifetime with an importantly increased prevalence in the elderly [3]. Chronic wounds will likely prevail more importantly along with the population's age or the presence of aetiologies such as diabetes and venous and arterial insufficiencies. People over the age of 60 are more likely to experience leg ulcers, which are chronic wounds commonly found on the lower extremity below the knee. There are three main types of leg ulcers according to the aetiologies that cause them: vascular (venous and arterial), diabetic (neuropathic) and pressure ulcers. Most patients with leg ulcers either have vascular or diabetic problems; and leg ulcers affect 1% of the adult population and 3.6% of people above 65 years [5]. Figure 2.1 demonstrates examples of two chronic leg ulcers of patients from Hospital Kuala Lumpur, Malaysia.

The healing process of chronic ulcers is not predictable and the chronic ulcers keep on evolving slowly over time. Healing may prolong usually due to underlying aetiologies, such as venous insufficiency, arterial perfusion, prolonged pressure and diabetes that cause inflammation

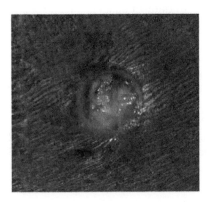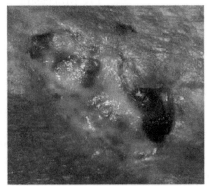

Figure 2.1 Chronic leg ulcer images collected at Hospital Kuala Lumpur.

and accumulation of debris and foreign materials and impair the natural course of healing. Hence, an accurate and thorough assessment of the ulcer is important to provide baseline information on the ulcer severity status and to determine the appropriate course of treatment [6,7]. Misdiagnosis of ulcer's condition can cause improper clinical decisions and lead to long periods of treatment, which reflect on the effectiveness of ulcer care and management in terms of time and cost of treatment. There are several ulcer assessment parameters that need to be thoroughly analysed by clinicians such as the physical appearance of the ulcer, the condition of the surrounding skin, the odour and pain associated with the ulcer as well the amount and characteristics of the exudates on the ulcer surface. The patients' medical history of previous ulcers and their corresponding treatments are also needed to acquire a full analysis of the ulcer condition.

The physical appearance of the ulcer, in particular, plays a significant role in determining the ulcer's severity status and monitoring its healing progression. Four main types of tissues exist on the ulcer surface: necrotic tissue, slough, granulation tissue and epithelial tissue. The ulcer's surface appearance changes gradually throughout the treatment course, as depicted in Figure 2.2 [8]. The ulcer can initially appear covered with a layer of black necrotic tissue (stage 1) or overlying layers of black necrotic tissue and yellow slough (stage 2), depending on how severe the ulcer is. As the healing progresses, red granulation tissue starts to grow from the base of the ulcer gradually replacing the black necrosis and yellow slough in effect filling the wound cavity and reducing its volume (stage 3). Granulation tissue consists of a collagen-based extracellular matrix combined with newly formed blood capillaries. The ulcer's healing progress is

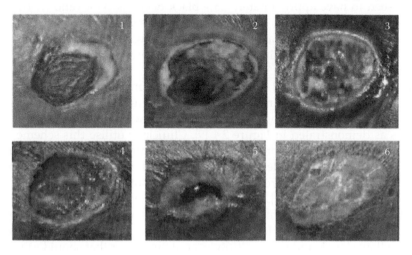

Figure 2.2 Typical healing stages of an ulcer. (From R. Goldman and R. Salcido, *Advances in Skin and Wound Care*, vol. 15, no. 5, pp. 236–245, 2002.)

indicated by the growth of granulation tissue and therefore demonstrates that the patient is positively responding to the treatment. At later stages of ulcer healing, pink epithelial tissue starts to grow from the edges of the ulcer, in effect slowly covering the granulation tissue and eventually closing the ulcer (stage 6).

The surface of the ulcer provides valuable information on healing progression or regression throughout the treatment course. At any one time during the course of the treatment, all four types of tissues may exist on the surface of the ulcer. It is generally well known and acceptable to recognise and measure the amount of each tissue (especially granulation tissue) in order to assess the healing progression or regression of ulcer.

2.1.2 Ulcers healing assessment

In most wound care clinics, the use of noninvasive assessment methods is preferred to avoid any contact with the ulcer, which may cause pain or discomfort to the patients and expose the ulcer to the risk of infection. Most of the assessment methods implemented currently are based on simple visual inspection utilising several schemes based on the colours of the tissues [8,9].

Some developed schemes have been designed to describe the percentages of colour of each type of tissue at the ulcer surface such as the red/yellow/black scheme [10]. Using this scheme, ulcers' surface tissues are described as estimated percentages of red, yellow and black colours, which refer to granulation, slough and necrosis, respectively. Figure 2.3 demonstrates a chronic ulcer that has been assessed utilising this scheme; it is seen to have approximately 25% black necrosis, 35% yellow slough and 40% red granulation. The more the shift towards the red colour is, the better the ulcer is healing. This scheme is widely used in hospitals and clinical settings and is normally recorded on the patient assessment chart.

Gray et al. developed the wound healing continuum (WHC), which identifies the tissue colours on the ulcer surface and associates them to a colour spectrum extending from black till pink with intermediate gradations as demonstrated in Figure 2.4 [9]. Clinicians utilise this scheme to make clinical decisions on ulcer status by identifying the ulcer colour, which is furthest to the left and determining the appropriate treatment and ulcer management procedures, which promote healing and shift the ulcer colour to the right [9]. For example, if an ulcer is described as yellow/ red using this scheme, this refers to an ulcer that contains both slough and granulation tissues. Hence, ulcer management should aim to remove the yellow slough and create a fully granulating ulcer that should gradually be covered with pink epithelial tissue following the normal course of healing.

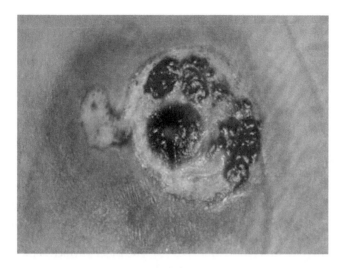

Figure 2.3 An ulcer with approximately 25% black, 35% yellow and 40% red. (From Care of the Wound Bed Assessment and Management Algorithm, pp. 10–38, 2009.)

These assessment methods are simple and widely used in clinical settings to evaluate the ulcer status and progression towards healing. However, they are based on subjective, inaccurate and inconsistent human vision perception, resulting in inability to perform quantitative tissue analysis. Moreover, chronic ulcers change slowly over time as they heal and hence recognising small changes with simple visual inspection is difficult. Inaccurate assessment of the ulcer's severity status leads to improper clinical decisions regarding treatment and may prolong the healing duration or worsen the ulcer condition in some cases. Therefore, monitoring the healing of chronic ulcers requires an objective and quantitative method that provides accurate and reproducible assessment of ulcer condition and healing progression.

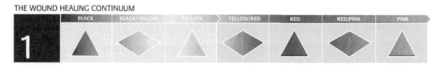

Figure 2.4 Wound healing continuum. (From D. Gray et al., *Applied Wound Management Supplement: The Wound Healing Continuum—An Aid to Clinical Decision Making and Clinical Audit.* Wounds UK: United Kingdom, pp. 9–12, 2004, with permission from Wounds UK.)

2.1.3 The role of digital photography

In most dermatology clinics, colour images of chronic ulcers are acquired at successive visits to provide chromatic data that help clinicians determine how severe the ulcer is and the healing progression throughout the treatment process [8]. The use of digital imaging in medicine enables data to be easily acquired in remote locations and transmitted to the main reference where clinicians can perform ulcer analysis and assessment [11]. This ensures providing quality healthcare regardless of the geographical location of the medical personnel.

Colour has been utilised as the key element for analysis in colour image processing in the application of wound assessment for most of the work that has been developed so far. Previously developed methods for wound tissue classification and segmentation performs single colour channel analysis on digital images in traditional colour models such as HIS and RGB (red, green and blue) [12–15]. The ulcer surface typically comprises mixture of different tissues and hence the use of only one colour channel is not adequate to classify each type of tissue fully. Studies demonstrated that for a particular type of ulcer tissue, the clusters of pixels in RGB colour model forms a uniquely shaped three-dimensional (3D) cloud that distinguishes three types of tissues: necrotic, slough and granulation; and hence colour pixels are considered in all colour channels in the image to be able to classify different ulcer tissues [16–18]. Segmentation-based classification of wound tissues utilising colour and texture attribute was also proposed [19,20]. The method utilises unsupervised segmentation to segment colours from wound images into several regions. The method eventually extracts the colour and texture descriptors from the coloured images so that automatic classification and labelling can be done to those regions.

The different environment conditions when acquiring images, such as type of camera used, quality of illumination in the room or the type of flashlight used, can cause the interpretation of colour content in the image to be inconsistent. These varying conditions alter the colour quality and scales in images that leads to inaccurate results, which poses the main shortcoming of the analysis based on colour features and attributes.

2.2 Research hypothesis and implemented approach

The existence of granulation tissue at the ulcer indicates the first stage of healing. If the ulcer is responding to the treatment, healing would be promoted by the increase of the granulation tissue on the ulcer's surface provided that there are no underplaying aetiologies that delay healing. However, if the current treatment is not effective, the granulation tissue will not grow and unhealthy black necrosis and yellow slough will be present on the ulcer's surface as a result of infection. Detecting small tissue changes that reflect early stages of healing accurately would enable the clinicians to determine the efficacy of the current treatment and make appropriate clinical decisions such as the medicine applied, the type of ulcer dressing and so on. This reflects on the effectiveness of the ulcer care and management in terms of time and cost of treatment.

The colours of ulcer's tissues are created due to the human's perceived vision of the light reflected from ulcer's surface. Majority of the light enters into the ulcer and skin tissues; and goes through a complex path where it interacts with different interior structures and pigments and gets reflected back from the ulcer [21]. These interactions (mainly absorption and scattering) are responsible of changing the spectral composition of light, which reflects the optical properties of the ulcer tissue structures and pigments. The reflected light can be registered with cameras producing colour digital images. Hence, an understanding of the colour image formation would reveal diagnostically important facts about the internal structure and composition of the skin ulcers and the prominent causes of the changes during the process of ulcer healing [22]. Detecting these causes can provide a more comprehensive study on wound tissues.

As shown in Figure 2.5, visible light spectrum (i.e., from violet at about 380 nm to red at about 750 nm) being captured by the retina provides colours to the eyes. This is caused by the different reflectance ranges for different colour modules within the visible spectrum. The red colour falls within wavelengths between 620 and 740 nm in the visible light spectrum.

Granulation tissue appears as red when viewed under the visible light due to the pigment haemoglobin present in the newly formed blood capillaries within the tissue [23]. This is because the haemoglobin pigment (both oxy-haemoglobin and deoxy-haemoglobin) gives off a reflection of the light in the range of 600 nm and above, as shown in Figure 2.6, which corresponds to the red colour component in the visible light spectrum [21].

Studies have demonstrated that haemoglobin contains certain optical attributes that can be identified in colour images and used to demonstrate their substance inside human skin [24,25]. Therefore, this study focuses on utilising the optical attributes of the pigment haemoglobin and determining its content inside and below the visible surface of ulcers. It is hypothesised that identified regions of haemoglobin distribution can be utilised as image markers to identify regions of granulation tissue indicating the

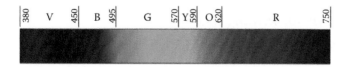

Figure 2.5 Visible light spectrum.

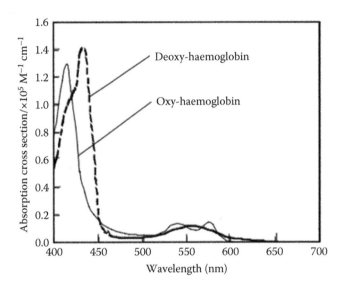

Figure 2.6 Absorption spectra of oxy-haemoglobin and deoxy-haemoglobin. (From R. R. Anderson and J. A. Parrish, *Journal of Investigative Dermatology*, vol. 77, no. 1, pp. 13–19, 1981.)

ulcer healing progression. The approach is to apply data transformation utilising independent component analysis (ICA) to excerpt source grey-level images that demonstrate the distribution of pigment haemoglobin. Extracted pictures of haemoglobin show regions of haemoglobin spreading that reflect area of granulation tissue on ulcer surface. This approach is fundamentally unique in a way that it does not focus on colour image features and attributes directly from the colour images like previous works in this field; instead it draws an understanding of tissue histology utilising a physics-based interpretation of the image colour.

Identifying and quantifying the amount of granulation tissue gives an indication of the healing progression, which reflects on the efficacy of the ulcer management and treatment. This is very significant in detecting early stages of ulcer healing especially in ulcers where granulation tissue is spreading slowly over the ulcer surface and cannot be detected using simple visual inspection.

2.3 Detection of granulation tissue regions for healing assessment

2.3.1 Data collection and acquisition of ulcer images

Colour pictures of various types and aetiologies of chronic leg ulcers that contain a mixture of tissues were collected from Department of

Dermatology and at the Outpatient Department in Hospital Kuala Lumpur, Malaysia. The action of collecting data from actual specimens is very important to this work as it ensured analysis on ulcer images taken from real conditions.

2.3.1.1 Acquisition settings

Ulcers may cause serious agony and discomfort to the patients and there is a high chance of bacterial infections if these ulcers are not managed properly during data acquisition sessions. Hence, it is crucial that the data acquisition device does come in contact with the ulcer and the overall acquisition process is noninvasive. Furthermore, the selected acquisition device should produce high-resolution images to ensure an accurate assessment and analysis. A handheld digital single lens reflector (DSLR) camera, Nikon D300, with a resolution of 12.3 megapixels is utilised to capture the colour images of the chronic ulcers. A Nikon SB-900 flashlight is utilised to give sufficient reproducible lighting for image capturing. The flashlight is further equipped with a diffuser dome to avoid harsh lighting and shadows.

The ulcer images are acquired at the dressing room where the ulcers were examined by the attending nurses. During the acquisition process, colour casts were created because of the combined effect of several light sources and the flashlight reflected back from the surrounding walls in the dressing room. Hence, a white sticker of size 9 × 13 mm (white point) was put next to the ulcer during the photographing process, to give a reference so that any colour shifts that may occur during the acquisition session can be corrected.

2.3.1.2 Data acquisition procedure

The data acquisition procedure involves three main steps:

1. *Fulfilling inclusion/exclusion criteria*: The target population for this study is adult patients above 18 years with chronic leg ulcers attending the ulcer clinics at the Department of Dermatology and the Outpatient Department at Hospital Kuala Lumpur during the study period. All ulcers of different types and aetiologies that contained a mixture of several tissues are included in the study. However, there are ulcers that are excluded from this study such as large ulcers that extended around the leg curvature or ulcers located in challenging positions such as between the toes. Ulcers that contain heavy exudates would cause severe specular reflections when photographed with flashlight and hence are excluded from the study as well.
2. *Obtaining patient consent*: Before acquiring the ulcer images, patients are informed as to the nature and objective of the study. A written

consent on participation in the study as well as acquisition of the
ulcer image is then obtained from the patients.

3. *Acquisition of ulcers images*: Colour pictures of the ulcers are acquired
   using a high-resolution handheld DSLR camera. The camera is placed
   perpendicular to the ulcer to ensure the inclusion of the whole ulcer
   wound within the field of the view of the camera. The flashlight is
   directed to either the wall or the ceiling to provide a more diffused
   illumination to avoid specular reflections. Several images are acquired
   of the same ulcer from different sides. Overall, 75 ulcer images that
   have met the inclusion criteria and provided the optimum view of the
   ulcers under ideal lighting conditions are used in the study.

2.3.2 Pre-processing and ulcer dataset preparation

2.3.2.1 Correcting for colour shifts

During ulcer images acquisition, the digital camera is calibrated so that
it produces equal RGB values for a white patch under flashlight (white
illumination) photography to correct for colour shifts. However, due to
the variety of light sources constituting the ambient illumination in the
dressing room, colour shifts that could not be easily corrected using the
camera settings are still produced. Hence, there is a need to correct for
these colour shifts before processing the ulcer images.

Since the dominant illumination source used in this study is white
flashlight, a white point estimation algorithm, or "max white," has been
implemented to correct for colour shifts. The white point algorithm assumes
that there is a white reference in the image through which the chromatic-
ity scaling factors are calculated. These scaling factors are determined
based on the assumption that the maximum of each of the RGB channels in
the image are found in this reference point and correspond to pure white
[26,27]. By scaling the RGB channels of the ulcer image using the calculated
scaling factors, the corrected image is obtained. Figure 2.7 shows an ulcer
image corrected using the developed colour shifts correction algorithm.
Figure 2.7a shows the ulcer image before colour correction and Figure 2.7b
shows the ulcer image after colour correction had been applied.

2.3.2.2 Selecting regions of interest

After colour correction has been applied on the acquired ulcer images,
two main regions of interest (ROIs) are manually selected from the
images. The first region is the "ulcer region," which includes the ulcer and
some of the surrounding skin. Ulcer regions should be excluded from the
background, which might contain unwanted regions of the surroundings
such as other parts of the patient's body and the wall of the room. These
unwanted regions could affect the algorithm performance and produced
inaccurate results.

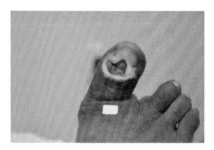 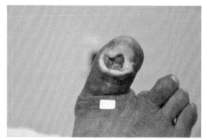

Figure 2.7 Ulcer image corrected using developed colour shifts correction algorithm.

The second region selected from the image is the "reference patch region," which includes the pre-determined size white reference sticker. This is needed to calculate the size of the identified regions of the granulation tissue. Figure 2.8 illustrates the two selected regions from the colour corrected ulcer image.

2.3.3 Data transformation to determine granulation tissue

Figure 2.9 is a flow chart of the created algorithm to extract the images of the haemoglobin distribution. The approach is to apply data transformation on the acquired and pre-processed ulcer images to excerpt grey-level pictures that demonstrate the spreading of pigment haemoglobin. A detailed explanation of the algorithm is given in the following sections.

2.3.3.1 Creating observation input dataset

Each coloured picture of ulcer can derive three grey-level pictures portraying the RGB channel in the spectral band, respectively. These pictures represent three characteristics of linear combinations of the original

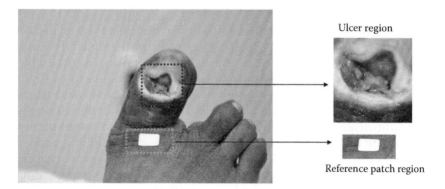

Figure 2.8 Selection of ROIs from colour corrected ulcer image.

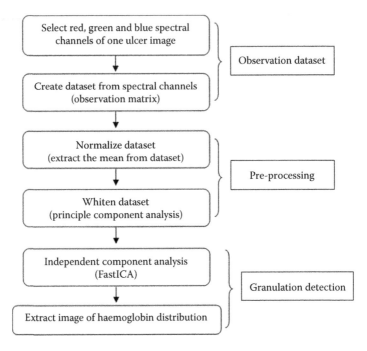

Figure 2.9 Flow chart of the data transformation algorithm.

coloured image source. For each grey-level picture of ulcer, the selected bands are used to create column vectors of a data matrix deriving an observation dataset (observation matrix) as shown in Figure 2.10. The observation matrix X contains observations of the colour ulcer image. Each column of X corresponds to a set of intensity values from each of the RGB colour channels (three observations). Each row of X corresponds to intensity amounts of RGB channels of one particular pixel location.

2.3.3.2 Pre-processing of input dataset

As depicted in Figure 2.9, pre-processing of the observation dataset involves two steps. First, each spectral band is being excerpted the mean value to normalise the dataset to centre on a zero point. The data whitening process is then applied using the Principle Component Analysis (PCA), which is a mathematical approach used to identify the most meaningful basis to re-express complex multidimensional datasets as simple lower dimensions datasets to filter out noise and extract useful hidden information underlying within the original datasets [28]. PCA is applied to convert the observation dataset linearly in order for its components to be uncorrelated and their variances become unity. These pre-processing steps are taken to streamline the ICA algorithms and lessen the parameters to be predicted.

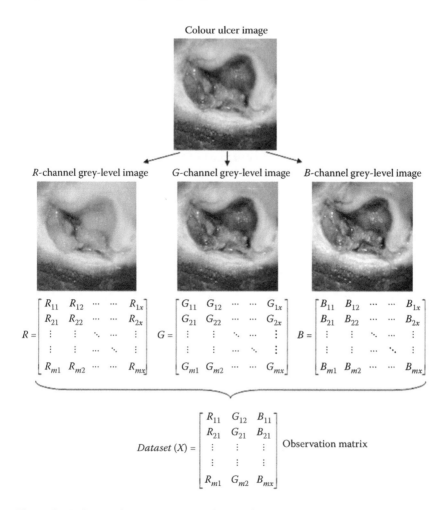

Figure 2.10 Create observation input dataset from colour ulcer image.

2.3.3.3 Detection of haemoglobin distribution

ICA is applied on the observation dataset to excerpt the source grey-level images that demonstrate the spread of the pigment haemoglobin representing the regions of granulation tissue in the colour images of chronic ulcers. ICA is a multivariate data analysis approach used to recover source signals from their observed linear combinations. ICA assumes that the observed signals, in this case the RGB data vectors of each picture of ulcer, are generated by linearly mixing original source signals with an unknown mixing matrix [29,30]. ICA estimates the source images assuming that they are statistically independent, which is achieved when their probability density function can be derived as the outcome of their marginal independent distributions [30]. In this study, ICA is implemented using the FastICA that is referencing on a fixed-point iteration, which utilises maximisation of non-Gaussianity as a measurement of independence in order to project the independent components [29,31–33]. In this method, an approximation of negentropy, which is Newton's iterative approxima-tion, is used to measure non-Gaussianity and estimate the independent source images.

The algorithm has been created so that it predicts all the independent source images concurrently. The outcome of the ICA algorithm is a matrix that comprises row vectors of independent components equalling the amount of observations, which were three observations in this case. The row vectors are reorganised as matrices, each representing a grey-level picture of a predicted independent source. One of the predicted source images was an image that demonstrated regions of the haemoglobin spreading representing the current regions of the granulation tissue on the ulcer's exterior. Figure 2.11 demonstrates a coloured ulcer picture and the corresponding predicted independent source pictures. Figure 2.11c demonstrates the second independent source picture, which represented the regions of an important range of intensity value (dark area in the pic-ture) that could be obviously recognised from the rest of the picture. The mentioned regions indicated haemoglobin spreading that reflected the areas of granulation tissue.

2.4 Clustering-based segmentation of granulation tissue

Segmentation is a type of image processing approach whereby an image is subdivided into regions. It is needed to isolate ROIs from the rest of the image for further processing and analysis. Segmentation normally results in a binary image with only two possible intensity values; 0 (black) or 1 (white). In this study, the identified regions of the granulation tissue on each extracted haemoglobin picture are segmented from the rest of the picture. The segmented regions of the granulation tissue can be mea-sured and utilised as an objective measure to monitor the ulcer healing progression.

The input images to the segmentation algorithms are the grey-level images that are extracted from colour images of the ulcers using the data transformation algorithms as explained in Section 2.3. These images, referred to as "haemoglobin images" in the remainder of this text, indicate the spreading of pigment haemoglobin reflecting the identified regions of the granulation tissue, which emerge with an outstanding range of inten-sity values that could clearly be detached from the rest of the picture, as shown in Figure 2.11c.

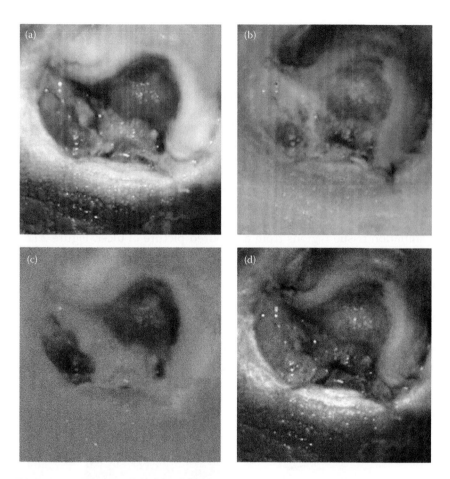

Figure 2.11 Excerpted independent sources from observed picture of colour ulcer. (a) Original colour ulcer image, (b) 1st independent component, (c) 2nd independent component and (d) 3rd independent component.

Segmentation based on clustering is used in this study to segment the identified areas of granulation tissue on the excerpted haemoglobin pictures. Particularly, soft clustering utilising fuzzy c-means algorithms is used on the haemoglobin pictures to classify the granulation regions referencing on their range of intensity values. The classified granulation regions are then segmented from the rest of the pictures accordingly.

2.4.1 Granulation region reference image

Before elaborating further on the clustering-based segmentation approach used in this study, it is important to describe the granulation region reference image, which is used to select the optimum amount of clusters necessary to correctly classify the areas of granulation tissue on the excerpted haemoglobin pictures.

The pictures of ulcer enclosed in this study are demonstrated to two dermatologists* at Hospital Kuala Lumpur who are requested to trace the area of the granulation tissue manually by drawing a line about the granulation tissue area's boundary. The traced regions done by the two dermatologist are consolidated together to create an optimum tracing reference of the granulation tissue regions for each ulcer image. The traced areas of the granulation tissue from the entire ulcer pictures are utilised to create binary images that contain the segmented areas of the granulation tissue, referred to as granulation assessment reference images, which are used as references for further analysis. Figure 2.12 shows a granulation assessment reference picture produced from the manual tracing of the granulation tissue regions from a coloured picture of ulcer. Figure 2.12a shows the colour ulcer image with the traced granulation regions indicated with a green boundary. Figure 2.12b shows the binary assessment reference picture produced from the tracing.

The granulation assessment reference images are utilised to determine the ideal amount of clusters. The ideal amount of clusters to classify the granulation regions in the extracted haemoglobin image is as shown in the following section. They are also used to compare the amount of the detected granulation tissue using the developed algorithm with the

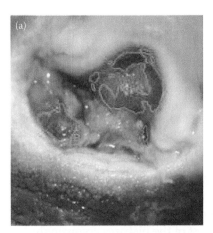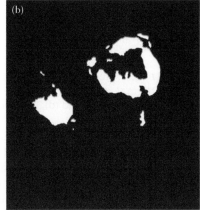

Figure 2.12 Granulation assessment reference picture collected from manual tracing of granulation tissue. (a) Traced granulation tissue region and (b) granulation region reference image.

* Dermatologists who participated in this study are Dr. Adawiyah Jamil and Dr. Felix Yap Boon Bin – Department of Dermatology – Hospital Kuala Lumpur.

amount traced manually by the dermatologists to calculate the amount of the region overlap for the agreement analysis discussed later.

2.4.2 Classifying and segmenting granulation tissue regions

Fuzzy c-means clustering is the method of soft clustering employed in this study to assign membership grades to each pixel in the extracted haemoglobin images. These membership grades determine the extent to which each pixel belongs to a certain amount of clusters referencing on the Euclidean distance of each pixel value to the mean of the cluster centre [34]. Depending on the number of clusters k, each cluster is assigned a number 1, 2, ... , k. After performing fuzzy c-means clustering, the membership grades of all the pixels for each cluster are determined. The pixels are then assigned to each cluster 1, 2, ... , k according to the highest membership grades corresponding to each cluster. The granulation tissue appears as a distinctive dark region in the extracted haemoglobin image. Hence, the cluster with the minimum cluster centre value is regarded as the granulation cluster and assigned the cluster number 1 accordingly. Figure 2.13 illustrates an example of the classification of the regions in the extracted haemoglobin image utilising the fuzzy c-mean clustering algorithm. Figure 2.13a shows the extracted haemoglobin image while Figure 2.13b shows corresponding classified image where the pixels were assigned to different regions according to the highest membership grades. The classified granulation tissue regions in the image are indicated by the arrows in the figure.

The classified picture is then transformed into a binary picture referencing on the intensity values of the clustered granulation tissue. The segmentation algorithm scours the classified picture resulting from being

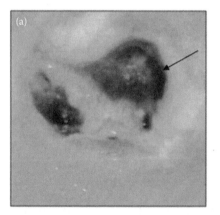
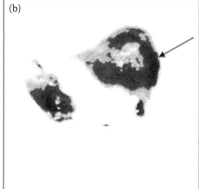

Figure 2.13 Classification of regions in extracted haemoglobin image. (a) Extracted haemoglobin image and (b) regions in haemoglobin image.

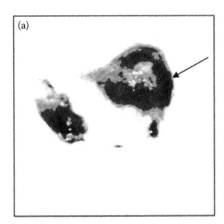
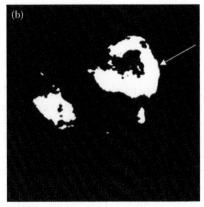

Figure 2.14 Segmentation of clustered granulation tissue in classified picture. (a) Clustered regions in haemoglobin image and (b) segmented granulation tissue regions.

applied the clustering algorithm for values of pixels that belonged to cluster number 1 (clustered granulation tissue) and converts them to value 1 (white) while preserving all other pixels with value 0 (black). This process produces a binary picture where the identified granulation tissue emerges as a black region detached from the rest of the picture, which emerges as a white background. Figure 2.14 illustrates an example of the granulation tissue segmentation in the classified image. Figure 2.14a shows the classified haemoglobin image and Figure 2.14b shows the corresponding binary picture with arrow indicating the segmented granulation tissue.

2.4.3 Selection of amount of clusters

The selection of the amount of clusters k is crucial to the clustering algorithm performance and output accuracy. In order to determine the ideal amount of clusters necessary for segmentation of the granulation tissue, the segmentation algorithm using fuzzy c-means is used iteratively on each excerpted haemoglobin picture with parameter k from the range of $k = 2$ until $k = 10$. The iteration process starts with $k = 2$ because the developed algorithm was expected to classify at least two clusters: the granulation tissue cluster and the cluster for the rest of the ulcer parts.

At each kth iteration step, the segmentation performance is computed by taking the difference between the detected granulation tissue regions using the developed clustering-based segmentation algorithms for each number of clusters with the traced granulation region in the granulation assessment reference image obtained from the dermatologist's tracing. Figure 2.15 illustrates an example of the computation of the difference between the assessment image and the algorithm image. Figure 2.15a

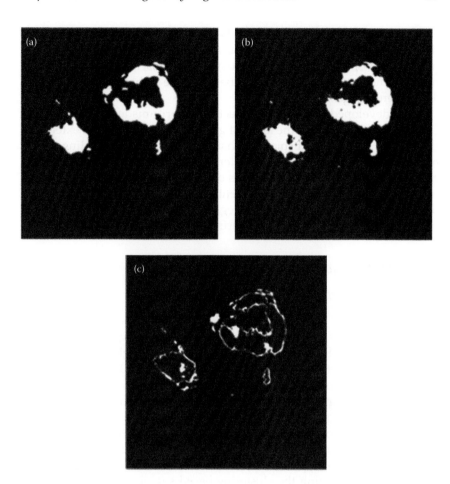

Figure 2.15 Computing the difference between the granulation regions detected using the developed algorithm and the granulation region traced by dermatologists. (a) Granulation tissue reference, (b) identified granulation and (c) granulation tissue.

shows the granulation assessment reference image, Figure 2.15b shows the image resulted from the algorithm segmentation of the granulation tissue and Figure 2.15c shows the difference image.

As shown in Figure 2.15c, the difference image contained wrongly segmented pixels, which are either granulation pixels in the assessment image not detected in the algorithm image or vice versa. The segmentation difference error Er is then attained by calculating the amount of white pixels (wrongly segmented pixels) in the difference image as follows:

$$Er = \frac{\sum_{i=1}^{n} x_i}{N} \qquad (2.1)$$

where n is the amount of white pixels (wrongly segmented pixels) in the difference picture and N is the total amount of pixels in the difference picture. The optimum number of clusters k is chosen based on the minimum segmentation difference error between the algorithm image and the assessment image.

The developed granulation detection algorithms are applied on the 75 ulcer images to detect the areas of granulation tissue on the exterior of the ulcers. First, grey-level pictures that demonstrate the spreading of haemoglobin on the ulcers' surfaces, referred to as haemoglobin images, are extracted from the coloured pictures of the chronic ulcers using the data transformation algorithms. The identified regions of the haemoglobin distribution, or granulation tissue regions, are then segmented from the haemoglobin images utilising clustering-based segmentation algorithms.

2.5 Results and discussion

2.5.1 Optimum number of clusters for clustering-based segmentation

The clustering-based segmentation algorithm using fuzzy c-means clustering is used iteratively on each excerpted haemoglobin picture with the amount of clusters k ranging from $k = 2$ until $k = 10$ to determine the optimum number of clusters needed for the segmentation of the granulation tissue. The segmentation difference error at each kth iteration step is computed using Equation 2.1 and plotted for all of the ulcer images. The optimum number of clusters is then determined as the cluster number at which the minimum segmentation difference error occurred. Figure 2.16 demonstrates an example of a plot of the segmentation difference error obtained from applying the clustering-based segmentation on one ulcer image iteratively for $k = 2$ till $k = 10$. The optimum number of clusters was chosen as $k = 5$ whereby the difference error is at the minimum as seen from Figure 2.16.

In some cases, the difference error reaches a certain value at a specific cluster number and does not change much after that with increasing the cluster number resulting in an L-shaped curve, as indicated in Figure 2.17. In this case, the optimum number of clusters is chosen to be the cluster number after which the change in the error value between two consecutive cluster numbers was very small and almost constant. This point occurs normally at the knee of the graph, as shown in Figure 2.17.

Figure 2.18 shows the minimum segmentation difference error obtained when applying the clustering-based segmentation algorithms for each ulcer image. Figure 2.18 also indicates the optimum number of clusters at which the minimum segmentation difference error occurred for each ulcer image.

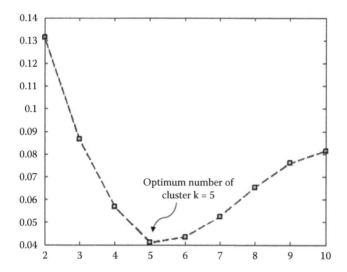

Figure 2.16 A plot of the segmentation difference error obtained from applying the clustering-based segmentation on one ulcer image iteratively for $k = 2$ till $k = 10$.

Figure 2.19 shows the frequency at which the optimum number of clusters occurred among all the cluster numbers from $k = 2$ till $k = 10$ for all of the ulcer images. It can be noted from Figure 2.19 that the optimum number of clusters at which the granulation tissue is successfully segmented with the minimum difference error is between $k = 3$ and 5 with

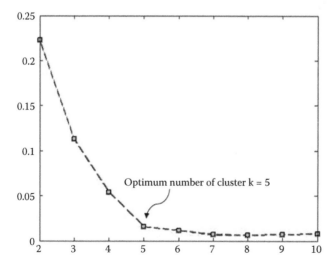

Figure 2.17 A plot of the segmentation difference error obtained from applying the clustering-based segmentation on one ulcer image iteratively for $k = 2$ till $k = 10$.

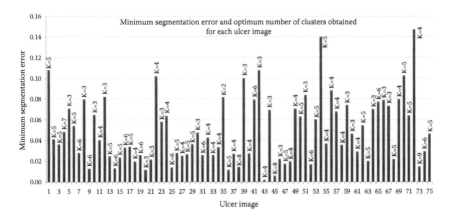

Figure 2.18 Minimum segmentation difference error and optimum number of clusters obtained for each ulcer image.

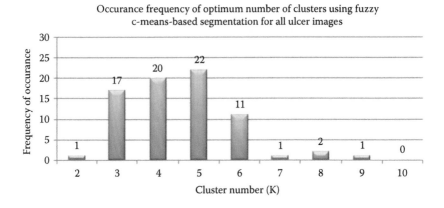

Figure 2.19 Frequency of optimum cluster number.

most cases occurring at $k = 4$ and 5. This can be explained by the fact that the surface of most ulcers contains a mixture of granulation, slough and necrotic tissues along with some damaged tissues or foreign materials that may exist on the surface. Hence, in order to segment and separate the granulation tissue from other tissues and regions on the surface and the surrounding skin, a cluster number of $k = 4$ or 5 is most appropriate. A few ulcers may have more foreign materials or damaged tissues within the ulcer surface and may subsequently need bigger cluster numbers, such as $k = 6$ to segment the granulation tissue from the rest of the haemoglobin picture, as indicated in Figure 2.19.

Eventually, the granulation tissue detection algorithms developed utilising both data transformation algorithms and clustering-based segmentation algorithms are applied on all 75 ulcer images included in this study. The clustering-based segmentation of the identified granulation regions is employed on each extracted haemoglobin image using fuzzy c-means clustering-based segmentation with the optimum number of clusters determined for that particular image as explained above.

2.5.2 Correlation and overlap analysis

The developed granulation detection algorithms have been applied on the 75 ulcer images to identify and segment the areas of the granulation tissue on the ulcers' surfaces. The amount of the detected granulation tissue is then measured from the overall ulcer region and compared with the amount of granulation tissue traced by the dermatologists in the granulation assessment reference images. Figure 2.20 represents a scatter plot of the amount of the detected granulation tissue using the developed granulation detection system versus the amount of granulation tissue traced by the dermatologists. Generally, it is noted from Figure 2.20 that there is a strong similarity between the amount of granulation tissue detected by the developed system and the one traced by the dermatologists.

In order to measure the relationship between the system's detection and dermatologists' tracings of the granulation tissue, the Pearson correlation coefficient is used. The Pearson correlation coefficient, which is denoted as r, was used to calculate the linear dependency between two measures or variables. It is described as the covariance of the variables divided by the outcome of their standard deviation. Given two samples X and Y, the Pearson correlation coefficient is calculated as follows:

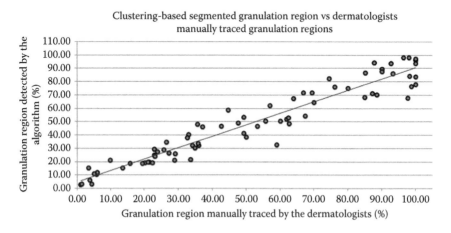

Figure 2.20 Scatter plot of detected granulation tissue using the developed granulation detection system versus the amount of granulation tissue traced by the dermatologists.

$$r = \frac{\sum_{i=1}^{n}(X_i - \bar{X})(Y_i - \bar{Y})}{\sqrt{\sum_{i=1}^{n}(X_i - \bar{X})^2}\sqrt{\sum_{i=1}^{n}(Y_i - \bar{Y})^2}} \qquad (2.2)$$

where n is the number of data points in the sample and $\bar{X}$ and $\bar{Y}$ are the sample means. The value of the correlation coefficient ranges from 0 to (+)1 or (–)1 with values near (+)1 and (–)1 indicating strong correlation. In this study, the Pearson correlation coefficient was calculated using Equation 2.2. The correlation value obtained is 0.961 indicating a strong positive relationship and similarity between the amount of the granulation tissue detected by the system and the amount traced by the dermatologists.

The high correlation value obtained indicated a strong relationship and similarity between the system detection and the dermatologists' tracing (dermatologists' assessments) of the granulation tissue. However, it was important to inspect the actual amount of overlap (regions shared) between the granulation tissue detected by the system and the amount traced by the dermatologists for further analysis. The overlap between both amounts of granulation tissue was calculated as follows:

$$\text{overlap} = \left(\frac{2*TP}{TP + TP + FN + FP}\right)*100 \qquad (2.3)$$

The amount of overlap between the system's detection and dermatologists' assessments of the granulation tissue was calculated using Equation 2.3 for all 75 ulcer images. The results obtained can be divided into three main cases:

Case one: Here, both amounts of the detected granulation tissue and the assessed granulation tissue are quite similar with a high percentage of overlap between the two regions. Such cases occur mostly in ulcers where the granulation tissue covered most of the ulcer as one whole region or as a few regions with defined boundaries. Dermatologists found it quite easy to trace the granulation regions and draw lines around their boundaries to separate them manually from the rest of the ulcer when creating the granulation tissue reference images. Subsequently, the amount of detected granulation regions would be similar to the assessed ones within similar locations on ulcer surface, which results in a high percentage of overlap.

In this study, this case has occurred in 16 ulcer images, as shown in Figure 2.21, where both amounts of detected and assessed granulation

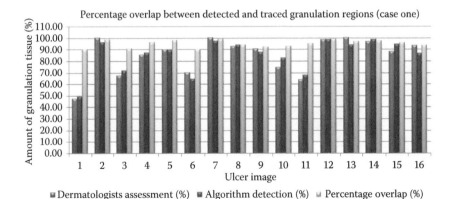

Figure 2.21 Percentage overlaps between detected and traced granulation tissue regions (case one).

regions were similar with a high percentage of overlap values. The difference range between the two regions in these cases was found to be within 0.0%–7.53% while the amount of the overlap between both regions was found to be within 89.84%–98.80% of overlap.

Figure 2.22 shows an example of this case (case number 13 in Figure 2.21). Figure 2.22a shows the original ulcer image in which the granulation tissue appeared to cover the whole ulcer surface with well-defined boundary that could be easily traced. Figure 2.22b shows the extracted haemoglobin image with the granulation tissue region identified with a distinctive intensity range (darkest region). Figure 2.22c shows the traced region of the granulation tissue while Figure 2.22d demonstrates the detected region of granulation tissue. Both regions occupied the same location with similar amounts, which led to a high percentage of overlap. The calculated percentage of overlap in this case was 96.78% with a difference of 6.2% between both regions.

> *Case two*: Here, both the amount of the detected granulation tissue and the amount of the assessed granulation tissue are quite similar but with a low percentage of overlap between the two regions. Such cases occur mostly in ulcers where the granulation tissue was scattered everywhere in the ulcer area while being assimilated with other tissues especially with slough tissue. Dermatologists found it quite difficult to discern the regions of the granulation tissue and draw lines along their boundaries to separate them manually from the rest of the ulcer when creating the granulation tissue reference pictures. This results in either over segmentation or under segmentation of the granulation tissue in the reference images particularly in regions where the granulation tissue was

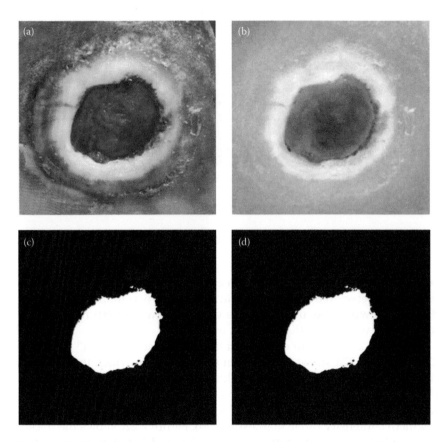

***Figure* 2.22** Example of granulation tissue detection (case one). (a) Original colour ulcer image, (b) extracted haemoglobin image, (c) granulation tissue reference image and (d) detected granulation region image.

heavily mixed with slough and could not be discerned visually. Subsequently, this lead to regions of granulation tissue that exist in the reference images not being detected by the system (over segmentation of granulation tissue in reference image) or vice versa. In either case, the amount of the detected granulation regions could be similar to the assessed ones but would occupy quite different locations on the ulcer's surface, which results in a low percentage overlap.

In this study, this case has occurred in 22 images, as shown in Figure 2.23, where both amounts of the detected and assessed granulation regions were similar but with a low percentage of overlap. The difference range between the two regions in these cases was found to be within

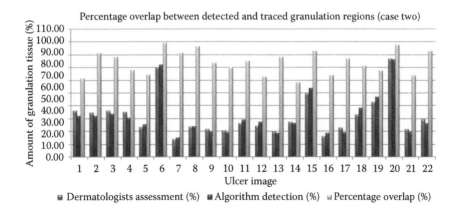

Figure 2.23 Percentage overlaps between detected and traced granulation tissue regions (case two).

0.1%–5.0% while the amount of the overlap between both regions is found to be within 58.05%–88.62% of overlap.

Figure 2.24 shows an example of this case (case number 9 in Figure 2.23). Figure 2.24a shows the original ulcer image in which the granulation tissue emerged to be scattered everywhere in the ulcer exterior assimilated with slough and other foreign materials, which made it difficult to be traced visually. Figure 2.24b shows the extracted haemoglobin image with the granulation tissue region identified with a distinctive intensity range (darkest region). Figure 2.24c shows the traced region of the granulation tissue while Figure 2.24d demonstrates the detected region of the granulation tissue using the developed system. The green arrow in Figure 2.24c indicates an example of a region that contained slough mistakenly identified as part of granulation region by the dermatologists. This region, however, was correctly identified as non-granulation by the system and did not appear in the system detection image as shown in Figure 2.24d. The red arrow on the other hand indicates an example of the granulation tissue regions detected by the system in Figure 2.24d but not traced by the dermatologists in Figure 2.24c. Subsequently, this would lead to both regions having similar amounts but occupying different locations in some parts on the ulcer's surface, which would lead to a low percentage overlap between both regions. The calculated percentage of overlap in this case was 73.19% with a difference of 2.3% between both regions.

Case three: Here, both the amount of the detected granulation tissue and the amount of the assessed granulation tissue are not the same with a low percentage of overlap between the two regions. There are two categories in this case:

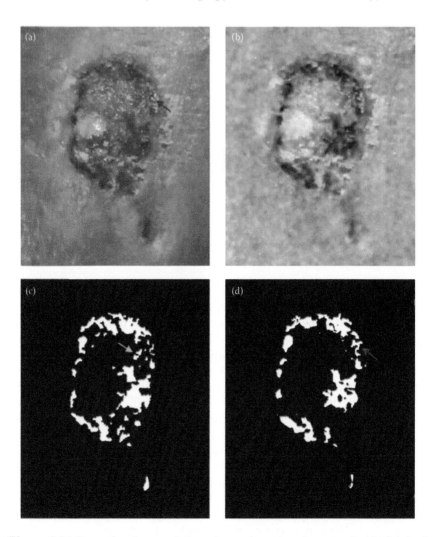

Figure **2.24** Example of granulation tissue detection (case two). (a) Original colour ulcer image, (b) extracted haemoglobin image, (c) granulation tissue reference image and (d) detected granulation region image.

Case three-one: The amount of the detected granulation tissue is more than the amount of the assessed granulation tissue. Such cases occur mostly in ulcers where the granulation tissue was scattered everywhere in the ulcer region assimilated with other tissues particularly with slough tissue. The dermatologists found it difficult to discern these regions visually. If slough was the dominant tissue type in the ulcer and was slightly mixed with granulation tissue, the dermatologists mistakenly marked the whole region as slough although there may have been some granulation tissue within the same region. The algorithm could detect those regions of granulation tissue and clearly separate them from the slough resulting in a larger number of detected granulation tissue regions compared to the assessed ones, which subsequently led to a low percentage of overlap.

In this study, this case has occurred in 16 images, as shown in Figure 2.25, where the amounts of the detected and assessed granulation regions are not similar with a low percentage of overlap. The difference range between the two regions in this case was found to be within 1.43%–14.03% while the amount of the overlap between both regions was found to be within 36.29%–86.87% of overlap.

Figure 2.26 shows an example of this case (case number 15 in Figure 2.25). Figure 2.26a shows the original ulcer image in which the granulation tissue appeared to be scattered everywhere in the ulcer exterior assimilated with slough and necrotic tissues, which made it difficult to trace visually. Figure 2.26b shows the extracted haemoglobin image with the granulation tissue region identified with a distinctive intensity range (darkest region). Figure 2.26c shows the traced region of the granulation tissue while Figure 2.26d shows the detected region of the granulation tissue. It was noted that the amount of the detected granulation tissue was more than the amount of assessed granulation tissue due to some regions of the mixed granulation and slough perceived as slough by the dermatologists as explained earlier. The system, however, detected the regions of the granulation tissue and clearly separated those (indicated

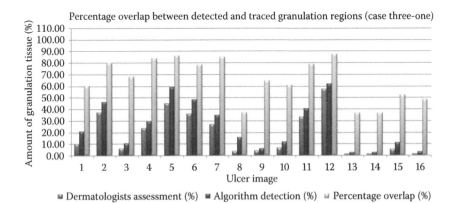

Figure 2.25 Percentage overlaps between identified and traced granulation tissue regions (case three-one).

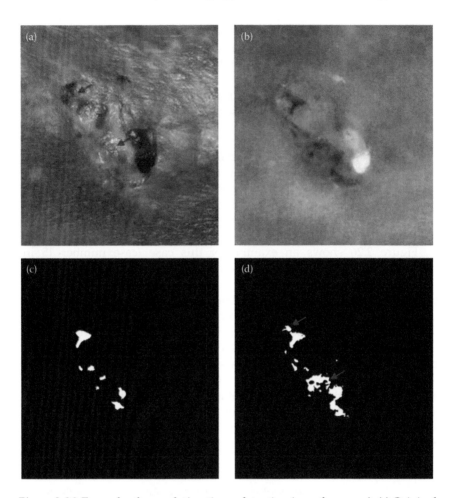

Figure 2.26 Example of granulation tissue detection (case three-one). (a) Original colour ulcer image, (b) extracted haemoglobin image, (c) granulation tissue reference image and (d) detected granulation region image.

by the red arrows in Figure 2.26d) from the regions of slough, which resulted in larger amounts of detected granulation tissue compared to the assessed ones and subsequently lower percentage of overlap. The calculated percentage overlap in this case was 52.33% with a difference of 5.50% between both regions.

Case three-two: The amount of the detected granulation tissue is less than the amount of the assessed granulation tissue. Such cases occur mostly in ulcers where the granulation tissue was scattered everywhere in the ulcer region assimilated with other tissues particularly slough tissue. The dermatologists found it difficult to discern these regions visually. If granulation tissue was the dominant tissue type in the ulcer and was slightly mixed with slough or other tissues, the dermatologists mistakenly marked the whole region as granulation tissue although there may have been some slough within the same region. The algorithm could detect those regions of granulation tissue and clearly separate them from the slough resulting in a fewer detected granulation tissue regions compared to the assessed ones, which subsequently led to a low percentage of overlap.

In this study, this case has occurred in 21 images, as shown in Figure 2.27, where the amount of the detected and assessed granulation regions were not similar with a low percentage of overlap. The difference range between the two regions in this case was found to be within 1.59%–30.03% while the amount of the overlap between both regions was found to be within 55.19%–91.37% of overlap.

Figure 2.28 demonstrates an illustration of this case (case number 5 in Figure 2.27). Figure 2.28a demonstrates the original ulcer image in which the granulation tissue appeared to be scattered everywhere in the ulcer exterior assimilated with slough tissue, which made it difficult to trace visually. Figure 2.28b shows the extracted haemoglobin image with the granulation tissue region identified with a distinctive intensity range (darkest regions). Figure 2.28c demonstrates the traced region of the granulation tissue while Figure 2.28d demonstrates the detected region of the granulation tissue. It was noted that the amount of the assessed

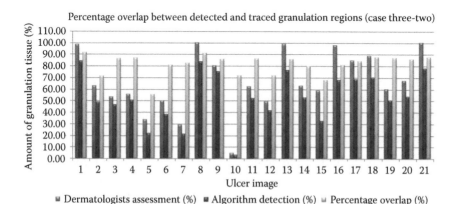

Figure 2.27 Percentage overlaps between detected and traced granulation tissue regions (case three-two).

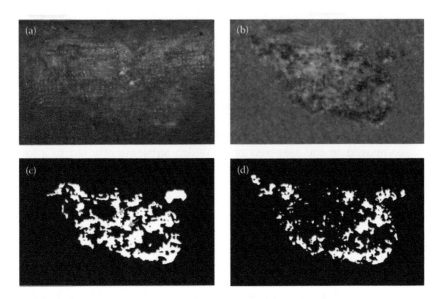

Figure 2.28 Example of granulation tissue detection (case three-two). (a) Original colour ulcer image, (b) extracted haemoglobin image, (c) granulation tissue reference image and (d) detected granulation region image.

granulation tissue was more than the amount of the detected granulation tissue due to some regions of mixed granulation and slough perceived as granulation by the dermatologists as explained earlier. The system detected the regions of the granulation tissue and separated them from the slough (indicated by the green arrows in Figure 2.28c), which resulted in a lesser amount of detected granulation tissue compared to the assessed ones and subsequently a lower percentage of overlap. The calculated percentage of overlap in this case was 55.19% with a difference of 11.93% between both regions.

From the correlation and overlap analysis discussed above, it can be generally concluded that the developed granulation detection algorithms are able to identify regions of granulation tissue that could be difficult to discern visually on real ulcer surfaces using coloured pictures of chronic ulcers. The identified areas of the granulation tissue can be clearly contrasted and segmented from other non-granulation areas on the ulcer's exterior. The amount of the detected granulation tissue, in terms of surface area, can also be measured using the developed system during consecutive visits throughout the course of treatment and used to monitor the healing progression. If the current treatment is effective, the amount of the detected granulation tissue should increase throughout the course of the treatment.

2.6 Conclusion

This research work aims to develop algorithms that are able to identify regions of granulation tissue on the exterior of ulcers and utilise them to provide an objective assessment of the severity condition and healing condition of chronic ulcers. Identifying and quantifying the amount of granulation tissue gives an indication of the healing progression, which reflects on the efficacy of the ulcer management and treatment. This is very significant in detecting early stages of ulcer healing especially in ulcers where granulation tissue is spreading slowly over the ulcer surface and cannot be detected using simple visual inspection. The identified granulation tissue regions can be segmented from the rest of the ulcer picture and their surface area can be measured to provide an objective measure of ulcer healing progression.

This work focuses on utilising the optical characteristics of the pigment haemoglobin and determining its content within and below the visible surface of ulcers. Identified regions of haemoglobin distribution can be utilised as image markers to identify areas of granulation tissue indicating the ulcer healing progression. The approach utilised in this work was to apply data transformation utilising the ICA to excerpt source greylevel pictures that demonstrate the spreading of pigment haemoglobin. The extracted haemoglobin pictures identify the regions of the granulation tissue, which appeared with a distinctive range of intensity values that could clearly be contrasted and detached from the rest of the picture. Clustering-based segmentation was employed in this study to segment the identified areas of the granulation tissue on excerpted haemoglobin pictures. This approach is fundamentally unique in a way that it does not focus on colour image features and attributes directly from the colour images like previous works in this field; instead it draws an understanding of tissue histology utilising a physics-based interpretation of the image colour.

The developed granulation detection algorithms were applied on 75 images of chronic leg ulcers of different types; vascular (venous and arterial), pressure and diabetic ulcers that contain a blend of tissues collected at Hospital Kuala Lumpur, Malaysia, to detect the regions of the granulation tissue on the ulcers' surfaces. The algorithms extracted the haemoglobin images from the coloured pictures of ulcers that highlight the areas of the granulation tissue with a range of intensity values that could be contrasted from the rest of the image. Clustering-based segmentation utilising fuzzy c-means technique was applied on the extracted haemoglobin images to segment the granulation tissue regions from the rest of the image. The optimum number of clusters k at which the granulation tissue was successfully segmented with the minimum segmentation difference error occurred mostly at $k = 4$ and 5.

The amount of the detected granulation tissue was measured and compared with the amount of the granulation tissue traced by the dermatologists at Hospital Kuala Lumpur. It was found that there was a strong positive relationship and similarity between the amount of the granulation tissue detected by the algorithms and the amount traced by the dermatologists as indicated by the obtained high Pearson correlation coefficient value of 0.961. Furthermore, the actual amount of the overlap between the granulation tissue detected by the algorithms and the amount traced by the dermatologist was inspected. It was found that granulation tissue appeared mixed with slough and other tissues in most of the ulcer cases, which made it difficult for the dermatologists to identify those regions based on visual inspection. The difference between the amount of the granulation tissue detected by the developed algorithms and the amount traced by the dermatologists is due to the algorithms' ability to identify and clearly separate the regions of the granulation tissue that could be difficult to discern visually from the rest of the non-granulation regions on the ulcers' surfaces. This is very significant in detecting early phases of ulcer recovery that is indicated by the growth of the granulation tissue on ulcers' surfaces that could not be detected using simple visual inspection. The amount of detected granulation tissue, in terms of surface area, can be measured during consecutive visits throughout the course of the treatment and used to monitor the ulcer healing progression.

It is hoped that this study will open the door for possible avenues of more research works that focus on investigating the optical characteristics of ulcer tissues based on their histology and cellular composition and utilising them to detect their content in coloured pictures of chronic ulcers. Ultimately, the aim is to develop a new unbiased and noninvasive scheme to gauge the recovery progression of chronic ulcers in a more accurate and dependable way.

References

1. A. Shai and H. I. Maibach, *Wound Healing and Ulcers of the Skin – Diagnosis and Therapy – The Practical Approach*. Berlin: Springer, 2005.
2. R. F. Diegelmann and M. C. Evans, Wound healing: An overview of acute, fibrotic and delayed healing, *Frontiers in Bioscience*, vol. 9, no. 4, pp. 283–289, 2004.
3. F. Werdin, M. Tennenhaus, H.-E. Schaller and H.-O. Rennekampff, Evidence-based management strategies for treatment of chronic wounds, *Eplasty*, vol. 9, pp. 169–179, 2009.
4. C. Pearson, How wounds heal: A guide for the wound-care novice, *Wound Care Canada*, vol. 4, no. 2, pp. 10–14, 2006.
5. N. J. M. London and R. Donnelly, ABC of arterial and venous disease: Ulcerated lower limb, *British Medical Journal*, vol. 320, no. 7249, pp. 1589–1591, 2000.

6. *The Care of Patients with Chronic Leg Ulcer—A National Clinical Guideline*, no. 26, Scottish Intercollegiate Guidelines Network, pp. 1–19, 1998.

7. G. Gethin, The importance of continuous wound measuring, *Wounds*, vol. 2, no. 2, pp. 60–68, 2006.

8. R. Goldman and R. Salcido, More than one way to measure a wound: An overview of tools and techniques, *Advances in Skin and Wound Care*, vol. 15, no. 5, pp. 236–245, 2002.

9. D. Gray, R. White, P. Cooper and A. Kingsley, *Applied Wound Management Supplement: The Wound Healing Continuum – An Aid to Clinical Decision Making and Clinical Audit*. Wounds UK: United Kingdom, pp. 9–12, 2004.

10. Care of the Wound Bed Assessment and Management Algorithm, pp. 10–38, 2009.

11. M. Romanelli, G. Gaggio, M. Coluggia, F. Rizzello and A. Piaggesi, Technological advances in wound bed measurements, *Wounds*, vol. 14, no. 2, pp. 58–66, 2002.

12. M. Herbin, A. Venot, J. Y. Devaux and C. Piette, Color quantitation through image processing in dermatology, *IEEE Transactions on Medical Imaging*, vol. 9, no. 3, pp. 262–269, 1990.

13. M. Herbin, F. X. Bon, A. Venot, F. Jeanlouis, M. L. Dubertret, L. Dubertret and G. Strauch, Assessment of healing kinetics through true color image processing, *IEEE Transactions on Medical Imaging*, vol. 12, no. 1, pp. 39–43, 1993.

14. A. Hoppe, D. Wertheim, J. Melhuish, M. Horris, K. G. Harding and R. J. Williams, Computer assisted assessment of wound appearance using digital imaging, in *23rd Annual International Conference of the IEEE Engineering in Medicine and Biology Society*, 2001, pp. 25–28.

15. A. A. Perez, A. Gonzaga and J. M. Alves, Segmentation and analysis of leg ulcers color images, in *International Workshop on Medical Imaging and Augmented Reality (MIAR'01)*, 2001, pp. 262–266.

16. W. P. Berris and S. J. Sangwine, A colour histogram clustering technique for tissue analysis of healing skin wounds, in *Proceedings of the 6th International Conference on Image Processing (IPA97)*, no. 443, pp. 693–697.

17. H. Zheng, L. Bradley, D. Patterson, M. Galushka and J. Winder, New protocol for leg ulcer tissue classification from colour images, in *Proceedings of the 26th Annual International Conference of the IEEE EMBS*, 2004, pp. 1389–1392.

18. J. R. Mekkes, W. Westershof, J. R. Mekkes and W. Westershof, Image processing in the study of wound healing, *Clinics in Dermatology*, vol. 13, no. 4, pp. 401–407, 1995.

19. H. Wannous, S. Treuillet and Y. Lucas, A complete 3D wound assessment tool for accurate tissue classification and measurement, in *15th International Conference on Image Processing, ICIP 2008*, 2008, pp. 2928–2931.

20. H. Wannous, S. Treuillet and Y. Lucas, Supervised tissue classification from color images for a complete wound assessment tool, in *29th Annual International Conference of the IEEE EMBS*, 2007, pp. 6031–6034.

21. R. R. Anderson and J. A. Parrish, The optics of human skin, *Journal of Investigative Dermatology*, vol. 77, no. 1, pp. 13–19, 1981.

22. E. Claridge, S. Cotton, P. Hall and M. Moncrieff, From colour to tissue histology: Physics based interpretation of images of pigmented skin lesions, in T. Dohi and R. Kikinis (Eds.), MICCAI 2002, LNCS 2488, 2002, pp. 730–738.

23. K. P. Nielsen, L. Zhao, J. J. Stamnes, K. Stamnes and J. Moan, The optics of human skin: Aspects important for human health, in *Solar Radiation and Human Health*, E. Bjertness (Ed.). Oslo: The Norwegian Academy of Science and Letters, 2008.

24. N. Tsumura, H. Haneishi and Y. Miyake, Independent component analysis of skin color image, in *The 6th Color Imaging Conference: Color Science, Systems and Applications*, vol. 1, 1999, pp. 177–180.

25. H. Nugroho, A. M. H. Fadzil, S. Norashikin and H. H. Suraiya, Determination of skin repigmentation progression, in *IEEE Engineering In Medicine And Biology Society*, 2007, pp. 3442–3445.

26. V. C. Cardei, B. Funt and K. Barnard, White point estimation for uncalibrated images, in *The IS& T/SID Seventh Color Imaging Conference*, 1999, pp. 97–100.

27. B. Funt, K. Barnard and L. Martin, Is machine colour constancy good enough?, in *5th European Conference of Computer Vision*, 1998, pp. 455–459.

28. J. Shlens, *A Tutorial on Principal Component Analysis*. Center for Neural Science, New York, 2009.

29. A. Hyvärinen and E. Oja, Independent component analysis: Algorithms and applications, *Neural Networks*, vol. 13, pp. 411–430, 2000.

30. S. Roberts and R. Everson, *Independent Component Analysis – Principles and Practice*. Cambridge, United Kingdom: Cambridge University Press, 2001.

31. A. Hyvärinen and E. Oja, A fast fixed-point algorithm for independent component analysis, *Neural Computation.*, vol. 9, pp. 1483–1492, 1997.

32. D. Langlois, S. Chartier and D. Gosselin, An introduction to independent component analysis: InfoMax and FastICA algorithms, *Tutorials in Quantitative Methods for Psychology*, vol. 6, no. 1, pp. 31–38, 2010.

33. A. Hyvärinen and E. Oja, Fast and robust fixed-point algorithms for independent component analysis, *IEEE Transactions on Neural Networks*, vol. 10, no. 3, pp. 626–634, 1999.

34. J. C. Bezdek, R. Ehrlich and W. Full, FCM: The fuzzy c-means clustering algorithm, *Computers & Geosciences*, vol. 10, no. 2, pp. 191–203, 1984.

chapter three

Skin image analysis for vitiligo assessment

*Ahmad Fadzil Mohamad Hani, Hermawan Nugroho,
Norashikin Shamsudin and Suraiya H. Hussein*

Contents

3.1 Skin anatomy and vitiligo disorder

3.1.1 Skin anatomy

Skin is the largest organ of the human body. It is made up of multiple layers of epithelial tissues, which protect muscles and organs. Skin functions are insulation and temperature regulation, sensation, vitamin D and B synthesis, and protection against pathogens. Skin has three primary layers: epidermis, dermis and hypodermis (subcutaneous tissue) (Rosebury, 1969). The epidermis provides protection against infection. The dermis serves as location for the appendages of skin. The hypodermis serves as the basement of skin membrane. The epidermis consists of keratinocytes, melanocytes, Langerhans cells and Merkel cells. There are no blood vessels in the epidermis and it is nourished by diffusion from the dermis. Epidermis is divided into five sublayers (strata), which are (from superficial to deep) strata corneum, strata lucidum, strata granulosum, strata spinosum, and strata basale. Epidermis cells are formed through mitosis at the innermost layers (Figure 3.1).

Skin has a pigment melanin that absorbs some of the potentially dangerous ultraviolet radiation in sunlight. Melanin is a colour pigment found in skin, eyes and hair. It is produced by melanocytes through processes called melanogenesis. Melanocytes are epidermis cells that are located in the bottom layer of the epidermis, as shown in Figure 3.2. The density of melanocytes in skin does not vary among different ethnic origins; however, skin pigmentation differs due to variations in the rate of melanin production.

The dermis is the second primary layer of skin and is located beneath the epidermis. It is connected to the epidermis by a basement membrane. There are many sensors and glands located in the dermis. The nerves that

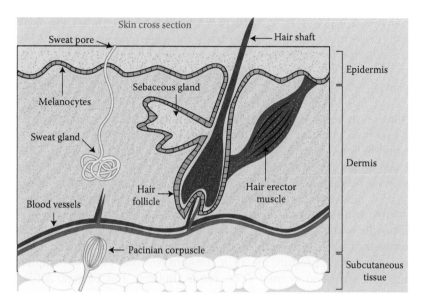

Figure 3.1 Anatomy of skin. (Taken from www.enchantedlearning.com.)

are related to sense of touch and heat, hair follicles, sweat glands, sebaceous glands, apocrine glands and blood vessels are all located in the dermis. The blood vessels in the dermis provide nourishment and removes waste.

The hypodermis is the last layer of skin and lies below the dermis. It attaches the skin to underlying bone and muscle, and supplies skin with

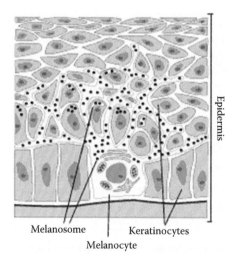

Figure 3.2 Melanocyte. (Reproduced from Turkington and Dover, 2007.)

blood vessels and nerves. It consists of loose connective tissue and elastin. The hypodermis contains 50% of body fat, where fat serves as padding and insulation for the body.

3.1.2 Vitiligo disorders

Vitiligo is an acquired, idiopathic pigmentary disorder characterised by depigmented macules that result from damage to and destruction of epidermal melanocytes. The prevalence of vitiligo varies from 0.1% to 2% in various global populations without any sex, racial, skin types or socioeconomic predilection. Onset may occur at any age but 50% of patients acquire it before the age of 20 years. The loss of melanocytes alters both structure and function of skin, mucous membranes, eyes and hair bulbs, and results in the absence of pigment melanin. Melanin, the pigment that determines colour of skin, hair and eyes is produced in melanocytes. If these cells cannot produce melanin, the skin becomes paler or completely white in contrast to normal skin colour (Roberts and Lesage, 2003), as shown in Figure 3.3.

Theories concerning the cause of vitiligo have concentrated on four different mechanisms: autoimmune, autocytotoxic, neural and genetic (Tonsi, 2004). In autoimmune theory, the extent of skin depigmentation is correlated with the incidence and level of antibodies against melanocytes. It is found that there is increased occurrence of vitiligo in certain autoimmune diseases such a thyroid disease (Hashimoto thyroiditis and Graves disease), Addison disease, pernicious anaemia, insulin-dependent diabetes mellitus and alopecia areata. In autocytotoxicity theory, it is reported that an intermediate or metabolic product of melanin synthesis causes destruction of melanocytes. A second mechanism by which autocytotoxicity occurs is through the inhibition of thioredoxin reductase enzyme. In neural theory, it is believed that a neurochemical mediator destroys melanocytes or inhibits melanin production. In genetic theory, melanocytes have an inherent abnormality that impedes their growth and differentiation in conditions that support normal melanocytes.

Most patients find vitiligo irritating. Vitiligo can have a major impact on patients' psychology, particularly for dark-skinned patients (Porter, 1979). Vitiligo can also increase the risk of developing autoimmune disease, such as thyroid disease, Addison disease, pernicious anaemia and alopecia areata.

3.1.3 Vitiligo treatment procedures

Vitiligo can be treated in many ways but generally, it can be categorised by the following three types of treatment: medical treatment, surgical and UVB (ultraviolet B)/laser treatment, as shown in Table 3.1.

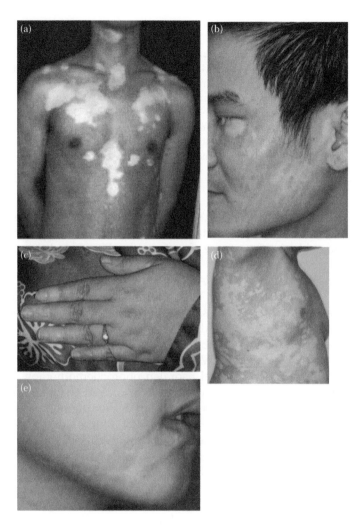

Figure 3.3 Samples of vitiligo lesions: (a) generalised vitiligo, (b) segmental vitiligo, (c) acrofacial vitiligo, (d) universal vitiligo and (e) focal vitiligo.

3.1.3.1 Medical treatment

In topical and systemic corticosteroids therapy, topical corticosteroids are used. Topical corticosteroids are effective repigmenting agents. It has been reported that optimal success of treatment with topical corticosteroids requires applications for 3–4 months or longer (Tonsi, 2004). Mid- or lower-potency corticosteroids may be preferable to avoid the toxicity associated with long-term applications of corticosteroids. Corticosteroid cream is applied to depigmented skin once daily for 3–4 months and the

Table 3.1 Vitiligo treatments

Medical treatment	Surgical	UVB/laser therapy
1. Topical and systemic corticosteroids 2. Psorelen with exposure to UVA radiation therapy 3. Depigmentation therapy with monobenzylether of hydroquinone 4. Tacrolimus ointment	1. Mini grafting 2. Transplantation of cultured melanocytes 3. Transplantation of noncultured melanocytes	1. Narrow band UVB therapy 2. 380 nm laser 3. Depigmentation with QS ruby laser

response is monitored with Wood's lamp examination at 6-weeks interval. Therapy is continued if repigmentation occurs, but the therapy is stopped if there is no evidence of response after 3 months. Photographs may assist in evaluating progress.

Psoralen-ultraviolet A (PUVA) is a repigmentation therapy using medication known as psoralen. This chemical is able to make human skin very sensitive to light. The skin is then treated with a special type of ultraviolet light. Treatment with PUVA is reported to have a 50%–70% chance of returning colour on the face, trunk, upper arms, and upper legs. There are two types of PUVA therapy: oral psoralen photochemotherapy and topical therapy. Oral psoralen photochemotherapy is used for patients with more extensive vitiligo or for patients who are unmanageable with topical therapy. It is found that darker pigmented patients respond better to PUVA therapy because of the increased tolerance to greater cumulative UVA (ultraviolet A) dosage. Vitiligo on the trunk, proximal extremities and face respond well to PUVA therapy, although distal extremities and periorificial areas do not. The potential side effects include burn, erythema, pruritus, xerosis, carcinogenicity, pigmented lesions, cataracts and aging. Topical therapy psoralen photochemotherapy is another PUVA therapy used for patients with limited vitiligo lesion areas (less than 20% of the body surface) or for children older than 5 years with localised vitiligo.

Heliotherapy is a repigmentation therapy using a combination of trisoralen and sunlight. Trisoralen is a photosensitiser used to increase skin tolerance to sunlight and enhance pigmentation. It darkens the skin and thickens skin layers.

Depigmentation therapy is a treatment of vitiligo to remove the remaining pigment melanin of normal skin and make the whole body an even white colour. This therapy is considered for patients with extensive involvement or patients with more than 50% involvement of the skin and has demonstrated therapeutic resistance. This treatment could be done by using 20% monobenzoether or hydroquinone applied to the skin once or twice daily for 1–3 years. The pigment removal is permanent and irreversible, resulting in permanent photosensitivity.

For some cases, patients have poor clinical response to topical steroid and PUVA therapy due to undesirable side effects. For such cases, dermatologists will consider a treatment with vitamin D analogues (topical tacalcitol).

Tacrolimus ointment is an immunosuppressant that is derived from the fungus *Streptomyces tsukubaensis*. Topical tacrolimus offers several advantages in treating vitiligo. It is well tolerated in adults and children and prolonged use does not cause atrophy and adverse potential ocular side effects. There is also no limitation for application to facial and intertriginous areas. The efficacy of tacrolimus for vitiligo was first reported in a case series of six patients with generalised vitiligo. Five of the six patients achieved at least a 50% repigmentation of the affected areas (Lepe et al., 2003). Tacrolimus ointment has been found to be safe and efficacious in both adult and childhood vitiligo patients in North America, Mexico, Europe and India. In conjunction with this research, a study of efficacy and safety of tacrolimus ointment in Malaysia is conducted in Hospital Kuala Lumpur, Malaysia. The study concentrates on repigmentation evaluation using objective and subjective methods while our developed digital image analysis system is used as the objective method.

3.1.3.2 Surgical

There are two types of surgicals (mini grafting); micropigmentation (tattooing) and dermabrasion (van Geel et al., 2001). Micropigmentation involves tattooing vitiligo skin, in order to match the normal skin colour. However, an exact match of pigment is difficult to obtain. In dermabrasion, vitiligo skin areas are superficially dermabraded. It may result in a darker repigmentation.

In transplantation of cultured melanocytes, melanocytes are harvested from a small fragment of pigmented skin from patient. The melanocytes are then isolated and grown in cell culture for 3 weeks. It is found that in in vitro transplantation method, the repigmentation areas can be as large as 10 times from the donor areas. A method that resembles in vitro cultured melanocytes is transplantation of noncultured melanocytes.

3.1.3.3 UVB/laser therapy

In narrow band UVB therapy, a new device that produces focused beam of narrow UVB is used. The dose is gradually increased until 50% repigmentation is observed. Photographs of the patients are taken for helping the observation. Another therapy that resembles UVB therapy is the therapy using excimer laser with wavelength of 380 nm. For depigmentation cases, it is known that bleaching creams may have serious side effects.

Q-switched (QS) ruby laser could be used as an alternative for depigmentation (Kim et al., 2001).

3.2 Assessment of vitiligo

3.2.1 Subjective assessment of vitiligo

Assessment of therapeutic response of vitiligo has always been unsatisfactory as currently there is no objective way to measure and quantify the repigmentation response. The current scoring systems used to evaluate treatment outcome is largely arbitrary and is highly subjective with inter- and intra-observer variations. There is no validated quantitative scale that allows vitiligo to be characterised parametrically.

PGA (Physician's Global Assessment) scale is the current scoring system widely used by dermatologists. The scale is based on the degree of repigmentation within lesions over time. However, it is found that most of the studies on vitiligo treatments vary in width and number of points of the PGA scale with different authors. The degree of repigmentation that defines success has often been set somewhat arbitrarily at 50%–75% repigmentation based largely on the global impression of the overall response (Lepe, 2003). It is difficult to compare treatment outcomes given the differences in using PGA scale to assess repigmentation. Table 3.2 shows the PGA scale used in this work.

Furthermore, the treatment efficacy would still be largely dependent on the human eye and judgment to produce the scorings. As a result, the judgment varies with dermatologists and thus becomes subjective.

The progression of vitiligo treatment can be very slow and can take more than 6 months (Roberts and Lesage, 2003). It is observed that dermatologists find it visually hard to determine the areas of skin repigmentation due to this slow progress and as a result the observations are made after a longer time frame. It is also known that patients respond differently to the vitiligo treatment. Therapeutic response of a particular treatment could vary for different patients. It is therefore useful for dermatologists to know the efficacy of a particular treatment early, in order that treatment can be adjusted accordingly.

Table 3.2 PGA scale

Repigmentation (%)	Scale
0–25	Mild
26–50	Moderate
51–75	Good
76–100	Excellent to complete

3.2.2 Objective assessment of vitiligo

The assessment of vitiligo therapeutic response is based on the measurement of degree of skin repigmentation within vitiligo areas over time by dermatologists. The evaluation of vitiligo treatment outcome is largely dependent on the human eye and judgment to produce the scorings. To monitor the efficacy of the treatment, dermatologists observe the disease directly, or indirectly using digital photos. These digital skin images are manually analysed for the purpose of diagnosis by dermatologists. As a result, a large number of skin images are being taken that require manual analysis and diagnosis. At present, dermatologist analyses the disease by comparing patient's images before and after the treatment. A dermatologist studies the photographs and assesses the efficacy of the therapeutic response of vitiligo treatment. This requires a high degree of skill and experience as the dermatologist has to be trained to enable an accurate assessment to be made. However, the technique is still subjective as it is possible to have different assessments due to the varying degrees of experience of dermatologists.

During treatment for vitiligo, skin images are produced using a digital SLR (single-lens reflection) camera. Digital SLR camera provides many advantages compared to digital compact camera. The principal advantage of digital SLR cameras over other digital cameras is the defining characteristic of an SLR: the image in the optical viewfinder is parallax-free because its light is routed directly from the main lens itself, rather than from an off-axis viewfinder.

The skin images produced by the camera are presented as arrays of pixels having discrete intensity values. These intensity values are produced by the camera's CCD (charge-coupled device). CCD is an image sensor consisting of integrated circuits containing an array of coupled light-sensitive capacitors. It is reported that CCD and photographic film respond to 70% and 40% of the incident light, respectively, thus making CCD more efficient than photographic film (Peterson, 2001). In digital image camera, CCD sensors are equipped with Bayer mask to produce colour images. Bayer mask filters all of the incoming light into three colour light: red, green and blue (RGB) (Bayer, 1976).

In signal processing, digital skin image can be seen as a two-dimensional signal that contains information of skin. Using computing techniques, skin image can be analysed and used as a tool for assisting dermatologists. Moreover, with the decrease in cost and increase in computation power of personal computers, it is now reasonable to develop a sophisticated and cost-effective computer-based image analysis system. Computer-aided analysis of digital skin image offers quantitative and repeatable measurements, reducing the subjectivity of diagnosis. In addition, it also has the potential to enable dermatologist monitors vitiligo on a shorter time cycle.

3.3 Digital skin imaging for vitiligo assessment

3.3.1 Problem formulation and objective

As described in Section 3.2.1, the current therapeutic response assessment for vitiligo disease is PGA scale. However, these are subjective as it is possible to have different judgments due to the varying degrees of experience of dermatologists. In order to perform PGA scoring accurately, a dermatologist has to be trained extensively. Another problem is that most of the studies on vitiligo treatments have different PGA scale. It is hard to compare treatment outcomes given differences in the scoring systems used to assess repigmentation. In addition, the progression of vitiligo treatment is very slow (Roberts, 2003). During treatment, areas of repigmentation are found to be small and patchy. Dermatologists found it difficult to discern visually areas of skin repigmentation during treatment. As a result, the observation and assessment process is made after a longer time cycle.

Based on the aforementioned discussion, it is necessary to develop a qualitative digital imaging and analysis tool that is highly sensitive to assist dermatologists for monitoring vitiligo treatment outcome objectively. The system should be able to analyse, determine and quantify vitiligo skin and repigmentation areas efficiently and reliably. More importantly, it can provide objective efficacy assessment to assist dermatologist make accurate diagnosis and therapeutic response. The system is expected to provide dermatologist with an objective tool to determine repigmentation areas.

3.3.2 Proposed technique for objective assessment of vitiligo disorder

In the development of such digital imaging and analysis tool for vitiligo assessment, techniques that determine and quantify the repigmentation surface areas objectively over a shorter time frame, based on digital signal and image processing techniques, are developed and evaluated. A combination of signal, image processing and analysis techniques is proposed to convert the skin images into images that represent skin areas specifically due to pigment melanin followed by a segmentation process. Areas of repigmentation will further be measured by comparing images before and after treatment. The developed algorithm consists of a variety of image processing techniques such as image rotation, geometrical transformation, median cut segmentation, morphological operations and several signal processing techniques such as principal component analysis (PCA) and independent component analysis (ICA). The algorithms are to be implemented using MATLAB® 7.1 software and converted into a stand-alone system for use in the field.

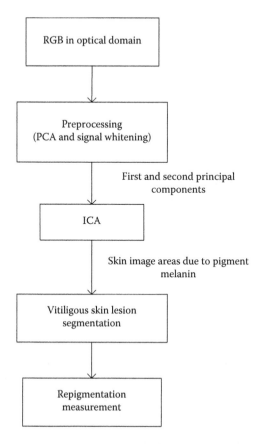

Figure 3.4 Process flow chart of vitiligo objective assessment system.

The process flow of the vitiligo objective assessment tool is as shown in Figure 3.4, comprising preprocessing, ICA estimation, image segmentation and repigmentation measurement. Each process in the process flow is elaborated in the following sections.

3.4 Development of vitiligo assessment tool

Visual cues play an important role in enabling dermatologists to make appropriate diagnosis. Visual descriptors of vitiligo lesion areas differ from normal skin in particular, vitiligo lesion areas are paler in contrast to normal skin. In addition, it is found that the appearance of skin due to repigmentation is similar to the appearance of normal skin.

In this research, the development of the vitiligo monitoring system is discussed. The performance and the limitation of the system are also studied. Digital colour skin images are analysed under several assumptions based on skin optic properties. The image processing analysis algorithm used in the system is based on PCA and ICA. PCA and ICA are used to transform digital colour skin images into skin images that represent skin areas due to melanin and haemoglobin only. The transformed skin images will enable the determination of melanin areas within skin image. The determination and quantification of repigmentation is investigated to enable treatment efficacy over a shorter time frame. The difference in the vitiligo surface areas before and after treatment will be expressed as a percentage of repigmentation in each vitiligo lesion. This percentage will represent the repigmentation progression of a particular body region.

To measure the performance and the limitation of the developed system, the image processing analysis is employed in the controlled environment. The controlled environment comprises skin colour models of healthy skin, vitiligo lesion, skin areas due to repigmentation and added noise. The complete process flow involved in vitiligo objective assessment is shown in Figure 3.4, and the process of developed system is shown in Figure 3.5.

In the following sections, details discussion is made.

3.4.1 Methodological approach for vitiligo assessment tool

3.4.1.1 RGB data set

In the case of skin surface, a small portion of the incident light will be reflected because of the difference in the index of reaction between the air and skin surface. It has been found that the surface reflectance is typically between 4% and 7% over the entire spectrum from 250 to 3000 nm. Most of the incident light penetrates into the skin and follows a complex path until it exits back out of the skin or gets attenuated by skin choromophores.

Skin choromophores absorb electromagnetic energy of the light. As shown in Figure 3.6, the primary choromophores in skin are pigment melanin, and haemoglobin (oxy-haemoglobin and deoxy-haemoglobin).

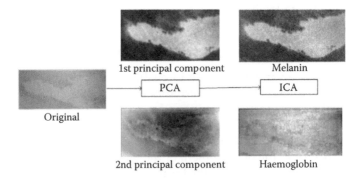

Figure 3.5 Process of vitiligo objective assessment tool.

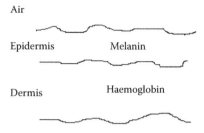

Air

Epidermis   Melanin

Dermis   Haemoglobin

Figure 3.6 Skin choromophores.

Due to the above process, information about skin choromophores can be extracted from the reflected light coming from skin. This reflected light is recorded by CCD sensor of a camera and forms a digital colour image. The digital colour image is created by combining three different spectral bands, namely, RGB.

3.4.1.2 Skin image model

The spatial distribution of melanin and haemoglobin in skin could be separated by employing linear ICA of a skin colour image (Tsumura et al., 1999). The analysis is based on the skin colour model with three assumptions. First, it is assumed linearity in the optical density domain of RGB channels. The second and third assumptions state that the spatial variations of skin image colour are caused by two skin choromophores, namely melanin and haemoglobin and their quantities are mutually independent, as shown in Figure 3.6. Figure 3.7 shows the skin model developed by Tsumura.

3.4.1.3 Principal component analysis

Figure 3.7 shows that skin colour distribution lies on a two-dimensional melanin–haemoglobin colour subspace. In order to determine repigmentation (due to pigment melanin), it is necessary to perform a conversion from RGB skin image to this two-dimensional colour subspace. Using PCA as a dimensional reduction tool, a two-dimensional subspace can be formed using the PCA first and second principal components. It is reported that the values of the RGB skin image can be adequately represented by using two principal components with an accuracy of 99.3% (Tsumura, 1999). In addition, it is also necessary to make the two-dimensional subspace zero mean and unit variance in order to get stronger independence condition. The stronger independence condition will make the results of ICA more accurate. The two-dimensional subspace zero mean is the two-dimensional subspace after subtracting the mean value from the data sets.

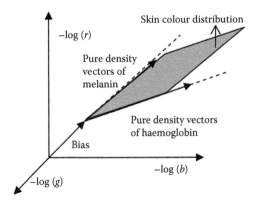

Figure 3.7 Skin colour model. (Reproduced from N. Tsumura et al., *Journal of the Optical Society of America A*, vol. 16, pp. 2169–2176, 1999.)

3.4.1.4 Independent component analysis

Skin colour distribution can be expressed as functions of pure density vector of melanin and haemoglobin. Let $s_1(x, y)$ and $s_2(x, y)$ represent the quantities of the two colour pigments on image coordinate, (x, y), which are independent variables. The colour vectors of the two pigments per unit quantity are denoted a_1 and a_2, respectively. It is also assumed that the compound colour vector $v(x, y)$ can be calculated using linear combination of the colour vectors as follows:

$$v(x, y) = a_1 s_1(x, y) + a_2 s_2(x, y) \tag{3.1}$$

This equation can be written as

$$v(x, y) = As(x, y) \tag{3.2}$$

$$A = [a_1 a_2] \tag{3.3}$$

Equation 3.3 is known as linear ICA, where A is a mixing matrix and s contains the independent components.

As depicted in Figure 3.8, the goal of ICA is to find a linear transformation W of the dependent sensor signals v that make the output independent as possible (Hvyarinen 2000) (Equation 3.4).

$$u = Wv, \quad u \gg s \tag{3.4}$$

In this work, matrix W is estimated using a method developed by Hyvarinen (1999, 2000). From this process, the two independent components of the skin image can be extracted. One is the image of skin areas due to melanin and the other is the image of skin areas due to haemoglobin only.

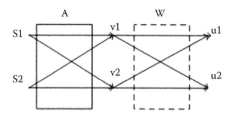

Figure 3.8 ICA model for colour skin image.

3.4.1.5 *Image segmentation*

Image segmentation method is performed on the image that represents skin areas due to melanin. The objective of the segmentation process is to separate vitiligo skin lesion from healthy skin. For this, we employed image segmentation technique based on thresholding.

Thresholding segments an image into regions of interest and removes all other regions deemed inessential. There are many segmentation techniques based on thresholding. In this particular research, the thresholding technique based on median cut algorithm is employed.

3.4.1.6 *Repigmentation measurement*

In the developed system, the difference in the vitiligo surface areas between skin images before and after treatment will be expressed as a percentage of repigmentation in each vitiligo lesion. This percentage will represent the repigmentation progression of a particular body region.

The dermatologists choose the vitiligo surface areas and the details of the position and locations of the lesions are recorded by the clinicians. This is to ensure the accuracy of the measurement by the developed system.

The calculation is explained as follows:

Let $a(K, L)$ be the logical image where vitiligo lesion and normal skin areas are represented by 1 and 0, respectively. $a(K, L)$ is defined as a processed image of the image segmentation of the developed system.

The vitiligo surface areas, *Area*, is measured as follows:

$$Area = \sum_{i=0}^{K} \sum_{j=0}^{L} a(i, j)$$

(3.5)

3.4.2 *Validation of developed vitiligo assessment tool*

3.4.2.1 *Reference model*

Reference model images are simulated images that represent healthy skin and vitiligo skin images. These images are modelled based on the distribution of colour combinations in the three spectral bands, namely RGB.

3.4.2.2 Distribution model

The distribution models are developed using samples of skin colour taken from historical data of four patients. These samples are chosen together with dermatologists to obtain valid reference model images. The distribution of each spectral value is modelled using Gaussian distribution.

$$f(x;\mu,\sigma) = \frac{1}{\sigma\sqrt{2\pi}} e^{-\frac{(x-\mu)^2}{2\sigma^2}} \tag{3.6}$$

where σ is the standard deviation and μ is the mean value.

The Gaussian distribution model is chosen based on studies of skin modelling by Caetano, Zhu and Chang (Caetano and Barone, 2001). In their works, it is reported that the skin colour distribution can be modelled by Gaussian distributions.

To employ reliable statistical parameters of normal distribution (mean and standard deviation), a good estimator is needed.

$$\bar{x} = \sum_{i=1}^{n} \frac{x_i}{n} \tag{3.7}$$

$$\sigma = \sqrt{\frac{1}{n-1} \sum_{i=1}^{n} (x - \bar{x})^2} \tag{3.8}$$

Equation 3.7 is used to measure the mean value of the distribution while Equation 3.8 estimates the standard deviation parameter. In this work, an estimator called minimum-variance unbiased estimator (MVUE) is used. MVUE is commonly used to estimate the parameters of normal distribution.

3.4.2.3 Healthy skin image model

The healthy skin image model is developed from simulated healthy skin images. Simulated healthy skin images are produced based on the statistical pixel distribution of healthy skin images. To establish the pixel distribution model, approximately 60,000 pixels are obtained from healthy colour skin images, sampled from four patients. Figures 3.9 through 3.11 show the pixel intensity distributions of RGB spectral bands. Gaussian

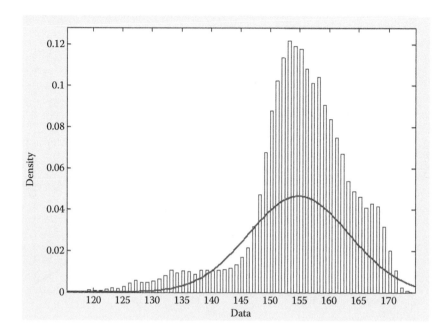

Figure 3.9 Pixel intensity distribution of red spectral band from healthy skin.

distribution models are obtained from the pixel intensity distributions and the parameters of the Gaussian distribution are then estimated. Table 3.3 shows the parameters of Gaussian distribution using MVUE.

Using these estimated parameters, the healthy skin image model is obtained. Figure 3.12 shows an example of 20-by-20 pixels of generated healthy skin.

3.4.2.4 Vitiligo lesion model

Vitiligo lesion model is a simulated vitiligo skin image. The simulated images are produced by the distribution model of vitiligo lesion. To develop the distribution model, we take approximately 40,000 pixels of healthy skin taken from four patients. Together with dermatologist, we grab samples of healthy skin from patients. These samples have approximately 40,000 pixels. Figures 3.13 through 3.15 show the distribution of the intensity value in the three different spectral bands. Parameters of Gaussian distribution are then estimated. Table 3.4 shows the parameters of Gaussian distributions for RGB spectral bands, respectively, using MVUE.

Figure 3.16 shows an example of 20-by-20 pixels of generated vitiligo lesion image using the vitiligo lesion model function.

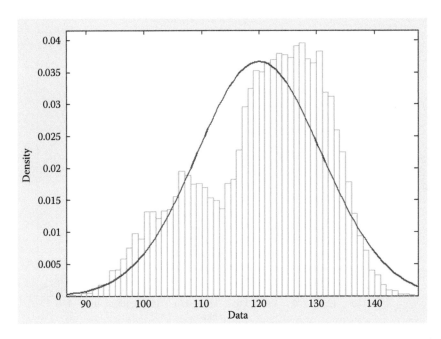

Figure 3.10 Pixel intensity distribution of green spectral band from healthy skin.

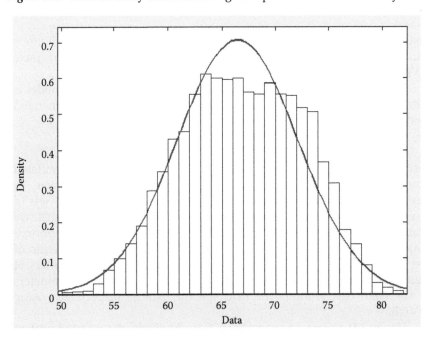

Figure 3.11 Pixel intensity distribution of blue spectral band from healthy skin.

Table 3.3 Estimated parameters of Gaussian
distribution from MVUE

Spectral colour	Mean	Standard deviation
Red	154.869	8.54991
Green	120.025	10.8663
Blue	66.476	5.63958

3.4.2.5 Reference model images

There are four reference images used in the development of the system, namely reference image A, B, C and D. Each reference image consists of 200-by-200 pixels. The size is constructed based on advice from the doctor and the size of vitiligo lesions found on the data.

Reference image A (Figure 3.17a) is constructed to model a skin image having vitiligo lesion. In this model, the size of image A is 200-by-200 pixels while the vitiligo lesion areas have 40-by-50 pixels. Reference image B (Figure 3.17b) is created similar to reference image A. However, in its vitiligo lesion areas we add three areas that represent skin areas due to repigmentation. The size of each repigmentation area is 5-by-5 pixels.

Reference image C (Figure 3.17c) and reference image D (Figure 3.17d) are created similar to reference image B. The differences of these reference images are on the size of the skin areas due to repigmentation. In reference image C, the size of the repigmentation areas is 3-by-3 pixels while in the reference image D, the size is reduced into 1-by-1 pixel.

Figure 3.12 Generated healthy skin.

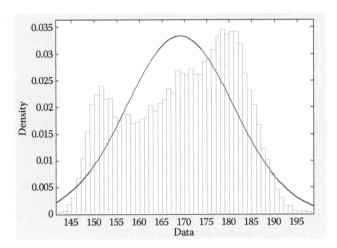

Figure 3.13 Vitiligo lesion distribution in red spectral band.

3.4.2.6 Noise generator

In this work, noise generator is used to add controlled noises to the reference model images in order to measure the performance of the developed system before applying it to the real data. The limitation of the developed system is analysed by employing the developed system to the reference images added by noise. Let I be the reference image and n is the noise. The reference image, R, after being added by noise can be written as

$$R = I + n \tag{3.9}$$

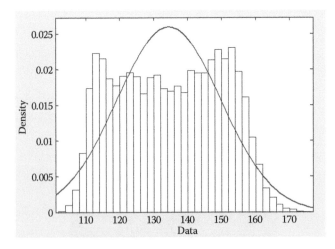

Figure 3.14 Vitiligo lesion distribution in green spectral band.

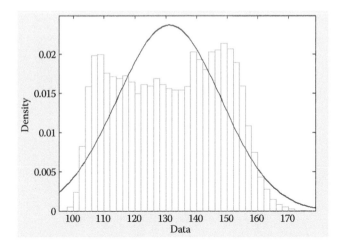

Figure 3.15 Vitiligo lesion distribution in blue spectral band.

where n is considered to be a white Gaussian noise defined as follows:

$$n(i;\mu,\sigma) = \frac{1}{\sigma\sqrt{2\pi}}e^{-\frac{(i-\mu)^2}{2\sigma^2}}$$ (3.10)

The added noise is controlled by the SNR (signal-to-noise ratio). SNR is the power ratio between a signal and the background noise.

$$SNR(dB) = 10\log\left(\frac{P_{signal}}{P_{noise}}\right) = 20\log\left(\frac{A_{signal}}{A_{noise}}\right)$$ (3.11)

where P is power and A the RMS (root mean square) value. The connection of RMS value and standard deviation of a data set x can be written as

$$A = x_{RMS}$$

$$x_{RMS}^2 = \mu_x^2 + \sigma_x^2$$ (3.12)

Table 3.4 Estimated parameters of Gaussian distribution

	Mean	Standard deviation
Red	169.016	11.9486
Green	134.417	15.3538
Blue	131.124	16.8001

Figure 3.16 Generated vitiligo lesion image.

where x_{RMS} is the RMS value of x, μ_x the mean value of x, and σ_x the standard deviation of x Equation 3.12 can be written as follows:

$$SNR(dB) = 20\log\left(\sqrt{\frac{\mu_{signal}^2 + \sigma_{signal}^2}{\mu_{noise}^2 + \sigma_{noise}^2}}\right) \tag{3.13}$$

If x is a zero mean data set, the RMS value of x is equal to the standard deviation. Equation 3.13 can be written as

$$SNR(dB) = 20\log\left(\sqrt{\frac{\sigma_{signal}^2}{\sigma_{noise}^2}}\right) = 20\log\left(\sqrt{\left(\frac{\sigma_{signal}}{\sigma_{noise}}\right)^2}\right) = 20\log\left(\frac{\sigma_{signal}}{\sigma_{noise}}\right) \tag{3.14}$$

Using Equation 3.14, we can generate Gaussian noise based on the SNR that we want to have.

$$\sigma_{noise} = \left(\frac{\sigma_{signal}}{10^{\frac{SNR(dB)}{20}}}\right) \tag{3.15}$$

Using Equation 3.14, noise, n of Equation 4.10 can be calculated. Then from Equation 3.9, image with noise, R, can be constructed.

3.4.2.7 Accuracy measurement result
Employing the developed system to all of the reference images, the developed system has been able to discern vitiligo lesion, the healthy skin

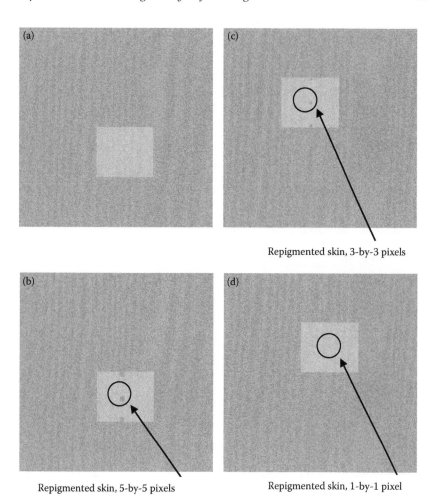

Repigmented skin, 3-by-3 pixels

Repigmented skin, 5-by-5 pixels

Repigmented skin, 1-by-1 pixel

Figure 3.17 Reference images: (a) skin image with vitiligo lesion, (b) image of vitiligo lesion with repigmented skin (5-by-5 pixels), (c) image of vitiligo lesion with repigmented skin (3-by-3 pixels) and (d) image of vitiligo lesion with repigmented skin (1-by-1 pixel).

and the skin repigmentation areas, as shown in Figure 3.18a through d. Moreover, it can detect skin repigmentation areas whose size is only 1-by-1 pixels, as depicted in Figure 3.18e.

3.4.2.8 Noise limitation measurement result

In this section, we test the limitation of the developed system by adding noise to the reference images. The range of SNR used for the test is from 20 to 1 dB. From the test, it is found that the developed vitiligo monitoring system can discern the vitiligo lesion, healthy skin and skin

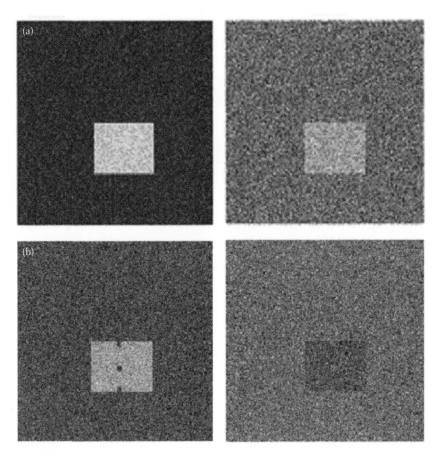

Figure 3.18 Results of the reference images. (a) Reference Image A: skin areas due to melanin (left) and skin areas due to haemoglobin (right). (b) Reference Image B: skin areas due to melanin (left) and skin areas due to haemoglobin (right).

(*Continued*)

repigmentation areas of reference image A, B and C even though the SNR is 1 dB, as shown in Figure 3.19a through c respectively.

However, for reference image D, it is found that if the SNR is less than 15 dB, the repigmentation areas located on the border of lesions and skin are starting to be blurring. Figure 3.20 shows the reference image D with SNR of 15 dB. It can be seen that the repigmentation areas located on the border are still discernable. The repigmentation areas located on the border are not visible.

To measure the accuracy of the vitiligo monitoring system, tests are performed involving reference models A, B, C and D. The method is able to discern vitiligo lesion, the healthy skin and the skin repigmentation

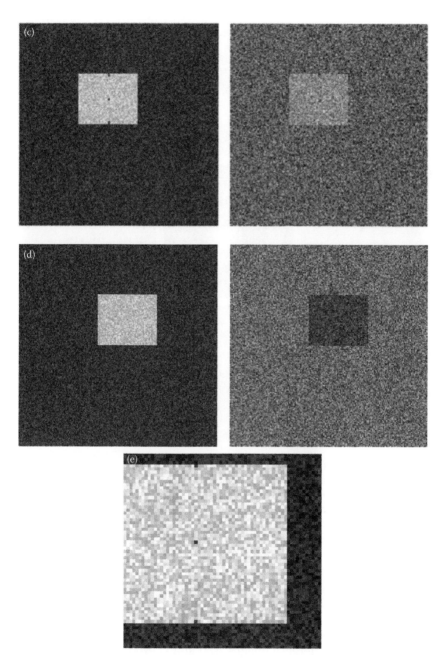

Figure 3.18 (Continued) (c) Reference Image C: skin areas due to melanin (left) and skin areas due to haemoglobin (right). (d) Reference Image D: skin areas due to melanin (left) and skin areas due to haemoglobin (right). (e) Reference Image A: skin areas due to melanin (left) and skin areas due to haemoglobin (right).

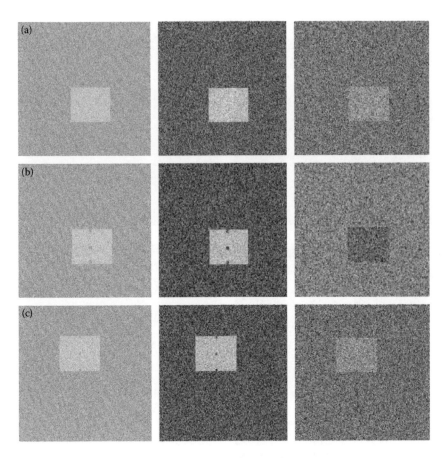

Figure 3.19 Results of reference images after adding noise. (a) The result of reference image A with noise (SNR = 1 dB) in left: skin areas due to melanin in middle and skin areas due to haemoglobin in right. (b) The result of reference image B with noise (SNR = 1 dB) in left: skin areas due to melanin in middle and skin areas due to haemoglobin in right. (c) The result of reference image C with noise (SNR = 1 dB) in left: skin areas due to melanin in middle and skin areas due to haemoglobin in right.

areas. Moreover, it can determine skin repigmentation area down to 1-by-1 pixel (Figure 3.18). Then, the reference images are added with noise before being analysed by the system. The range of SNRs used for the test is varying from 20 to 1 dB. It is found that the method is able to discern the repigmentation areas of reference images A, B and C even though the SNR is 1 dB. For reference image D, it is shown that if the SNR is less than 15 dB, the method cannot determine the repigmentation areas that are located on the border of vitiligo lesions and skin. The method is, however, still able to identify repigmentation area that are located in the centre of the

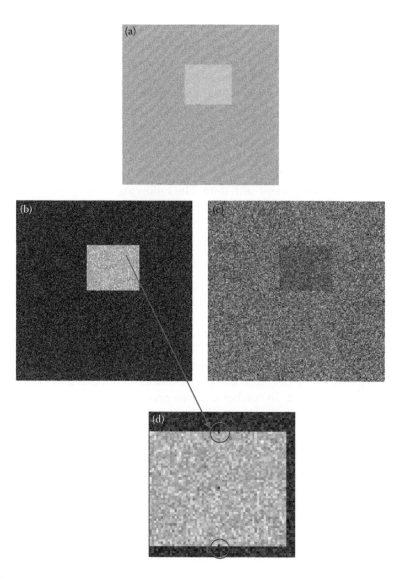

Figure 3.20 Results of (a) reference image D with noise (SNR = 15 dB); (b) skin areas due to melanin; (c) skin areas due to haemoglobin and (d) closed up of skin repigmentation areas. The repigmentation areas located on the border are still discernible.

vitiligo lesion area. The repigmentation area located in the centre of the vitiligo lesion area cannot be captured when the SNR is less than 10 dB as found from the measurements performed.

In summary, the method developed for vitiligo objective assessment works well with model skin images and its performance is measured by adding noise in controlled environment. Using this skin colour model, the developed vitiligo monitoring system converts RGB skin images into images that represent skin areas due to melanin and haemoglobin. The overall trend is that the system will deteriorate if SNR decreases. When SNR is low, the system cannot capture small repigmentation areas. The performance of the system also depends on the position of the repigmentation areas. The system tends to deteriorate more if the repigmentation areas are located on the border of the vitiligo lesion and normal skin.

After the successful implementation of the developed methods and its performance evaluation on skin model images, the developed method is employed on real patient skin data. The following sections describe the implementation of developed method on real patient skin data and results obtained.

3.5 Results and discussion

The developed vitiligo monitoring system based on the flowchart as shown in Figure 3.21 is applied on the real images obtained at Hospital Kuala Lumpur, Malaysia.

Patients are chosen by a dermatologist. The images of the vitiligo lesions are then taken using Nikon digital camera SLR D100. The study was divided into two phases: preliminary study and preclinical trial. For the first phase of the development of the vitiligo monitoring system, historical data were used. To further validate and improve the system, a second data set was taken during preclinical trial.

3.5.1 Preliminary assessment

The preliminary study involved images of vitiligo lesion taken from historical data of four different patients, taken before treatment and during treatment. The vitiligo monitoring system was used to determine the repigmentation by comparing the images. Figure 3.22 shows images of vitiligo skin samples from patient 1, patient 2, patient 3 and patient 4. The images refer to the same skin area and were taken during the course of treatment. As seen from the figures, the progression of the repigmentation is clearly visible for patient 1, patient 2 and patient 3 after more than 10 months of treatment. However, for patient 4, in which case the treatment has been going on for only 4 months, repigmentation is not visible from the figure.

The vitiligo monitoring system applied on the RGB skin images of patients 1, 2, 3 and 4 produced images that now represent the skin due to melanin and haemoglobin only, as shown in Figure 3.23. Once the melanin and haemoglobin components are extracted from RGB images of vitiligo skin lesion, segmentation of skin lesion is performed on the melanin

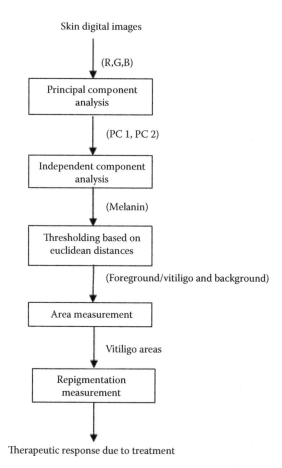

Skin digital images

(R,G,B)

Principal component
analysis

(PC 1, PC 2)

Independent component
analysis

(Melanin)

Thresholding based on
euclidean distances

(Foreground/vitiligo and background)

Area measurement

Vitiligo areas

Repigmentation
measurement

Therapeutic response due to treatment

Figure 3.21 (DOI: 10.1109/ITSIM.2008.4631635. Source: IEEE Xplore Conference: Information Technology, 2008. ITSim 2008. *International Symposium on,* Volume: 1.)

images as shown in Figure 3.23 (last column). The segmented images of melanin represent vitiligo lesion areas. The nonmelanin/vitiligo lesion areas after treatment can be seen to be smaller due to repigmentation, even for patient 4. In the historical data, the images that refer to the same lesion areas are assumed to have similar size. If the size is not the same, the images are adjusted accordingly. This is to ensure accuracy and objectivity of the system.

From the lesion area segmented using developed method, quantitative measurement as area of lesion in pixels are computed for all the four patients and listed in Table 3.5. Developed system quantifies that the vitiligo skin area for patient 1 is 26,263 pixels before treatment and 8,907

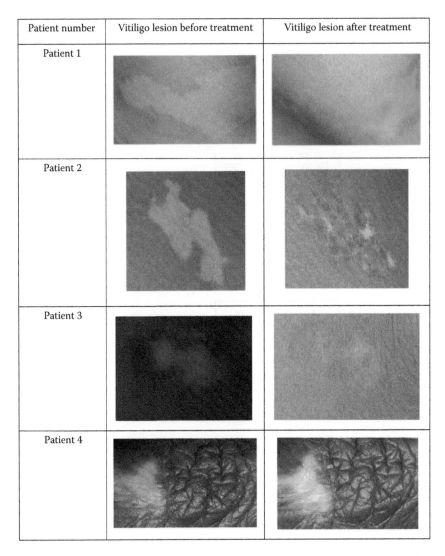

Patient number	Vitiligo lesion before treatment	Vitiligo lesion after treatment
Patient 1		
Patient 2		
Patient 3		
Patient 4		

Figure 3.22 Vitiligo lesions of patients before and after treatment for 10 months.

pixels after treatment, which indicate repigmentation progression of 66%. Similarly, for patient 2, patient 3, repigmentation growth is approximately 94% and 92%, respectively, while for patient 4 repigmentation growth is around 26% due to the less time of treatment duration. Obtained results are also compared with the dermatologist repigmentation score and scale based on PGA and it is found to be in moderate scale (51%–75% range) for patient 1, and mild (0%–25% range) for patient 4.

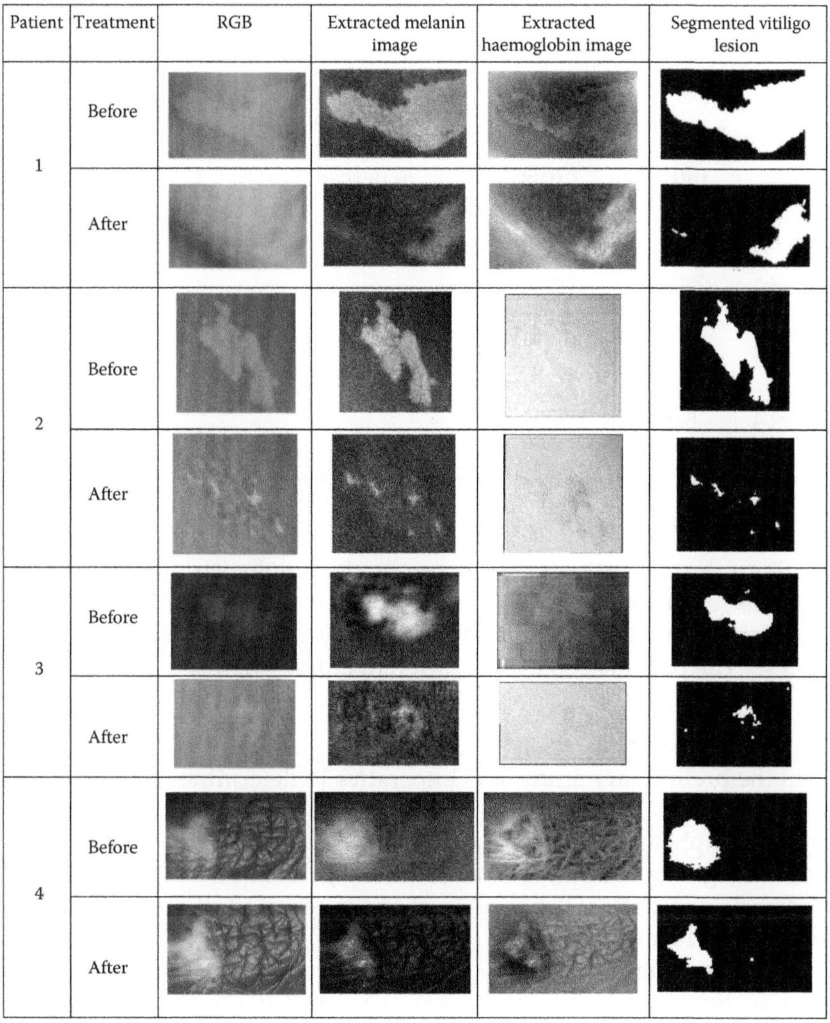

Patient	Treatment	RGB	Extracted melanin image	Extracted haemoglobin image	Segmented vitiligo lesion
1	Before				
	After				
2	Before				
	After				
3	Before				
	After				
4	Before				
	After				

Figure 3.23 Processed images of patients 1, 2, 3 and 4.

It is clearly seen that the percentages obtained using the vitiligo monitoring system are within the PGA ranges, except for the case of patient 4. In the case of patient 4, the images were taken within 4 months of treatment, therefore repigmentation has occurred on a smaller area. It is difficult for dermatologist to discern visually small repigmentation progression due to the treatment. The vitiligo monitoring system, however, is able to capture small repigmentation progression objectively and proves to be potentially superior as it allows monitoring on a smaller time frame.

Table 3.5 Determination of vitiligo skin areas using developed
method and PGA

	Treatment interval	Vitiligo skin areas (pixels)	Repigmentation measurement from development method in percentage (%)	Repigmentation measured using PGA (%)
Patient 1	Before	26,263	66	51–75
	After	8,907		
Patient 2	Before	20,848	94	76–100
	After	1,535		
Patient 3	Before	1,656	92	76–100
	After	133		
Patient 4	Before	585	26	0–25
	After	432		

3.5.2 Preclinical trial study

In this study, five patients are chosen by dermatologists as our data set.
The data set involves images of vitiligo lesion taken from four patients.
The images are taken before and after treatment with smaller interval of
6 weeks. The patients come from different ethnic origins.

3.5.2.1 Reference images

From the preliminary study, it is imperative to determine the true image
size and area to make accurate comparisons. Since the position or distance of the photographer from the patient is not necessity the same every
time during data collection, a reference image of known size and area is
needed during data collection. A reference object of a known size and
area is placed on the skin.

Gonzalez suggested having green colour as colour background in
order to focus solely on the region of interest (Gonzalez and woods,
2003). We use a rectangular green tape as a reference image of known
size on the skin under investigation. Figure 3.24a shows an example
of a reference image in the data. The actual of this reference image is
1.13×10^2 mm^2.

In order to determine the area represented by 1 square pixel, we segment the reference from the image. This is achieved by performing an
image segmentation process. From the green spectral band of image, the
green reference is segmented by employing Otsu's method. Figure 3.24b
shows the green spectral band of Figure 3.24a. The threshold selection
is then selected by maximizing between class variance within the histogram data as shown in Figure 3.24c. The result is a logical image, as shown
in Figure 3.24d. The reference image is found to have an area of 24,625

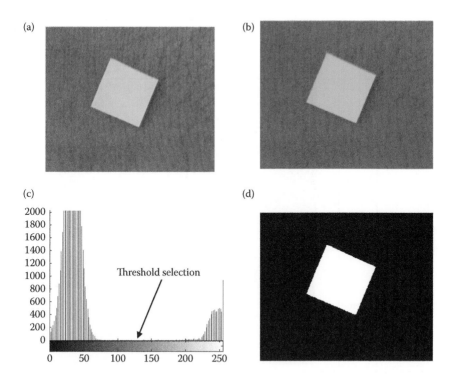

Figure 3.24 Preprocessing of reference image: (a) 1.13 × 102 mm² green tape as a reference, (b) green band of reference image, (c) histogram of reference image and (d) logical image of the reference image.

pixels. It can be concluded that in that particular image (Figure 3.24a), 1-by-1 pixel represents 4.5888×10^{-3} mm².

3.5.2.2 Patient data

Skin images of patients are taken with digital camera SLR Nikon D-100. The first RGB images are used as a baseline on the first time point. For treatment, all of the patients are given tacrolimus ointment. The second RGB images are then taken after 6 weeks of treatment. Figure 3.25 shows the sample images acquired from different body areas of patients with vitiligo before and after treatment. Some patients have vitiligo at one body area while others exhibit vitiligo lesions at multiple locations, as depicted in Figure 3.25.

Once the data are collected from all the patients, all the images were processed using the developed system in order to extract skin due to melanin and haemoglobin only as shown in Figure 3.26 where each of the image acquired further resulted in melanin and haemoglobin skin images. These resultant images are further utilized for segmentation and measurement of area in vitiligo lesion.

	Body Parts	Vitiligo Lesion	
		Before treatment	After treatment
Patient A	Face	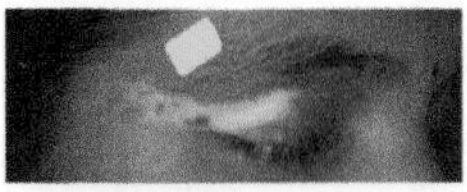	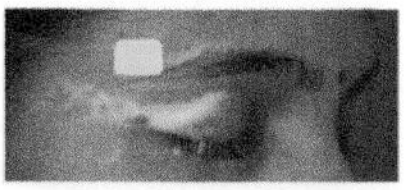
Patient B	Lower Limb		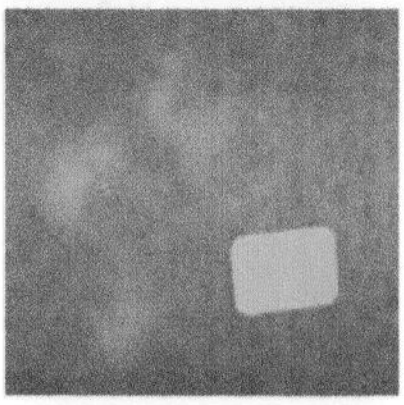
	Feet	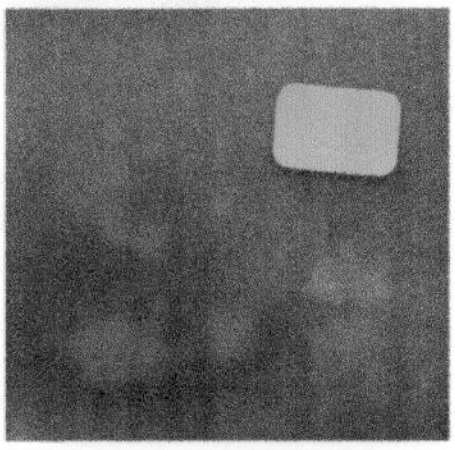	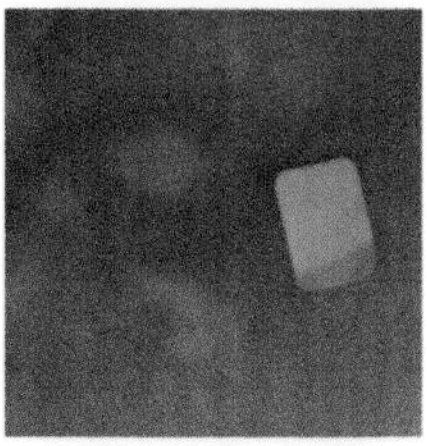
Patient C	Face	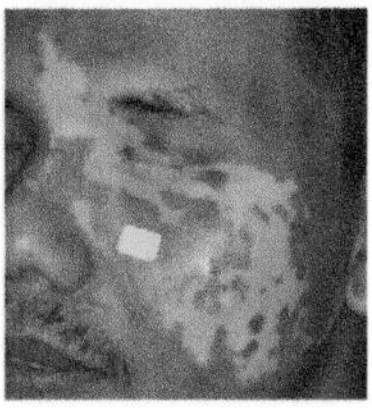	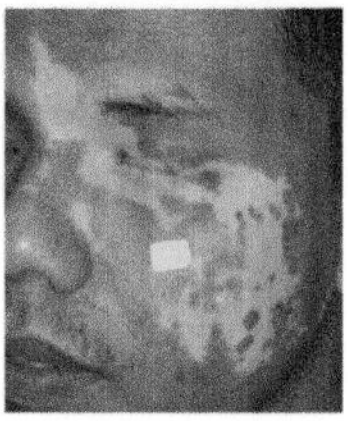

Figure 3.25 Image of patients acquired at different body areas.   (*Continued*)

3.5.3 *Segmentation of vitiligo skin lesion*

Segmented melanin images are shown in Figures 3.27 through 3.35. To ensure the accuracy of the system, the actual size of the pixel in each image is estimated using the reference image. For example 1 pixel in Figure 3.17a represents $113/45,972$ mm^2 or 2.458×10^{-2} mm^2, 1 pixel in Figure 3.17d represents $113/50,249$ mm^2 or 2.2488×10^{-2} mm^2 and so on. This process is performed in every preclinical image before we measure the vitiligo lesion area in the image.

It is found that for patient A, the determined nonmelanin area (vitiligo lesion area) on 17 July 2007 image is 170.3 mm^2 and on 28 August

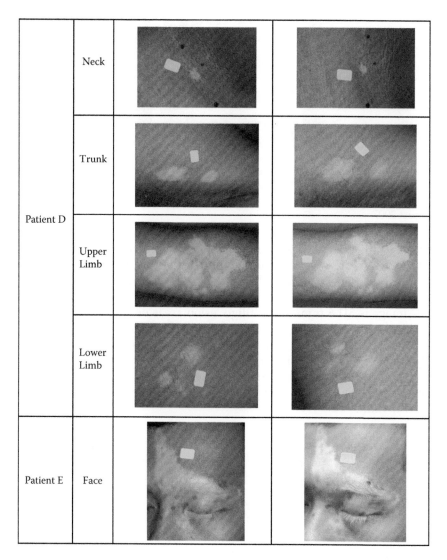

Figure 3.25 (Continued) Image of patients acquired at different body areas.

2007 image is 161.1 mm². For patient B, the nonmelanin area (vitiligo lesion area) on the lower limb on 17 July 2007 image is 217 mm² and on 28 August 2007 image is 161.1 cm². The nonmelanin area (vitiligo lesion area) on the feet on 17 July 2007 image is 177.9 mm² and on 28 August 2007 image is 121.2 mm². From Figure 3.29, the nonmelanin area (vitiligo lesion area) of patient C is found to be 2447.6 mm² on 17 July 2007 image and on 28 August 2007 image is 2227.4 mm². Patient D has four locations

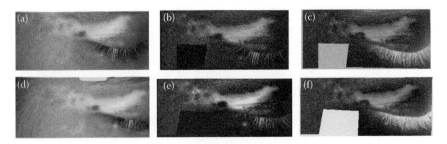

Figure 3.26 Processed images of lesions on the face of patient A: (a) RGB image—17 July 2007, (b) melanin—17 July 2007, (c) haemoglobin—17 July 2007, (d) RGB image—28 August 2007, (e) melanin—28 August 2007 and (f) haemoglobin—28 August 2007.

of vitiligo areas. For vitiligo lesion areas on the neck, the nonmelanin area (vitiligo lesion areas) is 66.9 and 54.3 mm^2 on 17 July 2007 and 28 August 2007, respectively. For vitiligo lesion areas on the trunk, the nonmelanin area (vitiligo lesion area) on July 17 images is 578 mm^2 and on 28 August 2007 image is 511.6 mm^2. For vitiligo lesion areas on the upper limb, the lesion area on July 17 images is 3632.5 mm^2 and on 28 August 2007 image is 3595 mm^2. For vitiligo lesion areas on the lower limb, the lesion area on July 17 images is 282.3 mm^2 and on 28 August 2007 image is 249.9 mm^2. From Figure 3.35, it is found that for patient E, the determined nonmelanin area is 3102.6 mm^2 on 17 July 2007 image and on 28 August 2007 image is 3049.7 mm^2.

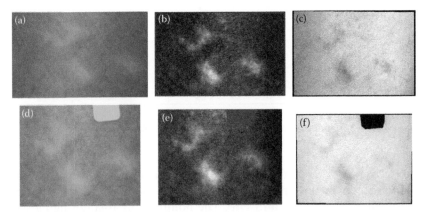

Figure 3.27 Processed images of lesions on the lower limb of patient B: (a) RGB image – 17 July 2007, (b) melanin – 17 July 2007, (c) haemoglobin – 17 July 2007, (d) RGB image – 28 August 2007, (e) melanin – 28 August 2007 and (f) haemoglobin – 28 August 2007.

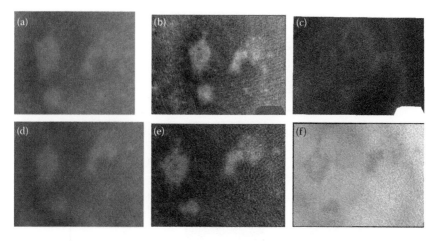

Figure 3.28 Processed images of lesions on feet of patient B: (a) RGB image – 17 July 2007, (b) melanin – 17 July 2007, (c) haemoglobin – 17 July 2007, (d) RGB image – 28 August 2007, (e) melanin – 28 August 2007 and (f) haemoglobin – 28 August 2007.

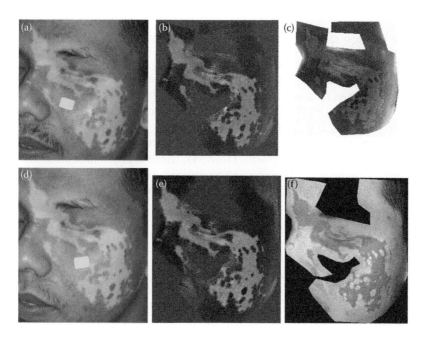

Figure 3.29 Processed images of lesions on the face of patient C: (a) RGB image – 17 July 2007, (b) melanin – 17 July 2007, (c) haemoglobin – 17 July 2007, (d) RGB image – 28 August 2007, (e) melanin – 28 August 2007 and (f) haemoglobin – 28 August 2007.

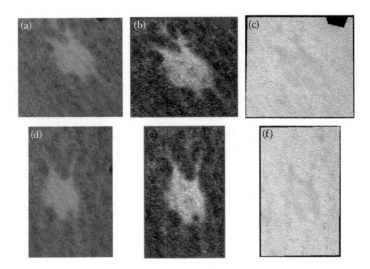

Figure 3.30 Processed images of lesions on the neck of patient D: (a) RGB image – 17 July 2007, (b) melanin – 17 July 2007, (c) haemoglobin – 17 July 2007, (d) RGB image – 28 August 2007, (e) melanin – 28 August 2007 and (f) haemoglobin – 28 August 2007.

3.5.4 *Vitiligo skin area measurement and assessment*

The measured vitiligo skin areas from the 17 July 2007 and 28 August 2007 lesion images are compared to obtain the differences and generate the system scores as tabulated in Table 3.6. PGA is the current scoring system used to evaluate the progression of vitiligo treatment and the scores are tabulated against the system's scores.

As seen in Table 3.6, repigmentation progressions are found for all cases after 6 weeks of treatment. However, these repigmentation areas as a result of therapeutic response to treatment, are so small (Figures 3.26 through 3.34) for dermatologists to discern visually from the images.

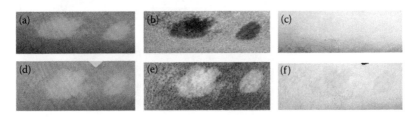

Figure 3.31 Processed images of lesions on the trunk of patient D: (a) RGB image – July 17, 2007, (b) melanin – 17 July 2007, (c) haemoglobin – 17 July 2007, (d) RGB image – 28 August 2007, (e) melanin – 28 August 2007 and (f) haemoglobin – 28 August 2007.

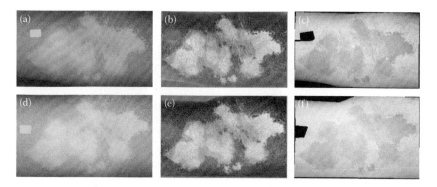

Figure 3.32 Processed images of lesions on the upper limb of patient D: (a) RGB image – July 17, 2007, (b) melanin – 17 July 2007, (c) haemoglobin – 17 July 2007, (d) RGB image – 28 August 2007, (e) melanin – 28 August 2007 and (f) haemoglobin – 28 August 2007.

The vitiligo monitoring system, however, has been able to quantify the repigmentation progression on the lesion areas objectively, as shown in Table 3.6. It is found that after 6 weeks of treatment, the vitiligo lesion areas are reduced. In comparison to PGA scores (Table 3.6), the percentages obtained using the developed method are within the PGA range except for the case of vitiligo lesion on feet of patient B.

In the case of patient B, there are areas of the vitiligo lesion that can be seen clearly from the melanin images of Figure 3.28, but in Figure

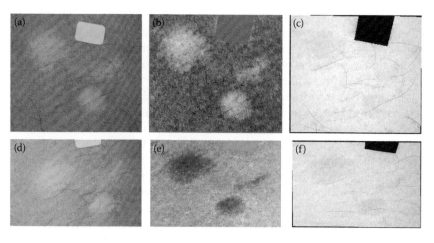

Figure 3.33 Processed images of lesions on the lower limb of patient D: (a) RGB image – 17 July 2007, (b) melanin – 17 July 2007, (c) haemoglobin – 17 July 2007, (d) RGB image – 28 August 2007, (e) melanin – 28 August 2007 and (f) haemoglobin – 28 August 2007.

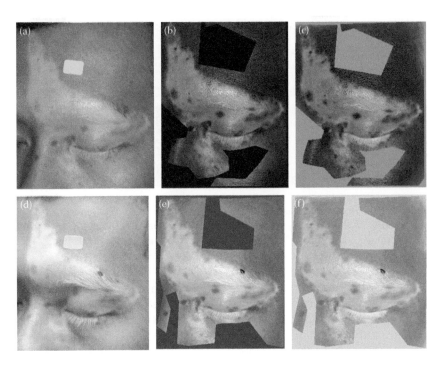

Figure 3.34 Processed images of lesions on the face of patient E: (a) RGB image – July 17, 2007, (b) melanin – 17 July 2007, (c) haemoglobin – 17 July 2007, (d) RGB image – 28 August 2007, (e) melanin – 28 August 2007 and (f) haemoglobin – 28 August 2007.

3.25 these areas are not so easy to discern visually. The developed system, however, is able to capture these areas (Figure 3.25). It is shown that the vitiligo monitoring system is superior as it is able to determine small changes in repigmentation areas.

In the processed images of Figures 3.26 through 3.34, it is possible to find dark and black areas on the images due to melanin and haemoglobin only. These are areas of reference (green tape) and reflective surfaces. From the study, the presence of reference (green tape) and reflective surfaces can affect the analysis of the vitiligo monitoring system. The effects of these areas are minimised by setting it aside from the process of the vitiligo monitoring system. The region of interest on every image has been chosen carefully with dermatologist.

Reflective surfaces are due to direct reflectance of light when the light comes into contact with the skin surfaces. The reflectance light is only 5% of the total light coming in contact with skin surfaces. It is found that most of the patients have oily skin surfaces on their face. Oily surfaces can affect the determination of melanin on skin. For the feet, the

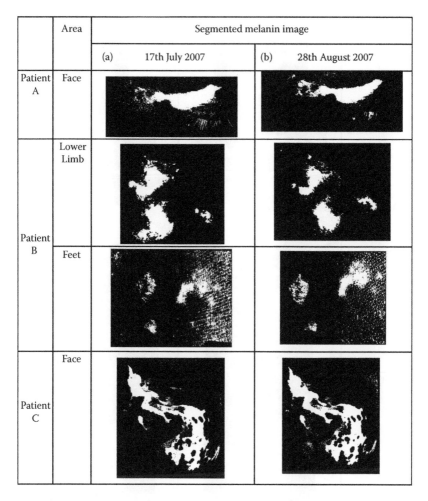

	Area	Segmented melanin image	
		(a) 17th July 2007	(b) 28th August 2007
Patient A	Face		
Patient B	Lower Limb		
	Feet		
Patient C	Face		

Figure 3.35 Patients A–E: (a) segmented melanin image on 17 July 2007, (b) segmented melanin image on 28 August 2007. *(Continued)*

reflective surfaces are due to the tibia bones. It is observed that in tibia bone area, the skin will look glossy and shiny on images. Generally, the reflective surfaces can affect the selection of regions of interest. Even dermatologists find it hard to determine regions of interest in these images. To overcome this problem, the selection of regions of interest are performed together with dermatologists when the patients coming for the evaluation to hospital.

The dark and black areas resulted by the selection process may affect the process transformation of RGB images to images due to melanin and haemoglobin only. However, this effect is eliminated by the PCA. PCA

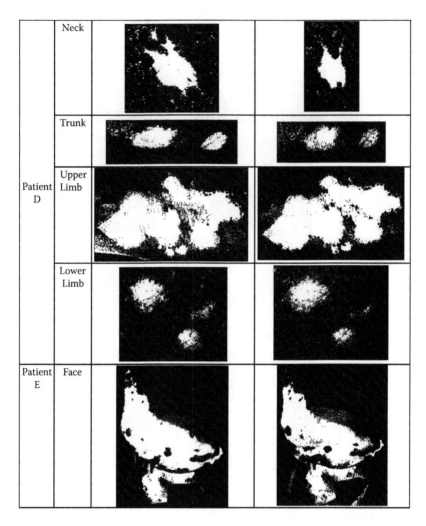

Figure 3.35 (Continued) Patients A–E: (a) segmented melanin image on 17 July 2007, (b) segmented melanin image on 28 August 2007.

transforms the data sets into new data sets such that the greatest variance by any projection of the data comes to lie on the first principal component of the new data sets, the second greatest variance on the second principal component of the new data sets and so on (Section 3.4). The dark and black areas have small variance in comparison to colour areas on the image. As a result, they will lie on the last principal component of RGB image data sets. Since the first and the second principal components are used due to PCA, we can conclude that dark and black areas do not affect the system.

Table 3.6 Determination of vitiligo skin areas using developed method

Body parts	Vitiligo skin areas (mm²)		Difference (mm²)	System score	PGA score
	17 July 2007	28 August 2007			
Patient A Face	170.3	161.1	9.2	5.4% (mild)	0%–25% (mild)
Patient B Lower limb	217	187.4	29.6	13.6% (mild)	0%–25% (mild)
Feet	177.9	121.2	56.7	31.87% (moderate)	0%–25% (mild)
Patient C Face	2447.6	2227.4	220.2	8.99% (mild)	0%–25% (mild)
Patient D Neck	66.9	54.3	12.6	18.8% (mild)	0%–25% (mild)
Trunk	578	511.6	66.4	11.49% (mild)	0%–25% (mild)
Upper limb	3632.5	3595	37.5	1% (mild)	0%–25% (mild)
Lower limb	282.3	249.9	32.4	11.5% (mild)	0%–25% (mild)
Patient E Face	3102.6	3049.7	52.9	1.7% (mild)	0%–25% (mild)

3.5.5 Analysis of vitiligo study

Overall, vitiligo lesions from 20 patients were obtained and analysed. Table 3.7 shows the vitiligo areas measured by the proposed image analysis algorithm based on two visits.

It is clearly shown that after 6 weeks of treatment, vitiligo areas, which have become smaller, can be measured by the system objectively. This measurement generate equivalent PGA scores that are useful to physicians in evaluating the efficacy of the treatment in a shorter time period.

Table 3.6 also compares the scores obtained using the proposed method that are found to be consistent with the PGA.

3.6 Conclusion

Vitiligo is a skin disorder that makes the skin areas paler in contrast to normal skin or completely white due to the lack of pigment melanin. Pigment melanin is a colour pigment found in skin, eyes and hair. It is produced by melanocytes through processes called melanogenesis.

Vitiligo treatment aims to repigment skin in order to obtain normal skin tone. To evaluate the therapeutic response of vitiligo, dermatologists currently employ PGA scale. This scale is based on the degree of

Table 3.7 Vitiligo areas measurements and assessments

Patients	Body area	Vitiligo areas (mm²)		System score	PGA score
		First visit	Second visit (after 6 weeks)		
1	Head	170.35	161.1	5.43% (Mild)	Mild
2	Head	2447.58	2227.4	8.996% (Mild)	Mild
3	Head	66.94	54.3	18.88% (Mild)	Mild
	Lower limb	282.3	249.9	11.48% (Mild)	Mild
	Trunk	577.7	511.6	11.44% (Mild)	Mild
	Upper limb	3632.5	3595	1.032% (Mild)	Mild
4	Head	3102.596	3049.7	1.705% (Mild)	Mild
5	Trunk	4021.67	3796.23	5.61% (Mild)	Mild
	Upper limbs	5666.8	5236.2	7.6% (Mild)	Mild
	Head	164.92	85.4	48.22% (Moderate)	Moderate
6	Trunk	2463.4	2142.37	13.03% (Mild)	Mild
7	Head	363.5	318.6	12.35% (Mild)	Mild
8	Feet	155.38	151.52	2.48% (Mild)	Mild
	Head	389.85	347.1	10.97% (Mild)	Mild
	Upper limbs	319.79	289.9	9.35% (Mild)	Mild
	Lower limbs	1010.24	1000.88	0.93% (Mild)	Mild
	Trunk	35.7	34.8	2.52% (Mild)	Mild
9	Hands	83.169	82.06	1.33% (Mild)	Mild
	Face	486.62	459.2	5.63% (Mild)	Mild

(Continued)

Table 3.7 (Continued) Vitiligo areas measurements and assessments

Patients	Body area	Vitiligo areas (mm²)		System score	PGA score
		First visit	Second visit (after 6 weeks)		
10	Feet	95.8	94.5	1.36% (Mild)	Mild
	Hand	61.8	57.6	6.8% (Mild)	Mild
	Face	272.7	223.12	18.18% (Mild)	Mild
	Upper limb	744.6	739.5	0.68% (Mild)	Mild
	Lower limb	813.47	809	0.55% (Mild)	Mild
11	Face	91.9	79.52	13.47% (Mild)	Mild
12	Lower limb	89.6	84.68	5.49% (Mild)	Mild
	Upper limb	47.09	37.8	19.73% (Mild)	Mild
13	Head	81.61	78.7	3.57% (Mild)	Mild
	Trunk	1882.7	1805.18	4.12% (Mild)	Mild
14	Feet	196.306	171.69	12.54% (Mild)	Mild
	Hand	175.9	164.05	6.7% (Mild)	Mild
	Head	98.2	77.29	21.29% (Mild)	Mild
	Lower limb	308.79	306.08	0.88% (Mild)	Mild
	Upper limb	302.11	265.4	12.15% (Mild)	Mild
15	Feet	141.61	134.7	4.88% (Mild)	Mild
	Trunk	420.2	334.1	20.49% (Mild)	Mild
	Upper limb	336.4	312.27	7.17% (Mild)	Mild
16	Head	41.95	38.52	8.18% (Mild)	Mild

(*Continued*)

Table 3.7 (Continued) Vitiligo areas measurements and assessments

Patients	Body area	Vitiligo areas (mm²)		System score	PGA score
		First visit	Second visit (after 6 weeks)		
17	Feet	87.9	82.9	5.69% (Mild)	Mild
	Hand	73.72	65.53	11.11% (Mild)	Mild
	Head	58.4	54.44	6.78% (Mild)	Mild
	Lower limb	128.77	113.34	11.98% (Mild)	Mild
	Trunk	591.36	580.4	1.85% (Mild)	Mild
18	Feet	677.7	611.29	9.8% (Mild)	Mild
	Hand	223.6	213.78	4.39% (Mild)	Mild
	Neck	69.74	69	1.06% (Mild)	Mild
	Lower limb	1695.14	1420	16.23% (Mild)	Mild
	Upper limb	457.1	448.8	1.82% (Mild)	Mild
19	Head	156.06	142.88	8.45% (Mild)	Mild
20	Head	1148.1	938.46	18.26% (Mild)	Mild

repigmentation within lesions over time. However, it is found that PGA is subjective as it has intra- and inter-variations. The objective of this chapter is to develop image processing algorithm and analysis that enable to determine and quantify the repigmentation progression objectively. This vitiligo monitoring system will be used as a tool for assisting dermatologist monitor vitiligo lesion during the course of treatment.

In this chapter, it is important to determine the reflectance of the skin in order to extract pigment melanin within the skin. Light reflections of skin could be defined by several components. Essentially, 5% of the incident light coming in contact with skin is directly reflected at the surface. Most of the incident light (nearly 95%) penetrates into skin and follows a complex path until it exits out of the skin or gets attenuated by skin chromophores (Preece and Claridge, 2004). The interaction of light within the dermis allows the light coming from skin to carry information of the composition within skin layers.

Essentially, skin colour is due to the combination of skin histological parameters, namely pigment melanin and haemoglobin. However, in digital imaging, colour is represented by three spectral bands: RGB. It is therefore necessary to find a robust algorithm to extract skin histological parameters from the RGB image. Here, statistical signal and image processing techniques are applied to determine melanin and haemoglobin from skin images.

ICA is employed on the two-dimensional colour space in order to separate sources due to melanin and haemoglobin only. Here, the Fast ICA algorithm developed by Aapo Hyvarinen (Hyvarinen, 1999, 2000) is applied in the vitiligo technique.

The PCA/ICA process produces skin images due to melanin and haemoglobin only. Segmentation of vitiligo lesion areas is then performed on image due to melanin. As mentioned earlier, vitiligo lesion areas are skin areas that lack pigment melanin. A threshold selection based on median cut algorithm is employed to segment nonmelanin areas and melanin areas on the image due to melanin only. The determined nonmelanin areas represent the vitiligo lesion areas.

The changes in the vitiligo surface areas of skin images before and after treatment are quantified by comparing the size of nonmelanin areas before and after treatment. The changes are expressed as a percentage of repigmentation to reflect the repigmentation progression of vitiligo lesion areas.

The performance of the vitiligo monitoring system is investigated in controlled environments. Here, we construct images of skin model and vitiligo lesion model. The skin and vitiligo model are developed using patients' data. It is assumed that the spatial distribution of skin and vitiligo lesion can be expressed by Gaussian distribution. These images are then distorted by controlled noise. The result shows the developed system is able to determine a vitiligo lesion down to 1-by-1 pixel in an image that has no noise. However, if we add noise to the image, the developed system is able to determine a 1-by-1 pixel vitiligo lesion area for SNRs 15 dB.

The vitiligo monitoring system is tested using real images provided by the Department of Dermatology, Hospital Kuala Lumpur. From the preliminary study, it is found that the percentages obtained using the developed method are within the PGA ranges. In patient 4, the repigmentation areas are small due the briefness of the treatment (4 months) compared to the other patients. It is difficult for dermatologists to discern visually small repigmentation progression due to the treatment. The vitiligo monitoring system is, however, able to capture small repigmentation progression objectively and thus can be potentially used as it allows monitoring on a shorter time frame.

In the preclinical trial study, initially the images are taken from 5 patients (patients A, B, C, D and E) and later increased to 20 patients (1–20). Each lesion areas on a patient have two images. The images are taken at different time (6 weeks different). The first images were taken on 17 July 2007 and the second images on 28 August 2007. There are repigmentation progressions on every case of the study. However, these repigmentation areas are so small, as a result, and dermatologists find it difficult to discern these areas visually in the images. The system, however, has been able to quantify the repigmentation progression on the lesion areas objectively. In comparison to PGA scores, the percentages obtained using the developed method are within the PGA range.

Bibliography

R. R. Anderson and J. A. Parrish, The optics of human skin, *Journal of Investigative Dermatology*, vol. 77, pp. 13–19, 1981.

B. E. Bayer, Color imaging array, US Patent US3971065 A, 1976.

T. S. Caetano and D. A. C. Barone, A probabilistic model for the human skin color. *Proceedings of 11th International Conference on Image Analysis and Processing*, Palermo, Italy, 2001.

S. Cooray and N. O'Connor, Facial feature extraction and principal component analysis for face detection in colour images. *Proceedings of the International Conference on Image Analysis and Recognition*, Porto, Portugal, 2004.

S. D. Cotton and E. Claridge, Developing a predictive model of human skin colouring. *Proceedings of the SPIE Medical Imaging*, Newport Beach, USA, 1996.

S. D. Cotton, E. Claridge et al. Noninvasive skin imaging, *Lecture Notes in Computer Science*, vol. 1230, pp. 501–506, 1997.

Z. Fan and B. Lu, An adjusted Gaussian skin-color model based on principal component analysis, *Proceedings of International Symposium on Neural Networks*. Advances in Neural Networks – ISNN 2004, Springer: Dalian, China, pp. 804–809.

S. Fischer, P. Schmid et al. Analysis of skin lesions with pigmented networks. *Proceedings of International Conference on Image Processing*, Lausanne, France, 1996.

R. C. Gonzalez and R. E. Woods, *Digital Image Processing*. Boston: Addison-Wesley Longman Publishing, 1992.

R. M. Gray and L. D. Davisson, *An Introduction to Statistical Signal Processing*. New York: Cambridge University Press, 2004.

A. Hyvärinen, Fast and Robust Fixed-Point Algorithms for Independent Component Analysis, *IEEE Transactions on Neural Networks*, vol. 10, no. 3, pp. 626–634, 1999.

A. Hyvärinen and E. Oja, Independent Component Analysis: Algorithms and Applications, *Neural Networks*, vol. 13, no. (4–5), pp. 411–430, 2000.

Y. J. Kim, B. S. Chung et al. Depigmentation therapy with Q-switched ruby laser after tanning in vitiligo universalis, *Dermatologic Surgery*, vol. 27, no. 11, pp. 969–970, 2001.

V. Lepe, B. Moncada et al. A double-blind randomized trial of 0.1% tacrolimus vs 0.05% clobetasol for the treatment of childhood, *Archives of Dermatology*, vol. 139, no. 5, pp. 581–585, 2003.

Y. W. Lim and S. U. Lee, On the color image segmentation algorithm based on the thresholding and the fuzzy c-means techniques, *Pattern Recognition*, vol. 23, no. 9, pp. 935–952, 1990.

Y. Ohno, CIE fundamentals for color measurements. *Proceedings of the IS&T NIP16 Conference*, Vancouver, CA, 2000.

N. Otsu, A threshold selection method from gray-level histograms, *IEEE Transactions on Systems, Man, and Cybernetics*, vol. 9, no. 1, pp. 62–66, 1979.

C. Peterson, How it works, the charged-coupled device or CCD. *Journal of Young Investigators*, vol. 3, 2001.

S. L. Phung, A. Bouzerdoum et al. Skin segmentation using color pixel classification: Analysis and comparison, *IEEE Transaction on Pattern Analysis and Machine Intelligence*, vol. 27, no. 1, pp. 148–154, 2005.

S. L. Phung, D. Chai et al. Adaptive skin segmentation in color images. *Proceedings of IEEE International Conference on Acoustics, Speech, & Signal Processing*, Hong Kong, 2003.

S. J. Preece and E. Claridge, Spectral filter optimization for the recovery of parameters which describe human skin, *IEEE Transaction on Pattern Analysis and Machine Intelligence*, vol. 28, no. 7, pp. 913–922, 2004.

G. X. Ritter and J. N. Wilson, *Handbook of Computer Vision Algorithms in Image Algebra*. Boca Raton, FL: CRC Press, 2000.

S. Roberts and R. Everson, *Independent Component Analysis: Principles and Practice*. Cambridge: Cambridge University Press, 2001.

N. Roberts and M. Lesage, Vitiligo: Causes and treatment, *The Pharmaceutical Journal*, vol. 270, pp. 440–442, 2003.

T. Rosebury, *Life on Man*. London: Secker & Warburg, 1969.

Rosenfeld and A. Kak, *Digital Picture Processing*. New York: Academic Press, 1982.

H. Sahbi and N. Boujemaa, Coarse to fine face detection based on skin color adaption. *Proceedings of the International ECCV 2002 Workshop Copenhagen on Biometric Authentication*, Copenhagen, Denmark, 2002.

P. Schmid and S. Fischer, Colour segmentation for the analysis of pigmented skin lesions. *Proceedings of the Sixth International Conference on Image Processing and Its Applications*, Dublin, Ireland, 1997.

H. Takiwaki, Measurement of skin color: Practical application and theoretical considerations, *Journal of Medical Investigation*, vol. 44, pp. 121–125, 1998.

P. Tichavský, Z. Koldovský et al. Performance analysis of the FastICA algorithm and Cramér–Rao bounds for linear independent component analysis, *IEEE Transactions on Signal Processing*, vol. 54, no. 4, pp. 1189–1203, 2006.

Tonsi; Vitiligo and its management update: A review. *Pakistan Journal of Medical Science*, vol. 20, no. 3, pp. 242–247, 2004.

N. Tsumura, H. Haneishi et al. Independent component analysis of skin color image, *Journal of the Optical Society of America A*, vol. 16, pp. 2169–2176, 1999.

N. Tsumura, H. Haneishi et al. Independent component analysis of spectral absorbance image in human skin, *Optical Review*, vol. 7, pp. 479–482, 2000a.

N. Tsumura, M. Kawabuchi et al. Mapping pigmentation in human skin by multivisible-spectral imaging by inverse optical scattering technique. *Proceedings of IS&T/ SID's 8th Color Imaging Conference, Color Science, Systems and Applications*, Scottsdale, USA, 2000b.

N. Tsumura, N. Ojima et al. Image-based skin color and texture analysis/synthesis by extracting hemoglobin and melanin information in the skin, *ACM Transactions on Graphics*, vol. 22, no. 3, pp. 770–779, 2003.

C. Turkington and J. Dover, *The Encyclopedia of Skin and Skin Disorders*. United States of America: Carol Turkington, 2007.

S. E. Umbaugh, *Computer Imaging: Digital Image Processing and Analysis*. Boca Raton, FL: CRC Press, 2005.

S. E. Umbaugh, G. A. Hance et al. Unsupervised color image segmentation with application to skin tumor borders, *IEEE Engineering in Medicine and Biology*, vol. 15, no. 1, pp. 104–111, 1996.

S. E. Umbaugh, R. H. Moss et al. Automatic color segmentation algorithms with application to skin tumor feature identification, *IEEE Engineering in Medicine and Biology*, vol. 12, no. 3, pp. 75–82, 1993.

N. van Geel, K. Ongenae et al. Surgical techniques for vitiligo: A review, *Dermatology*, vol. 202, no. 2, pp. 162–166, 2001.

N. van Geel, Y. Vander Haeghen et al. A new digital image analysis system useful for surface assessment of vitiligo lesions in transplantation studies, *European Journal of Dermatology*, vol. 14, pp. 150–155, 2004.

Q. Zhu, K. T. Cheng et al. Adaptive learning of an accurate skin-color model. *Proceedings of the Sixth IEEE International Conference on Automatic Face and Gesture Recognition*, Seoul, South Korea, 2004.

chapter four

Modelling and analysis of skin pigmentation

Ahmad Fadzil Mohamad Hani, Hermawan Nugroho,
Norashikin Shamsudin and Suraiya H. Hussein

Contents

4.1 Introduction

4.1.1 Pigmentation disorders

Pigmentation disorders are disturbances of human skin tone, either loss or reduction, which may be related to loss of melanocytes or the inability of melanocytes to produce melanin or transport melanosomes correctly. Pigmentary problems can be divided into two—those that are hyper-pigmented due to either increase in melanin (melanotic) or melanocytes (melanocytic), and those that are hypo-pigmented due to decrease or the

Table 4.1 Pigmentation disorders [1]

Pigmentation disorder	Characteristics	Treatment
Melasma (hyperpigmented)	Dark brown, symmetric patches of pigment on the face. During pregnancy, this is called the *mask of pregnancy*.	• Applying sun tan lotion and preventing sun exposure to prevent melasma from worsening. • Prescription creams to lighten the patches.
Albinism (hypopigmented)	This disorder is in the genes and skin loss of melanin in totality or fragmentary, comparing with the pigmentation of family members. Having white hair, pale skin and pink eyes.	• Albinism is not curable. • Avoiding sunlight.
Vitiligo (hypopigmented)	Smooth, white patches in the skin, vitiligo is due to the loss of pigment-producing cells in the skin (melanocytes). The white patches are very sensitive to the sun.	• Vitiligo is not curable. • Treatment such as covering smaller patches with long-lasting dyes or light-sensitive drugs. • Performing light therapy (ultraviolet A). • Applying corticosteroid creams. • Depigmentating the remaining skin.
Loss of pigment after skin damage (hypopigmented)	At times, after an ulcer, blister, burn, or infection, some of the pigment is not replaced to the skin.	• No treatment is needed. • Blemish can be covered using cosmetics.

absence of either melanin (hypomelanotic) or melanocytes (melanocytopaenic). Table 4.1 shows different types of pigmentation disorders.

Generally, pigmentation disorders cause the skin to appear lighter or darker than normal skin, as shown in Figure 4.1, and do not pose any serious physical effects. However, it is well recognized that the disease can have a profound effect on the self-image and self-esteem of the affected individuals [2]. Moreover, patients with pigmentation disorders will have an increased risk of developing autoimmune disease such as thyroid disease, Addison disease, pernicious anaemia and alopecia areata [3–5].

There are many types of pigmentation disorders. Most of these diseases do not have serious physical effects. However, there will be significant psychological effects and problems with personal relationships,

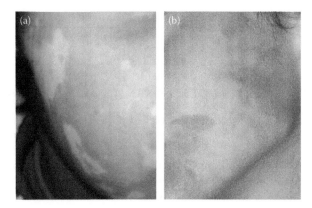

Figure 4.1 Pigmentation disorders in skin: (a) lighter skin patches and (b) darker skin patches. (Reproduced from C. Turkington and J. Dover, *The Encyclopedia of Skin and Skin Disorders*. United States of America: Carol Turkington, 2007.)

employment and sporting activity [6]. Generally, skin diseases have often been given low priority in comparison to other diseases (HIV [human immunodeficiency virus], tuberculosis) by international health authorities. The trends however have slowly changed. This is due to a global awareness that skin disease may be an early sign of more serious disease such as autoimmune disease [7]. Smith et al. and Laberge et al. reported that vitiligo can increase the risk of developing autoimmune disease such as thyroid disease, Addison disease, pernicious anaemia and alopecia areata [3,4]. It was also reported that melasma can increase the risk of developing autoimmune disease [5].

Pigmentation disorder can be treated in many ways. It can be categorized as three types of treatment: medical treatment, surgical and UVB (ultraviolet B)/laser treatment, as listed in Table 4.2.

Table 4.2 Treatments [1]

Medical treatment	Surgical	UVB/laser
• Topical and systemic corticosteroids	• Mini grafting	• UVB therapy
• Psorelen with exposure to ultraviolet	• Transplantation of cultured melanocytes	• Laser therapy
• Heliotherapy	• Transplantation of non-cultured melanocytes	• Q-switched ruby laser therapy
• Therapy with monobenzylether of hydroquinone		
• Ointment		

Although there are many available treatments for skin pigmentation disorder, changes to skin surface colour as a response to treatment takes time, affecting the ability of the dermatologists to assess the treatment efficacy. Moreover, the efficacy assessment process under Physician's Global Assessment framework only refers to visual conditions of skin surface. It does not assess the conditions of the underlying skin layers and pigments especially melanin types (eumelanin and pheomelanin) and concentration which are important to the resulting skin tone. The measurement process is not standardised, and thus can lead to inter- and intra-rater variability.

In dermatology, the evaluation of skin disease severity is essential in the diagnostic process as well as in treatment choice and in making the prognosis [8]. Ideally, the evaluation should be objective and reproducible. However, in spite of attempts to regulate a clinical evaluation, many wide variations both in assessment rules and in the interpretation exist, and as a consequence, intra- and inter-observer variations occur. Even judgments of the trained dermatologists may vary when attempting to diagnose the severity of the same clinical situation repeatedly. Moreover, not all treatments lead to prompt and complete clearance of skin diseases symptoms, but to a gradual reduction in clinical signs. In such cases, dermatologists need a longer time to discern these reductions of clinical signs. Therefore, there is a growing need for an objective measurement tool that is sufficiently accurate to assist dermatologist in the diagnostic process and to assess efficacy of the treatment.

Assessment of skin colour changes is important in dermatology. The changes, however, are not linear and hard to be discerned visually. In dermatology, human skin colour is cross-referred with skin phototype (SPT). Fitzpatrick skin type (FST) is a subjective format for assessing SPTs I–VI in human, as shown in Table 4.3 [9]. The FST is commonly used as a predictor of skin cancer [10].

In analysing human skin colour, two factors must be considered. First, skin surfaces may be classified into facultative skin colour (characterized as the colour of skin regions which are frequently exposed to sunlight) and constitutive skin colour (characterized as the colour of skin regions

Table 4.3 Fitzpatrick skin type [11]

SPT	Unexposed skin colour	Sun response history
I	White	Always burns, never tans
II	White	Always burns, tans minimally
III	White	Burns minimally, tans gradually and uniformly
IV	Light brown	Burns minimally, always tans well
V	Brown	Rarely burns, tans darkly
VI	Dark brown	Never burns, tans darkly

which are frequently hidden from the sun). The classification of skin surface into facultative and constitutive skin colour can influence estimation of its SPT. According to Choe [12], there is a connection between facultative skin colour and SPT. Nonetheless, this connection is less great compared to constitutive skin colour. Second, different modalities can yield different reflectance spectra as depicted in Galvan [13].

Skin pigmentation is connected with the creation of melanin. Melanin is the primary colour pigment that is created by melanocytes cells situated in epidermis through a procedure called melanogenesis. Through melanogenesis, two categories of melanin (eumelanin and pheomelanin) are integrated. Eumelanin is the dark brown-black insoluble polymer, while pheomelanin is the light red-yellow sulphur-containing soluble polymer [14].

Figure 4.2 shows the process of melanin synthesis during melanogenesis. Melanin synthesis begins with the catalysis of the substrates L-phenylalanine and L-tyrosine to produce L-DOPA via phenylalanine hydroxylase (PAH), tyrosinase, and partly tyrosinase hydroxylase 1 (TH-1). The process is then divided into eumelanogenesis to produce eumelanin or pheomelanogenesis to produce pheomelanin. The other melanogenic enzymes are TRP-2 (DCT) and TRP-1 for eumelanogenesis. So far, there has been no reported studies of the specific enzymes involved in pheomelanogenesis [11,12].

Today, there are many types of substances used in skin-brightening merchandizes, which perform as the depigmentation agents to reduce

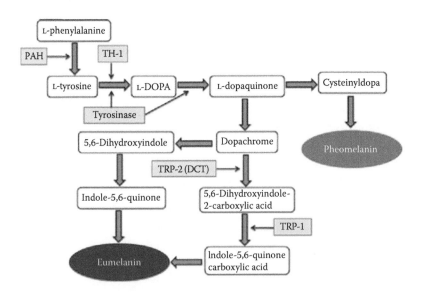

Figure 4.2 Melanin synthesis. (Reproduced from J. M. Gillbro and M. J. Olsson, *International Journal of Cosmetic Science*, vol. 33, no. 3, pp. 210–21, 2011.)

the level of pigmentation in skin [16–18]. Most of these agents have a tyrosinase-inhibiting effect leading to a reduced total melanin production. There are also molecules known to have an effect on the transfer of melanin from melanocytes to keratinocytes, leading to an overall lighter skin colour such as nicotinamide and soya bean. Substances that increase the loss of the skin are also used to remove excessive melanin content within the skin, for instance, retinoic acid. And, antioxidant enzymes are used to change the proportion between production of eumelanin and pheomelanin. For a paler skin, it will produce more pheomelanin than eumelanin [11,19].

Currently, cosmetic dermatology has no clinical rules and standard [20]. The evaluation of skin-brightening efficacy or other cosmetic operations depend mostly on the judgement, skills and experience of dermatologists—therefore creating inevitable intra- and inter-observer variations. Highly experienced dermatologist can even have varying judgement. Therefore, it is important to have an accurate and objective evaluation methodology to assess a treatment efficacy [8].

4.1.2 Emerging imaging technology for objective skin assessment

Visual cues play an important role in skin evaluation [21]. The visual evaluation of lesions is the first and the most frequently used procedure made by dermatologists in daily practice. The evaluation of lesion is performed based on the distribution, size, shape, border, symmetry and colour of the skin lesion. This evaluation, however, is subjective due to the dependency of visual perception of the human visual response to light as well as the light interaction with objects.

In signal and image processing, visual cues are actually a collective of light which is scattered and reemitted when encountering the skin. This reemitted light carries important information about the physical and optical tissue parameters. Currently, this phenomenon is mostly captured using digital colour camera system, which offers limited spectral information. It does not take advantage of the skin–light interaction, which occurs over the whole visible spectrum range. Optical coherence tomography (OCT), confocal scanning laser microscopy (CSLM), and ultrasound (US) systems (Figure 4.3) may provide extensive skin information but cannot provide spectral information. An imaging system, which can provide such information, is therefore required.

Several types of imaging systems that capture wider spectral information include multispectral camera (and hyperspectral camera) and spectroscopy, as shown in Figure 4.4.

Multispectral imaging (MSI) is an imaging technology, which measures light intensities at many spectral bands. It is able to provide the average light intensity spatially at spectral bands of wavelengths ranging

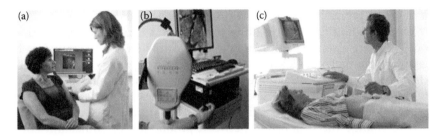

Figure 4.3 (a) OCT, (b) CSLM and (c) US. (Reproduced from V. Tuchin, *Anticancer Research*, vol. 30, no. 8, pp. 3215–3216, 2010.)

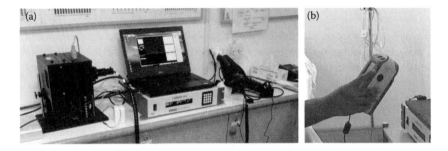

Figure 4.4 Skin imaging systems that capture wider spectral information of skin: (a) multispectral camera and (b) spectrophotometer.

from 320 to 1000 nm [23]. Spectrophotometry similarly measures average light intensity at spectral bands from visible to near-infrared but of a point area.

The measurement of a sample is linked to the physical light property over the entire light spectrum (UV [ultraviolet], VIS [visible], VIS + NIR, NIR [near infrared] and IR [infrared] spectral bands) [24]. More importantly, the measurement is not affected by ambient illumination (measurement area is concealed from external light). Compared to normal cameras, multispectral cameras and spectrophotometers provide wider spectral information of skin. In this work, such devices, which can provide a high spectral resolution, fast (and easy to use) measurement and easily available are preferred.

With the above imaging technologies, assessment of the pigmentation disorder is now evolving from subjective methods to objective methods, involving the use of imaging technologies that provide fast, reliable and objective measurement of pigmented lesion area. Moreover, imaging techniques are non-invasive and produce data that can be stored for future use. The conditions of the underlying skin layers and pigments can be objectively determined using the inversion procedure of skin–light interaction model.

A number of theorems of skin–light interaction have been created by researchers to analyse the skin–light interaction such as Kubelka–Munk (K–M) model, radiative transport equation, modified Beer–Lambert law and Monte Carlo (MC) simulation. These models simulate the spectral information of skin reflectance. To measure the skin optical characteristics, an inversion procedure can be employed. The procedure is the opposite of the actual procedure of working out reflection and transmission, using reflectance and transmittance values captured by skin imaging system as an input to determine the optical characteristics of the skin tissues.

4.2 Assessing pigmentation disorder

4.2.1 Current assessment of melanin

Ideally, skin assessment should be objective and reproducible. However, in spite of attempts to regulate a clinical evaluation, the assessment still depends on the judgement and the expertise of the dermatologists. As a consequence, intra- and inter-observer variations may occur. Moreover, not all treatments lead to prompt and complete clearance of skin diseases. In this case, dermatologists need a longer time to discern these reductions of clinical signs. Therefore, there is a growing need for an objective tool which can assist dermatologist in the diagnostic process, especially for pigmentation disorders.

Pigmentation disorder is a condition that causes the skin to appear lighter or darker than normal skin. This condition is due to abnormal melanin production by the skin. Melanin is the main colour pigment. There are two categories of melanin (eumelanin and pheomelanin) being integrated. Eumelanin is the dark brown-black insoluble polymer, while pheomelanin is the light red-yellow sulphur-containing soluble polymer. It is important to determine the condition of skin pigments such as for assessing treatment efficacy of skin pigmentation disorders and effects of whitening cream. At present however, the assessment of melanin types and their concentrations are invasive; skin biopsy is conducted for chemical analysis of skin samples. Alternative methods that are noninvasive are required.

Assessment of the pigmentation disorder can be performed objectively with the use of imaging technologies. Moreover, these imaging techniques are non-invasive and the recorded skin data (i.e., skin reflectance) can be stored for future use. The analysis of skin data, however, is not straightforward. The conditions of the underlying skin layers and pigments (melanin types and concentration) can be determined from the skin data using the inversion procedure of skin–light interaction model.

A number of theorems of skin–light interaction have been created by researchers with MC simulation and have been reported as the most accurate model. The simulation, however, requires a great deal of computation time and thus is computationally expensive. To enable the use of MC simulations in a clinical setting, an implementation of a fast MC simulation is required.

At present, the assessment of melanin types and their concentrations is essentially invasive, in which skin biopsy is conducted for chemical analysis of skin samples. In 1983, Ito and Jimbow quantitatively determined eumelanin and pheomelanin by analysing both pyrrole-2-3, 5-tricarboxylic acid (PTCA) as the biomarker of eumelanin while aminhydroxphenylalanine (AHP) as the biomarker of pheomelanin using high-performance liquid chromatography (HPLC) [25]. In 2002, Ito subsequently updated and elaborated a number of those biomarkers used in their method to determine the concentration of eumelanin and pheomelanin [26]. In 2003, Ito's method was used to determine the ratio of pheomelanin and eumelanin of normal and depigmented skin [27]. As reported in 2005, the method was also used to study some SPTs [28] and in 2009 was used to study the effect of simulated solar radiation in comparison to UVA and UVB radiation [29].

Earlier, Patil in 1984 determined pheomelanin concentration by analysing two of the hydroiodic acid (HI) degradation products, namely, α-amino-β- (4-hydroxy-7-benzothiazolyl) prop ionic acid and α-amino-β-(3-hydroxy-4-aminophenyl) prop ionic acid, as the biomarker of pheomelanin using high-performance liquid chromatography (HPLC) [30]. Panzella in 2006 proposed a number of different biomarkers to determine the concentration of eumelanin and pheomelanin [31]. In their article, pyrrole-2,3,5-tricarboxylic acid (PTCA) was proposed as the biomarker of melanin and 6-(2-amino-2-carboxyethyl)-2-carboxy-4-hydroxybenzothiazole (BTCA) and 1,3-thiazole-2,4,5-tricarboxylic acid as the biomarkers of pheomelanin. Kongshoj in 2006 reported the use of pyrrole-2,3,5-tricarboxylic acid (PTCA), as the biomarker of eumelanin and 1,3-thiazole-2,4,5-tricarboxylic acid (TTCA) as the biomarker of pheomelanin [32].

The methods of determining the underlying pigments (melanin types and concentration) are currently invasive and not all biochemists could perform such analysis. It is important to determine the condition of the underlying skin layers and the pigments for monitoring skin pigmentation that is required in diagnostics (e.g., treatment efficacy of skin pigmentation disorders) and skin care (e.g., effects of whitening cream).

From the above discussion, it is clear that there is a need to develop an *in vivo* and non-invasive method to measure accurately melanin types and its concentration in order to assess severity of skin pigmentation disorder and treatment efficacies.

4.2.2 Non-invasive in vivo skin pigmentation analysis

It is well understood that the dermatologists need an objective system for monitoring pigmentation disorders and a skin-whitening treatment outcome objectively. The system should be able to analyse, determine and quantify *in vivo* the melanin types and concentration before and after treatment in a non-invasive manner. In doing so, the system will provide objective efficacy assessment to assist dermatologist in making accurate diagnoses. Therefore, the objective is to develop such tool/system which is able to determine and quantify the melanin types and concentration in a clinical setting based on a digital signal processing approach.

The main pigment, melanin, consists of two subtypes, namely eumelanin and pheomelanin. Eumelanin is a dark brown-black pigment, whereas pheomelanin is a light red-yellow pigment [10,24,33]. In the treatment of pigmentation disease or skin whitening, the target of the treatment is to alter the production of melanin (to alter overall production of melanin or to alter the ratio between eumelanin and pheomelanin). In this work, a tool that gives the detailed examination of skin optical attributes (particularly pigment melanin categories and concentrations) using skin spectral information is produced and evaluated.

The proposed non-invasive system to assess and analyse skin pigmentation *in vivo* consists of a hand-held spectrophotometer and a computer workstation with Graphics Processing Unit (GPU). Hand-held spectrophotometer is utilized to produce spectral information (skin reflectance) of pigmented lesion and the surrounding normal skin. The skin reflectance spectral information is then examined in detail by applying the developed inverse procedure of MC simulation to obtain skin parameters such as pigments and their concentrations. The MC simulation runs on GPU workstation known as CUDA (compute unified device architecture). It is reported that CUDA provides a better performance per cost and per watt compared to the traditional central processing technologies application [34]. According to their reports, with the speedup factors achieved by implementing MC on GPU [33,35–37], it is now possible to use the inverse procedure based on MC simulation developed for clinical purposes. The developed inverse procedure also employs optimisation operator to achieve optimum results. The algorithm is implemented using C++ and MATLAB.

MC simulation has been reported as the most accurate approximation of skin–light simulation [33,38,39]. However, there has been no inverse procedure based on MC simulation developed for clinical purposes. This is because the simulation requires a great deal of computation time. Because of this downside, MC simulations have so far been utilized predominantly for forward modelling, which is to compute the photon density dispersion given skin tissue structures and their optical attributes. In order to solve inverse problems using MC simulations, an implementation of a fast MC simulation is required.

The skin pigmentation model is developed based on the realistic skin model (RSM) module of the Advanced Systems Analyses Program (ASAP®) software from Breault Research Organization (BRO) [40]. The estimated optical parameters obtained from the system from the skin data of participants were inputted into the RSM to model a simulated skin. It is envisaged that if the computational simulated skin produced by RSM is similar with the skin data of the participants, the inverse analysis method is thus proven to be correct. As reported in the literature, the RSM can be modified to generate data of skin and thus, it can be used as ground truth for validating the system [41,42].

To evaluate the performance of the system, two observational studies are conducted. In observational study I, the system is evaluated with skin data of normal participants having different skin tones based on Fitzpatrick classification [11]. In observational study II, the system is evaluated with skin lesion data of patients suffering from hypopigmentation and hyperpigmentation. The skin reflectance data of vitiligo and melasma lesion are collected to represent hypopigmentation and hyperpigmentation disorder, respectively.

4.3 Skin optics

4.3.1 Structure of skin

Skin is the largest body organ, commonly ranging from 12% to 16% of the total body mass and covering an area of about 1.2–2 m^2 in adults [43]. Its functions include insulation and temperature regulation, sensation and production of vitamin D and B synthesis and body protection against pathogens. As illustrated in Figure 4.5, skin comprises three layers, namely epidermis, dermis and subcutaneous fatty tissue [42], each of which, in turn, produces a noticeable purpose in the overall operations of the skin.

The epidermis consists of keratinocytes, melanocytes, Langerhans cells and Merkel cells. It has no blood vessels but is nourished by diffusion from the dermis. Melanocytes in this case are melanin-forming cells through melanogenesis [14] and located at the bottom layer of the epidermis, as shown in Figure 4.6. Among different ethnic origins, the density of melanocytes in skin is conformable. The difference in skin pigmentation is, however, due to the variations in the rate of melanin production.

The dermis is the second primary layer of skin beneath the epidermis. It is connected to the epidermis by a basement membrane. Contingent upon the area of the body, dermis is roughly 1–4 mm thick and made out of flexible collagen fibres, veins, nerves, lymph vessels, hair follicles and

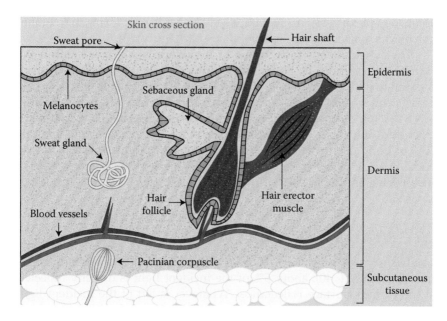

Figure 4.5 Anatomy of skin. (Reproduced from *Skin Anatomy* [Online]. Available: www.enchantedlearning.com. Accessed 12 January 2014.)

sweat glands. The dermis contains a lot of arteries and veins as well as capillaries for blood circulation. Here, blood carries pigment haemoglobin, which acts as the main absorber of light in dermis [38]. The microvasculature are concentrated on the uppermost layer of the dermis, called papillary plexus and the larger vessels are situated on a lower layer, called

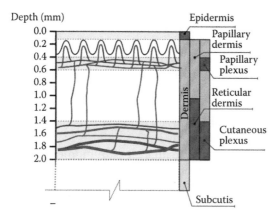

Figure 4.6 Skin dermis. (Reproduced from P. Valisuo, *Photonics simulation and modelling of skin for design of spectrocutometer*, Universitas Wasaensis, 2011.)

cutaneous plexus [45]. A layer between the papillary plexus and cutaneous plexus may contain fewer blood vessels (Figure 4.6).

The subcutaneous fatty tissue or hypodermis is a layer within the skin below the dermis. Functionally, hypodermis does not only attach the skin to underlying bone and muscle but also supplies skin with blood vessels and nerves. Consisting of loose connective tissue and elastin, this layer that binds the skin to underlying structures, insulates the body from cold, and stores energy in the form of fat. The hypodermis contains 50% of body fat in which fat serves as padding and insulation for the body. Because of the existence of the white fat deposits, a lion's share of the visible light going up to this tissue is bounced back to the upper layers [46].

4.3.2 Reflection model of skin

The Dichromatic Reflection Model of skin predicts that at incident angles near to normal (<40), about 5% of the incident light is directly reflected at the surface (surface reflectance). Whatever is left of the incident light (95%) enters the skin where it is absorbed or diffused within the skin's layers before being reflected back to the surface (diffuse reflectance). The retransmitted light or reflectance is a function of diffusion and absorption of light within various layers of skin.

In the epidermis, the pigment melanin mainly absorbs radiation over the entire visible range. In the dermis, the light is absorbed mostly due to pigment haemoglobin in blood. Other pigments are carotene and bilirubin. The subcutaneous fatty tissue contains 50% of body fat and due to the presence of these white fat deposits, most of the visible light reaching this tissue is reflected back to the upper layers [46].

Skin pigments are chemical compounds. Molar absorptivity is used to measure the strength of a chemical compound in absorbing light. A number of experiments have shown that molar absorptivity of skin pigments is a function of wavelength. Figure 4.7 shows the molar absorptivity of eumelanin and pheomelanin as the function of light wavelength. Figures 4.8 and 4.9 show the molar absorptivity of haemoglobin and bilirubin–carotene, respectively.

Because the molar absorptivity of skin pigments are different and is a function of the light wavelength, it is hypothesized that the spectral reflectance of skin can be utilized to analyse skin pigments (chromophores) to find out the concentrations of melanin categories and concentration noninvasively because reflectance spectrum is influenced by dermal absorption. The dermal absorption itself is defined as the sum of skin pigment absorption which is wavelength-dependent. In summary, by knowing the contribution of skin pigments to the dermal absorption and other factors (i.e., scattering coefficients, skin thickness and anisotropy factor) we can

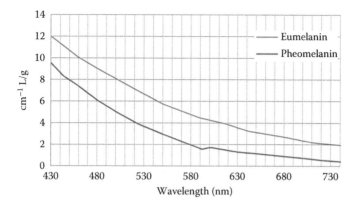

Figure 4.7 Eumelanin and pheomelanin molar absorptivity. (Reproduced from S. L. Jacques, *Advances in Optical Imaging and Photon Migaration*. Optical Society of America, 1996, pp. 364–370.)

determine melanin types and concentration in a non-invasive and objective manner.

4.3.3 Light–skin interaction

As discussed in Section 4.3.2, the reflectance of skin may be best portrayed by the Dichromatic Reflection Model shown in Figure 4.10. At incident angles near to normal (<40°), about 5% of the incident radiation is directly reflected at the surface (surface reflectance). The reflection happens because of the change in refractive index between air ($n_D = 1.0$) and

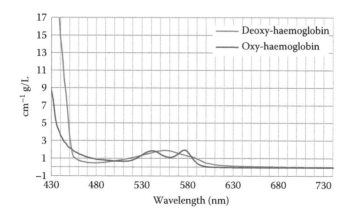

Figure 4.8 Haemoglobin molar absorptivity. (Reproduced from S. Takatani and M. D. Graham, *IEEE Transactions* on *Biomedical Engineering*, vol. 26, pp. 656–664, 1987.)

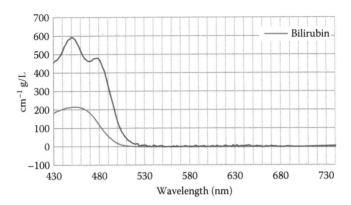

Figure 4.9 Bilirubin and carotene molar absorptivity. (Reproduced from H. Du et al. *Photochemistry and Photobiology*, vol. 68, pp. 141–142, 1998.)

stratum corneum ($n_D = 1.55$). Surface reflections increment for bigger incident angles is explained in Fresnel's equation [50]. Whatever is left of the incident radiation (95%) enters the skin where it is absorbed or diffused within the skin's layers. In Figure 2.8, this incident radiation is depicted as epidermal and dermal remittance. Both of the remittances constitute the body (diffuse) reflectance. The diffuse reflectance of the skin is a function of diffusion and absorption within its various layers through which the radiation enters.

In the epidermis, the pigment melanin mainly absorbs radiation over the entire visible range, although more absorption happens in the short wavelengths versus the long ones. In the dermis, the light is diffused and absorbed. The absorption is primarily because of the pigment

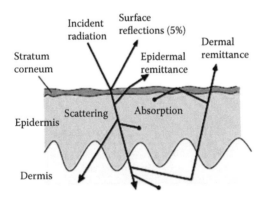

Figure 4.10 Optics of skin. (Reproduced from R. R. Anderson and J. A. Parrish, *Journal of Investigative Dermatology*, vol. 77, no. 1, pp. 13–19, 198AD.)

haemoglobin in the blood. Haemoglobin might be oxygenated (oxy-hae-moglobin), providing a reddish colour to the blood, or deoxygenated, providing a bluish colour to the blood [51]. Other pigments are carotene and bilirubin. Carotene has just about the same absorption as bilirubin [52]. For the most part, the optical characteristics of the dermis are assumed equivalent for every single human race [53].

The rest of the non-absorbed radiation is diffuse-reflected from collagen fibres and white fat. Preceding leaving the skin, it goes through again the dermal and epidermal while being absorbed and diffused at the same time. Figure 4.11 demonstrates a common reflectance spectrum curve of skin in the visible bands that can be obtained from measurements using spectrophotometer.

4.3.3.1 Light reflectance model

Reflectance spectroscopy is the study of light as a function of wavelength that has been reflected or scattered from a medium [54]. The reflectance spectrum measurement of human skin can provide valuable inputs to non-invasive analysis in diagnosing various skin diseases such as venous ulcers, psoriasis and pigmentation disorders [55]. To analyse the skin reflectance spectra, an in-depth understanding of skin optics is necessary.

Light is a type of electromagnetic radiation, which comprises not only the visible light but also microwaves and x-rays. Wavelength, λ, is a parameter utilized to recognise the different types of radiation, whereby the said wavelength is usually measured in nanometres (nm, 10−9 m). Electromagnetic radiation happens over an extensive range of wavelengths (λ) from gamma rays to long radio waves of kilometres. The wavelengths visible to humans are between x-rays and radio waves. They sit

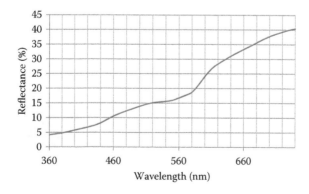

Figure 4.11 Reflectance spectrum of skin.

in the narrow band between violet at about 380 nm (1 nm = 10−9 m) and deep red at about 770 nm, as depicted in Figure 4.12.

Light can get in the way of matter, become directionally polarised and deviate a little when passing an edge [56]. The light-matter simulation includes three primary procedures: radiation, diffusion and absorption. At the atomic level these associations happen between photons of light and electrons and can be simplified into three fundamental activities: a photon moving from one location to another, an electron moving from one location to another and an electron radiating or absorbing a photon.

Radiation is the process by which the energy of a photon is released either by thermal or luminescent [57] radiation. Thermal radiations are caused by the material emitting extra heat energy in the form of light. However, luminescent radiations are caused by energy touching base from somewhere else, kept in the material and radiated (after a brief period) as photons. The incident energy causes the excitation of electrons of the material in the outer and incomplete inner shells move to a higher energy state within the atom. When an electron returns to the ground state, a photon is emitted. The wavelength of the emitted photon will depend on the atomic structure of the material and the magnitude of the incoming energy.

Diffusion is because of the deflection of light through impacts with molecules, particles or group of particles lessening the energy of the incident light at the same time. The diffusion procedure may be grouped into three: molecular diffusion, particle diffusion and surface/reflective–refractive diffusion [58–60]. Molecular scattering (Rayleigh scattering) happens when the wavelength of the light is larger than the size of the molecules/particles. Particle scattering (Mie scattering), meanwhile, happens when the wavelength of the incident light is comparable to the size

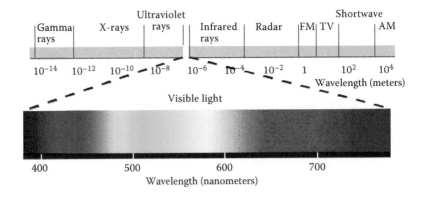

Figure 4.12 Spectrum of light.

of the molecules or particles. For some practical intent, the error in utilizing Rayleigh, rather than Mie theory, to small particles is less than 1% when the radius of the particle is smaller or equal to 0.03λ [59]. Moreover, reflective–refractive or geometrical optics diffusion happens when the size of the particles is much larger than the wavelength of incident light. This category of diffusion happens for a large portion of the internal diffusion in organic tissues, such as on human skin. It is fundamentally brought about by the arrangement of tissues, and the refractive differences, connected with the air-cell wall interfaces with respect to cells whose dimensions are quite larger compared to the wavelength of light. Due to its dependency on refractive differences, the variations across the spectrum are directly associated with the wavelength dependency of the refractive indices of the materials.

Light absorption may occur during the transmission of light into a medium. In a dielectric material such as skin, light absorption is caused by the absorptive elements inside the medium, such as pigments, the materials that exhibit both selective scattering and selective absorption [61]. The subsequent distribution spectrum of light performing an absorption procedure depends on the absorption spectrum of the absorptive component. The absorption spectrum, thus, is influenced by the categories of chromophore that are available in the component. In chromophore, electrons may be excited to higher states by just a moderately little measure of energy. When light with the right wavelength hits a chromophore, it is consumed through the electron excitation from its ground state into an energized state [60]. If the incident light does not have the correct wavelength, it will not be absorbed but diffused instead.

Numerous molecules found in living life forms have various elements that decrease the energy expected to energize their electrons, and in this manner gives their colour, which is dictated by the spectral distribution of the absorbed light [62]. Their atoms can comprise a transition metal, which is a group of metals that have unfilled electron orbits available for electron excitation (such as titanium, iron, cobalt, nickel and copper). For instance, iron in haemoglobin is in charge of the red colour of blood.

The absorption spectra of pigments, for example, haemoglobin, are typically quantified in their specific absorption coefficient (SAC), indicated by μ_{sac}. SAC can be acquired through direct measurements or by dividing the material's molar extinction or absorptivity coefficient, ε, by the material's molecular weight. Its units rely on the measurement methodology of the concentration of the material [22,63]. On account of inorganic materials such as water, the absorption spectra is quantified in their extinction coefficient. The extinction coefficient of certain inorganic materials like pure water is relatively low over the visible light spectrum. Thus, the absorption of visible light by these materials is usually assumed insignificant.

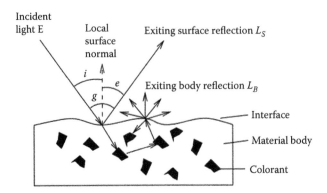

Figure 4.13 Dichromatic reflection model of skin. (Reproduced from J. van de Wijer and S. Beigpour, *International Joint Conference on Computer Vision, Imaging and Computer Graphics Theory and Applications*, 2006.)

The absorption of a particular pigment spectrum available in a tissue is typically acquired under in vitro conditions in which numerous methods such as implementing biochemical study on skin biopsy is used to extract the pigment from the tissue. Because of the distinctions in the encompassing environment, the distribution and condition of these pigments, their absorption spectra under in vitro conditions contrast from those pigments under in vivo conditions [64]. Regularly, in vivo pigments are uniformly distributed in the tissues. As a result, light transport models that use in vitro information to analyse pigments should take into consideration these changes to improve accuracy.

A light reflectance model is a model used to describe the interaction of light with a surface. Typically, the model is formulated regarding the properties of the surface and the properties of the incident light. Figure 4.13 shows a frequently used physics-based reflection model of skin called the Dichromatic Reflection Model as applied in the reflections of dielectric non-homogeneous materials [66–68]. The Dichromatic Reflection Model describes the reflected radiance or light, L as an additive mixture of the light, L_S reflected at the material's surface (surface reflection or surface reflectance) and the light, L_B reflected from the material's body (diffuse reflection or diffuse reflectance):

$$L(i,e,g,\lambda) = L_s(i,e,g,\lambda) + L_B(i,e,g,\lambda) \tag{4.1}$$

where e represents the viewing angle, g represents the phase angle and i represents the illumination direction angle. These are called photometric angles.

For skin, it was reported that the surface reflection, L_S, makes up 5% of the reflected light and the body light, L_B, makes up the rest (95%) [69]. The body reflection is the light reflected from the material body. It enters into the materials where it is diffused, partially absorbed at a specific wavelength and remitted out of the material.

The spectra of surface and body reflections from the dielectric materials are invariant to the illumination geometry – thus the surface and body reflections may be split into a geometrical scaling factor and a spectrum, respectively [70]:

$$L(\theta,\lambda) = m_S(\theta)c_S(\lambda) + m_B(\theta)c_B(\lambda) \tag{4.2}$$

where $m_S(\theta)$ and $m_B(\theta)$ are geometrical scaling factors, and $c_S(\lambda)$ and $c_B(\lambda)$ are the light spectra for the surface and body reflections, respectively.

4.3.3.2 Surface reflection

When the light beam crosses a boundary with differing refractive indices, the light is partly reflected from the surface. This reflection is called as specular reflection. A portion of the light may cross the boundary and its speed may change due to the difference in the refraction coefficients. According to Snell's Law, the change in the speed of light causes refraction resulting in a change of direction of the transmitted light.

The skin surface contains a thin lipid layer functioned to protect the excessive evaporation of water from the skin. The relative refraction index of this lipid layer is significantly different from that of air. Therefore, incident light is reflected at the air-lipid boundary, making the skin shinier. This specular reflection is weakly dependent on wavelength.

Fresnel formulated the strength of the surface reflection of a collimated light and the incident angle of which is normal to the skin surface. The derivation of the formula, known as the Fresnel equation, is shown in Equation 2.3 [50]. If a beam of light is collided orthogonally in the air-dielectric surface, the specular reflectance, R_f can be formulated as

$$R_f = \left(\frac{1-n}{1+n}\right)^2 \tag{4.3}$$

where n is the relative index of refraction of the dielectric. Figure 4.14 shows the surface reflectance as a function of the incident angle (with respect to the surface normal) at a planar interface of a material with refractive index $n_D = 1.55$.

Skin surfaces are not smooth due to wrinkles and pores, and therefore the specular reflection is dispersed resulting in an unevenly distributed illumination.

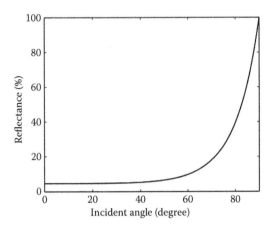

Figure 4.14 Surface reflectance and incident angle. (Reproduced from G. Poirier, *Human skin modelling and rendering*, University of Waterloo, 2003.)

4.3.3.3 Skin base absorption

The absorption in skin is mainly due to pigments deposited in epidermis or dissolved in blood located in the dermis. The total optical absorption coefficient of the epidermis and dermis depends on several minor factors (such as skin baseline absorption, water absorption and pigments bilirubin and carotene absorption) and dominant factors of melanin and haemoglobin absorption. Melanin is the most important factor behind the colour of the skin. The concentration of melanosomes does not have a direct relationship with absorption, but its size and structure will affect the production of melanin. Hence, the volume fraction of melanosome is often used as one of the optical characteristics of skin [72].

Similar to the epidermis, the dermis does not absorb much light. The haemoglobin dissolved in blood, however, is a strong light absorber. The iron complex of the haemoglobin molecule causes blood to appear as red colour by absorbing blue and green colour. The absorption spectrum of haemoglobin changes is based on how many oxygen atoms are bounded to the iron complex [73]. Other pigments like bilirubin and carotene contributes to the absorption of light photon. Nevertheless, most studies agree that the overall effect of carotene and bilirubin on skin reflectance can be considered negligible [42].

The skin baseline absorption is defined as the dermal absorption without melanin and haemoglobin [74]. The independent parameter specifying the absorption of skin baseline is the wavelength λ. The baseline absorption of both epidermis and dermis are approximated by Jacques [47]. The expression (Equation 4.4) is based on the measurements of bloodless rat skin using an integrating sphere.

$$\mu_{a.skinbaseline}\left(\lambda\right) = 0.224 + 85.3e^{\frac{-(\lambda-154)}{66.2}} \tag{4.4}$$

Another measurement for the baseline absorption was performed by Saidi [75]. Here, the function (Equation 4.5) is approximated by studying the baseline absorption of neo-natal skin. It is generated within vitro neo-natal skin samples using an integrating sphere after accounting for excess absorption due to residual haemoglobin and bilirubin in the samples.

$$\mu_{a.skinbaseline}\left(\lambda\right) = \left(7.84x108\right)\lambda^{-3.255} \tag{4.5}$$

Figure 4.15 presents the baseline absorption based on neo-natal skin. The graph is simulated from data obtained from Saidi [75].

4.3.3.4 Water spectral absorption

Water spectral absorption contributes to the overall dermal absorption coefficient, though small in nature [76]. Water absorption has to be considered for any applications using near-infrared light. It becomes visible after 900 nm. Related to this, some computational models of skin such as the Meglinski–Matcher model have included such absorption [77]. Figure 4.16 depicts the spectral absorption coefficient of water using the experimental data from Segelsten et al. [56].

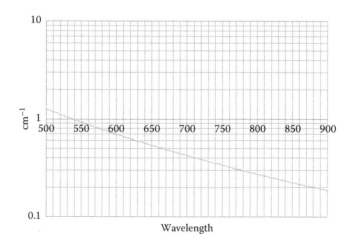

Figure 4.15 Baseline spectral absorption of skin.

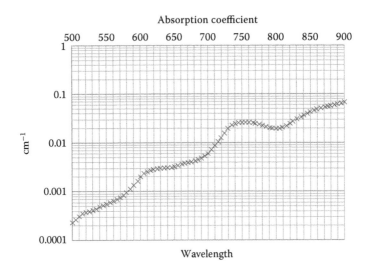

Figure 4.16 Water spectral absorption.

4.3.3.5 Stratum corneum absorption

The dermal absorption coefficient accounts for the presence of eumelanin, pheomelanin, oxy-haemoglobin, deoxy-haemoglobin, bilirubin and carotene. The total absorption coefficient for each layer is the sum of the absorption coefficients of each pigment in the layer, which is attained by multiplying the pigment's spectral extinction coefficient by its predicted concentration in the layer.

The stratum corneum total absorption coefficient, $\mu_{a.sc}(\lambda)$, is given by [78]

$$
\begin{aligned}
\mu_{a.epidermis}(\lambda) = &\, (\mu_{a.eu}(\lambda) + \mu_{a.ph}(\lambda))\upsilon_m \\
&+ (\mu_{a.skinbaseline}(\lambda) + \mu_{a.ce}(\lambda))(1 - \upsilon_m)
\end{aligned}
\tag{4.6}
$$

where $\mu_{a.cs}(\lambda)$ is the carotene absorption coefficient.

The carotene absorption coefficient $\mu_{a.cs}(\lambda)$ is given by [78]

$$
\mu_{a.eu}(\lambda) = \frac{\varepsilon_{eu}(\lambda)}{537} c_{eu}
\tag{4.7}
$$

where
$537 =$ molecular weight of carotene (g/mol)
$c_{cs} =$ carotene concentration in stratum corneum
$\varepsilon_{car}(\lambda) =$ molar absorptivity of carotene

The molar absorptivity is a measure of the amount of light absorbed per unit concentration. Molar absorptivity has units of L/mol cm. The absorption of a substance is expressed as an absorption coefficient, μ_a, which is the molar absorptivity of the chromophores, ε, multiplied by the concentration of the chromophores, c.

4.3.3.6 Epidermis absorption

The absorption coefficient of epidermis is determined by the presence of melanin (eumelanin and pheomelanin) and others pigments.

The epidermis total absorption coefficient, $\mu_{a.epidermis}(\lambda)$, is given by [79]

$$\mu_{a.epidermis}(\lambda) = (\mu_{a.eu}(\lambda) + \mu_{a.ph}(\lambda))v_m$$
$$+ (\mu_{a.skinbaseline}(\lambda) + \mu_{a.ce}(\lambda))(1 - v_m) \tag{4.8}$$

where

$\mu_{a.eu}(\lambda)$ = eumelanin absorption coefficient
$\mu_{a.ph}(\lambda)$ = pheomelanin absorption coefficient
$\mu_{a.ce}(\lambda)$ = carotene absorption coefficient in epidermis
v_m = volume fraction of epidermis occupied by melanosomes

The absorption coefficient for eumelanin is given by [79]

$$\mu_{a.eu}(\lambda) = \varepsilon_{eu}(\lambda)c_{eu} \tag{4.9}$$

where

$\varepsilon_{eu}(\lambda)$ = molar absorptivity of eumelanin
c_{eu} = eumelanin concentration in epidermis

The molar absorptivity of eumelanin is a measure of the amount of light absorbed per unit concentration of eumelanin. The molar absorptivity of eumelanin was estimated by Jacques [47]. Figure 4.17 shows the plot of molar absorptivity of eumelanin as a function of wavelength.

Similarly, the absorption coefficient for pheomelanin is given by [79]

$$\mu_{a.ph}(\lambda) = \varepsilon_{ph}(\lambda)c_{ph} \tag{4.10}$$

where

$\varepsilon_{ph}(\lambda)$ = molar absorptivity of pheomelanin
c_{ph} = pheomelanin concentration in epidermis

The molar absorptivity of pheomelanin was estimated by Jacques [47]. Figure 4.18 shows the plot of molar absorptivity of pheomelanin as a function of wavelength.

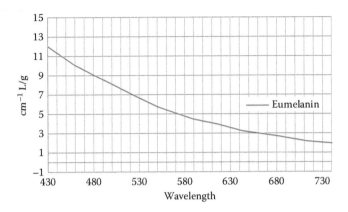

Figure 4.17 Molar absorptivity of eumelanin.

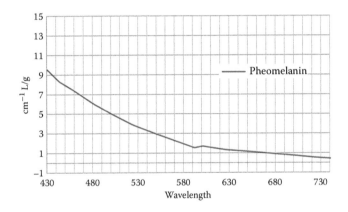

Figure 4.18 Molar absorptivity of pheomelanin.

In addition, the absorption coefficient $\mu_{a.ce}(\lambda)$ is attained by revising the concentration of carotene (c_{ce}) from the previous equation.

$$\mu_{a.ce}(\lambda) = \frac{\varepsilon_{car}(\lambda)}{537} c_{ce} \qquad (4.11)$$

where
  537 = molecular weight of carotene (g/mol)
  c_{ce} = carotene concentration in epidermis

4.3.3.7 Dermis absorption
The absorption coefficient of dermis is determined by the presence of hae-moglobin (both oxy-haemoglobin and deoxy-haemoglobin) and others pigments.

The dermis total absorption coefficient, $\mu_{a.dermis}(\lambda)$, is given by [80]

$$\mu_{a.dermis}(\lambda) = (\mu_{a.ohb}(\lambda) + \mu_{a.dhb}(\lambda) + \mu_{a.cd}(\lambda) + \mu_{a.bil}(\lambda))v_b$$
$$+ \mu_{a.skinbaseline}(\lambda)(1 - v_b) \tag{4.12}$$

where

$\mu_{a.ohb}(\lambda) =$ oxy-haemoglobin absorption coefficient
$\mu_{a.dhb}(\lambda) =$ deoxy-haemoglobin absorption coefficient
$\mu_{a.cd}(\lambda) =$ carotene absorption coefficient in dermis
$\mu_{a.bil}(\lambda) =$ bilirubin absorption coefficient in dermis
$v_p =$ volume fraction of dermis occupied by blood

The absorption coefficient for oxy-haemoglobin is given by [80]

$$\mu_{a.ohb}(\lambda) = \frac{\varepsilon_{ohb}(\lambda)}{66,500} c_{hb} * \gamma \tag{4.13}$$

where

$66500 =$ molecular weight of haemoglobin (g/mol)
$\varepsilon_{ohb}(\lambda) =$ molar absorptivity of oxy-haemoglobin
$c_{hb}(\lambda) =$ concentration of haemoglobin in the blood (g/L)
$\gamma =$ ratio of oxy-haemoglobin to the total haemoglobin absorption

The absorption coefficient for deoxy-haemoglobin is given by [80]

$$\mu_{a.dhb}(\lambda) = \frac{\varepsilon_{dhb}(\lambda)}{66,500} c_{hb} * (1 - \gamma) \tag{4.14}$$

where

$66500 =$ molecular weight of haemoglobin (g/mol)
$\varepsilon_{dhb}(\lambda) =$ molar absorptivity of deoxy-haemoglobin
$c_{hb}(\lambda) =$ concentration of haemoglobin in the blood (g/L)
$\gamma =$ ratio of oxy-haemoglobin to the total haemoglobin absorption

The oxy-haemoglobin (HbO_2) and deoxy-haemoglobin (Hb) have different spectra of molar absorptivity. The molar absorptivity was estimated by Meglinski [51]. Figure 4.19 shows the plot of molar absorptivity of oxy-haemoglobin and deoxy-haemoglobin as a function of wavelength.

The absorption coefficient $\mu_{a.cd}(\lambda)$ is attained by revising c_{cd} as the concentration of carotene in the skin layers.

$$\mu_{a.cd}(\lambda) = \frac{\varepsilon_{car}(\lambda)}{537} c_{cd} \tag{4.15}$$

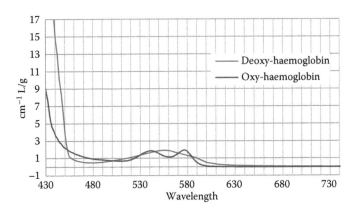

Figure 4.19 Molar absorptivity of oxy- and deoxy-haemoglobin.

where

c_{cd} = carotene concentration in epidermis

In addition, the absorption coefficient for bilirubin is given by [80]

$$\mu_{a.bil}(\lambda) = \frac{\varepsilon_{bil}(\lambda)}{585} c_{bil} \qquad (4.16)$$

where

585 = molecular weight of bilirubin (g/mol)

$\varepsilon_{bil}(\lambda)$ = molar absorptivity of bilirubin

$c_{bil}(\lambda)$ = concentration of bilirubin in dermis (g/L)

4.3.3.8 Scattering in skin tissues

Scattering occurs when a photon interacts with a particle in the medium where molecules are unordered, changing its direction, but not losing its energy. The change of direction of a photon can be described by a phase function of $p(\vec{s}, \vec{s}')$. Phase function provides the probability of the photon being scattered in the direction of $\vec{s}'$ when propagating in $\vec{s}$ before the scattering. Due to the scattering, some photons, which have already entered into the medium, may reverse their direction and exit the media from the side of the illumination. This reflection is called body reflectance or diffuse reflectance.

The human skin is a strong medium of light scattering. The stratum corneum in epidermis makes the light beam diffused, while the collagen and the elastine fibres in the dermis scatter light and so do the cytoplasm membranes. The size of the cells, mitochondria and collagen fibres are usually larger than 1000 nm, thus making them larger than the wavelength in the diagnostic–therapeutic window. When the diffusing particle is close to the wavelength of light, the scattering can be best modelled by Mie scattering [2,4,36,37,81]. The strength of the Mie scattering is roughly proportional to $\lambda{-}1.5$, where λ is the wavelength of radiation. The cell nucleus and membranes also scatter light, but much smaller than the wavelength. The scattering introduced by these small particles is often described using the Rayleigh scattering formula, which is more strongly wavelength-dependent, being proportional to $\lambda{-}4$.

The optical models of skin do not usually work at the individual cell level. The skin layers are assumed homogeneous, and the scattering sources are distributed evenly in each layer. The scattering of human skin is frequently modelled as a combination of Mie and Rayleigh scattering [82] as follows:

$$\mu_s(\lambda) = \mu_{s.Mie}(\lambda) + \mu_{s.Rayleigh}(\lambda)$$
$$\mu_s(\lambda) = 2.10^5.\lambda^{-1.5} + 2.10^{12}.\lambda^{-4.5}$$

$$(4.17)$$

where λ is visible light wavelength (nm). Figure 4.20 shows the plot of combination of Mie and Rayleigh scattering.

4.4 Skin computer models

4.4.1 Skin modalities

Understanding human skin reflectance can be useful in a number of applications [83]. For example, it gives an important aspect of photo-realistic rendering of human skin for game development and film production. In dermatology, it can provide valuable information of skin diseases [84]. In understanding skin reflectance, acquisition/measurement of the skin reflectance provides a foundation in analysing skin optical properties

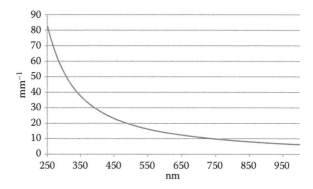

Figure 4.20 Scattering coefficient.

through a simulation of light–skin interaction model. The accurate acquisition of skin reflectance data, in turn, leads to improve both skin simulation and skin analysis methods [42].

A number of theorems of skin–light interaction has been created by researchers for many applications, such as in computer rendering for animation [9,67,85], dosimetry [86–88] and in diagnosis [89–94]. In diagnosis, the application of the light–skin models is used to analyse skin spectral information, leading to noninvasive determination of skin optical properties. The models simulate the spectral information (reflectance and transmittance) of skin tissues. To measure the properties, an inversion operation, an approach to determine biochemical and optical properties from *in situ* and non-invasive measurements, is utilized. The operation is an inversion of the real method of computing reflection and transmission, using reflectance and transmittance values captured by skin imaging tool as input to determine absorption and scattering properties of the tissues.

In dermatological practice and studies, certain visual cues can play an important role to enable dermatologists to make an accurate diagnosis [21]. In this case, visual evaluation of lesions is the first and most frequently used procedure made by dermatologists in daily practice that is by evaluating the lesion condition and recording its score in notes. In many instances, notes and lesion photography are referred in determining the evolution of the skin condition. An evaluation of lesion by dermatologist will be based on the distribution, size, shape, border, symmetry and colour of the skin lesion. However, the evaluation might be subjective due to the dependency of visual perception on the human visual response to light as well as light interaction with objects.

The retina of the human eye has two receptors namely, rods and cones. Rods are monochromatic and do not provide spectral information to the visual system. Cones consist of three different types, each of which has a selective wavelength response. The cones are named L, M and S with responses centred at long (564 nm), medium (534 nm) and short (420 nm) wavelengths, respectively [95]. Furthermore, the human eye does not have the same sensitivity for all wavelengths and among individuals [96]. The discriminant power is poor for the extremity of the spectrum but much higher in the wavelength range of 490 and 550 nm. This leads to dermatological diagnoses relying mainly on skin colour, and visual analysis to be subjective.

In response, a better and more accurate imaging system that can capture wider spectral information is sorely needed. A wide spectral information of skin can provide valuable information to non-invasive *in vivo* approach in diagnosing various skin diseases [55]. In the following sections, different modalities to obtain skin reflectance data are investigated and will cover skin modalities systems, models of light propagation in skin including the K–M model, radiative transport equation, the modified Beer–Lambert law and MC simulation.

4.4.1.1 Digital photography

Digital photography is a photographic method that stores the image digitally. A digital image is composed of arrays of pixels that generally have a discrete intensity value. These intensity values are produced by the camera's CCD (charge-coupled device), an image sensor consisting of integrated circuits that contain the array of coupled light-sensitive capacitors. In a digital camera, CCD sensors are equipped with a Bayer mask to produce colour images, as illustrated in Figure 4.21. The Bayer mask filters the incoming light into three colours of light red, green and blue [97]. These three primary colours (trichromatic model) represent the colour response and sensitivity of the eye [98].

With decreasing costs and increasing resolution and capacity storage over the last decade, digital imaging has been adopted in dermatological practise [99]. Most dermatologists consider that baseline photography is useful in the follow-up of skin lesions [100]. Digital photography offers a wide range of combination with different configurations, such as high spatial resolution (over 10 Megapixels), colour resolution (8, 16 or 24 bits), colour space representation (RGB, CMY, HSI, La*b*, etc.) and view (different lenses). Standardisation, however, is still a drawback in digital imaging due to a large number of technical factors in image quality such as camera sensor type, resolution, use of filters and type of lighting. Indeed,

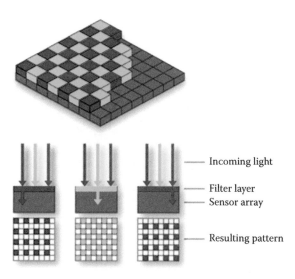

Incoming light

Filter layer
Sensor array

Resulting pattern

Figure 4.21 Bayer mask. (Reproduced from B. E. Bayer, *Color Imaging Array*, 555477, 1976.)

these multiple configurations have brought positive effects on the diagnosis accuracy [101]. Essentially, considering its practicality and availability, digital colour camera is a promising technology. However, the spectral bands of images acquired are not narrow enough to provide spectral information and thus set limits in the detection and identification of tissue. Appropriate illumination can improve clinical photography of skin lesions [102].

4.4.1.2 MSI system

MSI is an imaging technology, which measures light intensities at various spectral bands. In dermatology, MSI can provide spectral information of skin at spectral bands of wavelengths ranging from visible to near infrared one. Images of different spectral bands can be combined to generate a composite image. Such composite images produce colour patterns that can be used to distinguish surface features [7,20,103].

As shown in Figure 4.22, MSI systems acquire three-dimensional data consisting of two-dimensional spatial information (x, y) at spectral wavelength, λ. In comparison with digital photography, the innovation of MSI lies on the provision of spectral information at each pixel. The extended spectral capacity reduces the effect of metameric mismatches that may occur with different illuminations [105] and variability of the sensor spectral responses.

In MSI, the system contains several sensors, each of which records the intensity of light, I, in one spectral band defined by the bandwidths of the

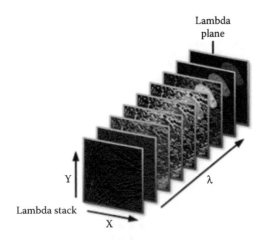

Figure 4.22 MSI images of skin. (Reproduced from K. Burton, J. Jeon, S. Wachsmann-Hogiu and D. Farkas, *Biomedical Optical Imaging*. Oxford University Press, 2009, pp. 1–44.)

light source, $I_0(\lambda)$, and the sensor, $S(\lambda)$ [38]. The reflectance of the sample is obtained by comparing the light intensity reflected from the sample with a light intensity from the white reference. The white reference is usually a special target with a number of known values, R_w. The reflectance of the sample, R, is given by

$$R = \frac{I_{sample}}{I_{white}} R_w = \frac{\displaystyle\int_\lambda I_0(\lambda)S(\lambda)R(\lambda)\,d\lambda}{\displaystyle\int_\lambda I_0(\lambda)S(\lambda)R_w\,d\lambda} R_w \qquad (4.18)$$

The characteristics of the sensor, $S(\lambda)$ and light source, $I_0(\lambda)$ define the bandwidth of the image. Based on acquisition technologies, MSI can be categorised into spectral scanning system and spatial scanning system.

Spectral imaging filters and camera are used in spectral scanning. There are two types of filter, namely fixed and tuneable filters (Figures 4.23 and 4.24). For fixed filters, the filters are usually placed in the optical path, performing a wavelength selection. A common solution is to incorporate a set of band pass filters into a filter wheel [107]. The recording is performed upon the synchronised rotation of the wheel with the camera acquisition. Spectral scanning is low cost and allows a large selection of filters. However, it is inflexible in terms of filter specifications and even though we have a large selection of filters, the filter wheel has a limited number of slots.

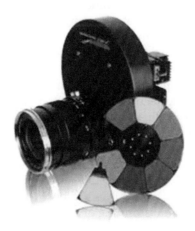

Figure 4.23 MSI with fixed filter. (Reproduced from J. Y. Hardeberg, F. Schmitt, and H. Brettel, *Optical Engineering*, vol. 41, no. 10, pp. 2532–2548, 2002.)

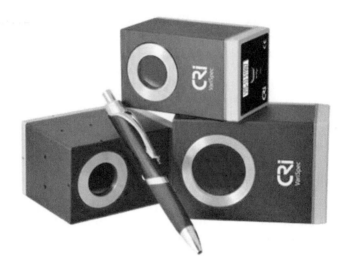

Figure 4.24 MSI with tuneable filter. (Reproduced from J. Y. Hardeberg, F. Schmitt and H. Brettel, *Optical Engineering*, vol. 41, no. 10, pp. 253–2548, 2002.)

In tuneable filters, a spectral transmission band can be shifted continuously along an electromagnetic spectrum at any wavelength λ within its ranges. There are two types of tuneable filters – liquid crystal tuneable filter (LCTF) and acousto-optic tuneable filter (AOTF). Liquid crystal tuneable filters (LCTFs) consist of a set of liquid crystal layers and each layer transmits a different band of frequencies [106].

Both LCTF and AOTF are not affected by mechanical constraints, image shift, speed limitation or vibration associated with the use of filter wheel but these filters have a weak transmission (often in the order of 30%), out of band rejection (wavelength leaking) and limited bandwidth. Strong illumination devices are used to compensate the weak transmission.

In spatial scanning, spectral information is acquired along a spatial dimension at a single time. Generally, the spatial information is obtained by scanning in spatial coordinates through the area of interest. There are two techniques of spatial scanning, namely single-slit spectrometer and multi-slit spectrometer [104].

A single slit can be used in point-scanning or line-scanning. The spectrometer of a single slit consists of a disperse element (example: a prism) and a linear detector array [108]. This will allow the system to capture spatial resolution (by x–y spatial scanning of a focused laser beam) with high spectral resolution (depends on the resolution of the disperse element used). As illustrated in Figures 4.25 and 4.26, the object is illuminated and the spectral information of a point or a line of the object is obtained using

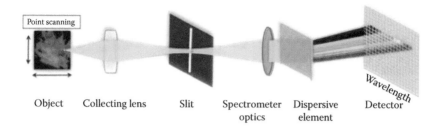

Figure 4.25 Point-scanning of a single slit system. (Reproduced from K. Burton et al. *Biomedical Optical Imaging.* Oxford University Press, 2009, pp. 1–44.)

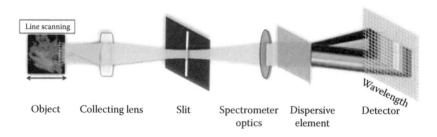

Figure 4.26 Line-scanning of a single slit system. (Reproduced from K. Burton et al. *Biomedical Optical Imaging.* Oxford University Press, 2009, pp. 1–44.)

a single-slit spectrometer with a disperse element and CCD detector. A complete image (a spectral cube) is obtained by scanning the object in the direction perpendicular to the excitation line.

Similar to a single-slit system, the spectrometer of a multi-slit system also consists of a disperse element (a prism) and a detector. The difference is that it employs a special mask known as Hadamard mask. Hadamard masks are made up of a pattern of reflective and transmissive slits of various widths constructed from a Hadamard matrix. A Hadamard matrix is a square matrix whose entries are either +1 or −1 and whose rows are mutually orthogonal. The spectral information is then generated from Hadamard transform [109]. As illustrated in Figure 4.27, the object is illuminated and spectral information is obtained using a multiple slit (Hadamard mask) spectrophotometer with a disperse element and a linear array of CCD detector. A complete image (a spectral cube) is obtained by varying the mask and performing Hadamard transform.

Limitations of these systems are due to the diffraction system employed. A single slit system offers a fast data capture but with limited spectral resolution. A multi-slit system offers high spectral resolution but slower data acquisition.

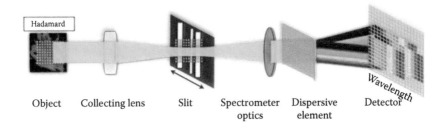

Object   Collecting lens   Slit   Spectrometer   Dispersive   Detector
                                      optics   element

Figure 4.27 Multi-slit system. (Reproduced from K. Burton et al., *Biomedical Optical Imaging.* Oxford University Press, 2009, pp. 1–44.)

4.4.1.3 Spectrophotometry

A spectrophotometer is a combination of a spectrometer and a photometer (Figure 4.28). Spectrometer refers to a light radiation system and photometer is a photon conversion system into an electrical (digital) signal. In a spectrophotometer, a prism or similar optical equipment is located between spectrometer and photometer and used to disperse the re-emitted light from the skin into numerous bands (Figure 3.8).

Spectrophotometry measures the light intensity as a function of wavelength in the form of a spectrum. The measurement here is directly linked to the physical light property over the entire spectrum (UV, VIS, VIS + NIR, NIR, IR spectral bands) of a sample studied and is not affected by illumination as the measurement area is concealed from external light. A number of researchers has demonstrated that measurements of skin colour via spectrophotometry are reproducible and not affected by ambient lighting [89,111]. Different optical spectroscopic techniques can be employed such as fluorescence spectroscopy, Raman spectroscopy and diffused reflectance spectroscopy.

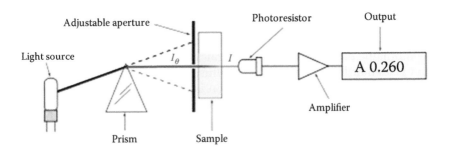

Figure 4.28 Spectrophotometry. (Reproduced from M. G. Gore, *Spectrophotometry and Spectrofluorimetry: A Practical Approach.* New York: Oxford University Press, 2000, p. 368.)

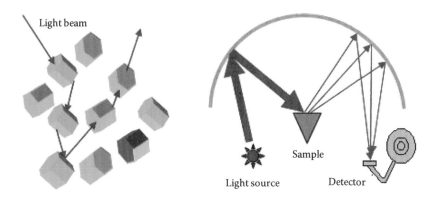

Figure 4.29 Diffused reflectance. (Reproduced from G. Zonios and A. Dimou, *Biomedical Optics Express*, vol. 2, no. 12, pp. 3284–3294, 2011.)

Diffuse reflectance spectroscopy (DRS) is a spectroscopy technique that measures the characteristic reflectance spectrum produced as light passes through a medium (Figure 4.29). The primary mechanisms are absorption and scattering, both of which vary in wavelength in order to produce a recorded reflectance spectrum. This spectrum contains information about the optical properties and structure of the medium being measured [24].

Generally, DRS uses white light source guided by optical fibres to the probe head in contact with the skin (in diameter of 0.2–0.4 mm for the optical fibre and 3–8 mm for probe head). The light illuminates and penetrates the skin sample area. The light will be partly reflected, absorbed, affected by multiple scattering and re-emitted. A reading optical fibre collects the diffuse light back to a spectrometer for an acquisition where the light will be converted into a digital signal in the form of an amount of light per wavelength (spectrum) by a spectrometer detector.

Spectrometer detector typically is a linear array sensor. The detectors are usually based on CCD silicon technology [89]. The wavelength is sampled by the relation of diffused light over the size of the array detector. The diffused light is split into wavelength by a diffraction grating (Figure 4.30). There are two possible positions to disperse the diffused light in the optical path. First, the diffraction grating can be located before the sample. In this way, the incident light illuminates the sample at a single waveband (monochromatic) and makes every band sequentially acquired. Second, it is positioned after the sample to allow acquisition in a single shot. At this point, the sample is illuminated by a light source covering a large spectrum (polychromatic illumination) and the illuminated sample light subsequently is dispersed into the detector.

Spectrophotometer measures a ratio value (between 0% and 100%) as shown in Figure 4.31. The reflectance value is obtained after a calibration

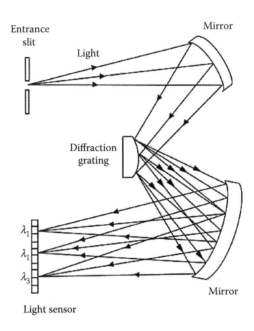

Figure 4.30 Diffraction grating. (Reproduced from G. Zonios and A. Dimou, *Biomedical Optics Express*, vol. 2, no. 12, pp. 3284–3294, 2011.)

step, which takes into account the intrinsic wavelength dependence of the detector as it has different efficiency over its wave range. A spectrum is a ratio of reflected sample light divided by the reflected light from a reference white surface.

After illuminating the skin, two types of light, namely specular light and diffused light are returned to the observer. The determination of the specular light is mainly conducted using the surface properties [41] and the diffused light is a result of the scattering and absorption properties of the skin, called diffuse reflectance. The diffuse reflectance from the skin is linked to the ratio of the scattering (μ_s) and the absorption (μ_a) coefficients of the chromophores within the skin.

Healthy skin and disease tissues are expected to have different reflectance spectra and thus can be used for diagnostic purposes. For this reason, diffuse reflectance should be measured instead of surface reflectance spectrum, which does not contain skin composition information. This type of measurement is achieved by choosing the right position and orientation of the light source to prevent a direct illumination on the skin surface only allowing diffuse light to be measured. For example, Minolta CM-2600C spectrophotometer (Figure 4.32) that has the orientation of 0° of light sensor and 45° of white light source, can offer high capability in capturing diffused light.

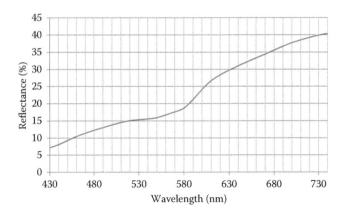

Figure 4.31 Reflectance of skin.

In addition to the general spectrophotometer, there are also dedicated spectrophotometer for specific purposes. As an example, the narrow-band spectrophotometer is designed specifically to measure melanin and haemoglobin. This kind of spectrophotometry is referencing on a model created by Diffey et al. [113]. These devices are usually portable, such as DermaSpect and DermaScan, and measure at specific wavelengths (absorption coefficient of melanin and haemoglobin) [8]. Both scanners only emit light at two wavelengths. Due to the limited information returned by this technique, narrow-band spectrophotometry systems generally are limited in their application.

The main advantage of DRS is the strong intensity of the signal (several orders of magnitude compared to fluorescence signal), which results in higher signal-to-noise ratios at a relatively moderate cost. This technique is fast (few milliseconds to few seconds), easy to set-up, and commercially available. However, it does not provide spectral information from a single location, that is, the diffuse reflectance spectrum is the average over an area.

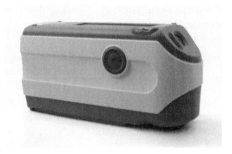

Figure 4.32 CM 2500C.

DRS has been widely used in dermatology either as a tool of the quantitative measure of melanin or the haemoglobin content of the skin [114,115]. Additionally, the device can be used to measure other chromophores [116]. The reflectance captured by the device can provide information about the light-scattering properties of the skin [117,118]. It also can be used to analyse skin colour [119], muscle [120], skin pigmentation disorder [121] and skin cancer [122–126].

4.4.1.4 Comparison of skin modalities

Table 4.4 presents a summary of the advantages and disadvantages of the aforementioned modalities systems used to obtain skin reflectance data.

In this work, a device, which can provide high spectral resolution and fast (and easy to use) measurement is required. It is preferred that the acquisition technology is already mature and easily available. Considering the aforementioned preferences, the DRS is most appropriate.

4.4.2 K–M skin model

The K–M theory was developed to study light propagation in parallel colorant layers of infinite extension in the x–y plane (Kubelka, 1948) [127]. The original theory assumed that the layer was homogeneous and the light distribution inside the layer was completely diffuse. Under these assumptions, the light propagation in the layer can be represented by two diffuse light fluxes through the layer – one is upward and the

Table 4.4 Advantages and disadvantages of imaging technique for skin analysis

Skin imaging	Advantages	Disadvantages
Digital photography	• Easily available • Practical	• Low spectral resolution Different illumination results indifferent acquired images
MSI—fixed filter	• High spectral resolution • Mature in technology, compared to tuneable-filter MSI	• Limited spectral information • Limited configuration
MSI—tuneable filter	• High spectral resolution	• Limited light transmission • Limited bandwidth selection • Probability of spectral leakage
DRS	• High spectral resolution • Strong signal intensity • Good signal-to-noise ratio • Fast	• Provides an average spectrum of an area • No spatial information

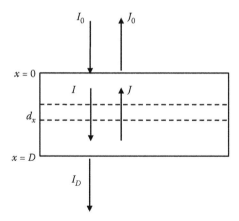

Figure 4.33 Assumption in K–M model.

other is concurrently downward. The theory was then extended by other researchers [128]. Kubelka, for example, reported the first application to inhomogeneous sample [129] and Mandel and Grossma, meanwhile, proposed a more generalized approach for inhomogeneous optical media [130].

In 1981, Anderson and Parrish reported the application of K–M theory to analyse the interaction between light and skin for computing the skin optical properties, particularly in the absorption and scattering coefficient of skin dermis [41]. As depicted in Figure 4.33, radiation within the skin samples can be divided into two opposing diffuse fluxes, I and J.

The skin scattering coefficient (μ_S) and absorption coefficient (μ_a) for diffuse radiation are defined as the fraction of diffuse radiation either back scattered or absorbed per unit differential path length of the sample. The K–M model is expressed mathematically as follows:

$$\frac{dI}{dx} = -\mu_S I - \mu_a I + \mu_S J$$

$$\frac{-dJ}{dx} = -\mu_S J - \mu_a J + s_s I$$

$$R = \frac{J_0}{I_0}$$

$$T = \frac{I_D}{I_0}$$

(4.19)

It is found that the use of integration and substitution of boundary condition can provide a particular condition, which can be arranged to express μ_S and μ_a in terms of R (reflectance) and T (transmittance). R and T are measureable quantities, thus the formula become

$$\frac{\mu_a}{\mu_s} = \left[\frac{(1+R^2-T^2)}{2R}\right] - 1 \tag{4.20}$$

If the skin tissue is thick enough, T approaches zero and the equation can be rewritten as

$$\frac{\mu_a}{\mu_s} = \frac{(R-1)^2}{2R} \tag{4.21}$$

In Equation 4.21, the reflectance of the thick tissue depends solely on the ratio of its absorption and scattering coefficients. Generally, skin dermis is quite thick for wavelengths less than 600 nm. In this way, its transmittance approaches zero. If μ_S is a known constant, μ_a can be estimated directly from R. The skin structure determines the scattering coefficients (μ_S), and the chromosphores present will determine absorption coefficients (μ_a). For any given layer of skin, μ_a is compositely determined by the concentration and distribution of those chromosphores present. This is convenient because certain chromosphores such as haemoglobin, bilirubin and melanin change rapidly in normal skin, causing changes in absorption coefficients whereas scattering coefficients should not change significantly.

Wan et al. reported the extension of the K–M light–skin model [131] in their work, whereby the K–M theory was used to study human epidermis over the UV and visible region. The model was applied to calculate the absorption and scattering coefficients of human epidermis *in vitro* and to estimate the epidermal transmittance under a simulated *in vivo* condition.

The application of K–M theory to human skin has also been proposed by Cotton [132,133] and Doi [46,67]. Cotton et al. proposed a mathematical model of colour formation by only using two pigments of melanin and blood, where the K–M theory was used only for the dermis layer. In the study, the dermis was categorised into upper papillary dermis, lower papillary dermis and reticular dermis. It was also hypothesized that through an understanding of the image formation process, a number of important facts about the internal structure and composition of the skin lesions could be derived from skin colour images. In the work, a physics-based model of tissue colouration was able to provide a cross-reference between image colours and the underlying histological parameter and could be used to analyse pigmented skin lesions. The model showed several histological parametric maps showing the concentration of dermal and epidermal

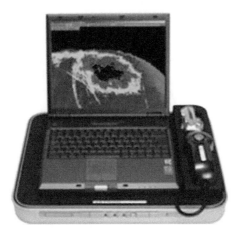

Figure 4.34 Siascope.

melanin, blood and collagen thickness across the imaged skin and used to aid early detection of melanoma with 80.1% sensitivity and 82.7% specificity. In 2006, they further proposed a new optical skin imaging method, called spectrophotometric intracutaneous imaging (Siascopy) in which the computationally reconstructed images determined either the concentration of epidermal melanin, concentration of dermal blood, thickness of the papillary dermis or, in pathological cases, the presence of dermal melanin [93]. The imaging system had taken a number of spectrally filtered images ranging from 400 to 1000 nm (Figure 4.34). The K–M method was then applied to measure its optical properties.

Meanwhile, Doi estimated a reflectance spectrum function for the human skin surface. The K–M theory was applied to calculate a transmission and a reflection within the skin tissue layers making the surface-reflectance spectrum predictable. Here, the optical process in human skin was estimated in detail by assuming the five pigments of melanin, carotene, bilirubin, oxy-haemoglobin and deoxy-haemoglobin (Figure 4.35).

In Doi's work, the skin consisted of two layers of epidermis and dermis. Here, multiple reflections in the interface between the epidermis (Layer 1) and the dermis (Layer 2) were considered. In the two-layer model, the total reflectance $R_{1,2}$ including the inter-reflection has been described as

$$R_{1,2} = R_1 + T_2^1 R_2 (1 + R_1 R_2 + R_1^2 R_2^2 + \ldots) = R_1 + \frac{T_2^1 R_2}{1 - R_1 R_2} \qquad (4.22)$$

where T_1 and R_1 represent the transmittance and reflectance of Layer 1, respectively, and R_2 represents the reflectance of Layer 2.

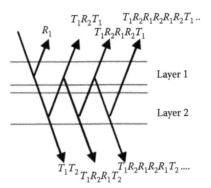

Figure 4.35 Two-layer skin model.

Doi compared the estimated reflectance with the direct measurement of skin reflectance that later showed the reliability of the estimation in all cases [134].

Romuald Jolivot reported the development of an image acquisition system called Asclepios [135]. The system was able to image a skin region of 32×38 mm within 2 s with a resolution of 33 pixels/mm. Furthermore, the tool creates a multispectral picture comprising 10 mono-band pictures. The system, in this case, could enhance a spectral resolution by rebuilding the hyper-spectral cube of skin reflectance using an artificial neural network-based methodology [136,137]. The hyperspectral cube was then analysed using K–M method in order to determine the percentage volume of melanosome and concentration of haemoglobin in dermis.

The K–M approach has indeed enabled a number of researchers to determine the skin optical properties in real time [136]. However, this approach still lacks the detailed analysis of the interaction between light and structure of skin that plays an important role in analysing the skin optical properties.

4.4.3 *Radiative transport equation: The inverse adding-doubling method*

Created by Van De Hulst, the inverse adding-doubling (IAD) method is a general, numerical solution of the radiative transport equation [138]. This method commonly comprises the following steps: (1) speculating a group of optical properties, (2) computing the reflection and transmission utilizing the adding-doubling methodology, (3) contrasting the computed values with the acquired reflection and transmissions and (4) reiterative until a match is found. The set of optical properties generating reflection and transmission values matching the acquired values can be used as the optical properties of the sample.

The term of doubling in IAD refers to the capacity of the reflectance and transmission of a layer used at a certain ingoing and outgoing angle to determine the reflectance and transmission of a layer with a thickness double that of the original. The term adding indicates that the doubling procedure may be extended to some heterogeneous layers to model multi-layer tissues [139].

The IAD has been extended to solve the one-dimensional transport equation in the layer geometry of skin [113]. The IAD technique assumes that the reflection and transmission for a light incident at a particular angle are established for one layer. The twice-thicker reflection and transmission of a layer can be predicted by putting two indistinguishable layers together and summing up the contributions of the reflection and transmission from each layer. The reflection and transmission for an arbitrary layer are computed by locating the reflection and transmission for a thin initial layer and thereafter doubling the said reflection and transmission until the aimed thickness is attained. The summation method extends the doubling technique to different categories of layers. Accordingly, layers with various optical properties can be put adjacent to each other to simulate layered media or internal reflection due to refraction differences index. Boundary conditions are executed in the adding–doubling technique by creating a layer, which mimics the reflection and transmission at a boundary. This layer is added to a layer so as to identify the reflection and transmission for a layer including the boundary conditions. Then, the algorithm compares the calculated values with the measured reflection and transmissions. Iteration is performed to get a match between simulated reflection and transmission and the measured reflection and transmission.

Troy and Thennadil used the IAD method to determine the optical properties of human skin in the near-infrared wavelength (1000–2200 nm) [140]. In their work, 22 samples were collected from 14 subjects. The absorption coefficient of skin within near-infrared wavelength closely resembled to the absorption coefficient of water and the scattering coefficients were found between 3 and 16 cm^{-1}.

The adding–doubling technique is appropriate to take care of iterative issues of the precise total reflection and transmission computations. In all computations, it is accepted that the distribution of light is independent of time, samples have uniform optical properties, the sample geometry is an infinite plane-parallel layer of finite thickness, the tissue has a uniform index of refraction, internal reflection at boundaries is within Fresnel's law and the light is not polarized.

IAD, in general, possesses a number of disadvantages that include (a) the low speed of algorithm in calculating internal fluencies, the flux integrated over time; (b) the limitation of the IAD method – only suitable for a layered geometry with uniform irradiation and (c) in the method, assumed that each layer has homogeneous optical properties.

4.4.4 *Diffuse reflectance approximation*

Diffusion approximation refers to the approximate solution of Boltzmann photon transport [141]. The Boltzmann equation for radiative transfer equation is written as follows:

$$\frac{\partial L(\vec{r},\hat{s},t)/c}{\partial t} = -s.\nabla L(\vec{r},\hat{s},t) - \mu_t L(\vec{r},\hat{s},t)$$

$$+ \mu_s \int_{4\pi} L(\vec{r},\hat{s},t)P(\hat{s}',\hat{s})d\Omega' + S(\vec{r},\hat{s},t) \tag{4.23}$$

where $L(\vec{r},\hat{s},t)$ represents radiance and $S(\vec{r},\hat{s},t)$ describes the light source. Radiance is defined as an energy flow per unit normal area per unit solid angle per unit time. C is the speed of light. $\mu_t = \mu_a + \mu_s$ is the extinction coefficient, $P(\hat{s}',\hat{s})$ is the phase function representing the probability of light with propagation direction $\hat{s}'$ being scattered into angle, $d\Omega$ around $\hat{s}$. In most cases, the phase function depends only on the angle between the scattered $\hat{s}'$ and incident $\hat{s}$ direction. In the diffusion theory, radiance is assumed to be largely isotropic. Only the isotropic and the first-order of anisotropic are used.

$$L(\vec{r},\hat{s},t) \approx \sum_{n=0}^{1}\sum_{m=-n}^{n} L_{n,m}(\vec{r},t)Y_{n,m}(\hat{s}) \tag{4.24}$$

where $Y_{n,m}$ represents a basis set of spherical harmonics and $L_{n,m}$ represents the expansion coefficients. Radiance is expressed into four terms; one for $n = 0$ (the isotropic term) and other three terms for $n = 1$ (the anisotropic terms). Using properties of spherical harmonics and the definitions of fluencies rate $\phi(\vec{r},t)$ and current density $\vec{J}(\vec{r},t)$, the isotropic and anisotropic terms can, respectively, be expressed as follows:

$$L_{0,0}(\vec{r},t)Y_{0,0}(\hat{s}) = \frac{\phi(\vec{r},t)}{4\pi}$$

$$\sum_{m=-1}^{1} L_{1,m}(\vec{r},t)Y_{1,m}(\hat{s}) = \frac{3}{4\pi}\vec{J}(\vec{r},t).\hat{s} \tag{4.25}$$

Hence, the radiance can be approximated as

$$L(\vec{r},\hat{s},t) = \frac{\phi(\vec{r},t)}{4\pi} + \frac{3}{4\pi}\vec{J}(\vec{r},t).\hat{s} \tag{4.26}$$

Substituting the above expression for radiance, it is obtained

$$S(\vec{r},t) = \frac{\partial \phi(\vec{r},t)}{c\partial t} + \mu_a \phi(\vec{r},t) + \nabla \vec{J}(\vec{r},t)$$

$$0 = \frac{\partial \vec{J}(\vec{r},t)}{c\partial t} + (\mu_a + \mu'_s)\vec{J}(\vec{r},t) + \frac{1}{3}\nabla \phi(\vec{r},t) \qquad (4.27)$$

The diffusion approximation is limited to systems where some reduced scattering coefficients are much larger than their absorption coefficients and have a minimum layer thickness of the order of a few transport mean free path. Gemert utilized a skin model referencing on the scattering estimation including a light propagation in turbid media to study a skin optic [113].

Farrell, on the other hand, highlighted a model referencing on a scattering theory to be utilized in the noninvasive identification of the absorption and diffusion characteristics of mammalian tissues [117] in which he simplified the formula into

$$R_f(r) = \frac{a}{4\pi}\left[\frac{1}{\mu'_t}\left(\mu_{eff} + \frac{1}{r_1}\right)\frac{\exp(-\mu_{eff}r_1)}{r_1^2} + \left(\frac{1}{\mu'_t} + \frac{4A}{3\mu'_t}\right)\left(\mu_{eff} + \frac{1}{r_2}\right)\frac{\exp(-\mu_{eff}r_1)}{r_1^2}\right]$$

$$(4.28)$$

where r represents the distance from the incident point, a represents the transport albedo ($a = \mu_s'/(\mu_a + \mu_s')$) and μ_{eff} represents the effective attenuation coefficient ($\mu_{eff} = [3\mu_a(\mu_a + \mu_s')]^{1/2}$). μ'_t is the total interaction coefficient ($\mu_t' = (\mu_a + \mu_s')$), r_1 and r_2 are the distances from the observation point at the interface to the isotropic source and the image source.

In 2009, Tsumura developed an analytical solution of skin reflectance from works of Ishimada [119]. The analytical solution was formulated as

$$R = \frac{1}{2}\exp\left(-\sqrt{\frac{3\mu_a}{\mu_a + \mu'_s}}\right)x\left[1 + \exp\left(-4A\sqrt{\frac{3\mu_a}{3(\mu_a + \mu'_s)}}\right)\right] \qquad (4.29)$$

where μ_a and μ_s are the absorption and the reduced scattering coefficients, respectively and A is the constant value calculated from the refractive index of media. Tsumura also has proposed an empiric model for a single layer skin as

$$[-\log_{10}(R)]^{2.38} = 2.79\frac{\mu_a}{\mu'_s} \qquad (4.30)$$

The drawback of diffusion approximation is that when the absorption coefficient of a turbid medium is not significantly smaller than the scattering coefficient, the diffusion theory will come to be a weak estimation for the photon transport equation [142].

4.4.5 Modified Beer–Lambert law skin model

The Beer–Lambert law relates the absorption of light to the properties of the material through which the light is travelling. The law formulates that there is a logarithmic dependence between the transmission, T, of light through a substance and the product of the absorption coefficient of the substance, α, and the distance the light travels through the material (i.e., the path length), ℓ. The application of Beer–Lambert law and its modification for skin have been reported by Shimada [69,143,144]. This technique uses the spectral distortion induced by multiple scattering via a linearised equation relating the general tissue attenuation to the tissue absorption coefficient, μ_a. The absorbance, A, is defined from the reflectance, R, of the skin, which is regarded to be a semi-infinite medium.

$$A = -\log_{10} R \qquad (4.31)$$

The absorbance, A, of a uniformed diffuse medium, with molar absorption and molar concentration are ε and C can be computed as follows:

$$A = \varepsilon C \overline{l}(C) + G \qquad (4.32)$$

where G and $\overline{l}(C)$ are scattering loss and mean path length, respectively. For a non-uniformed scattering medium, the absorbance, A, for each wavelength reformulated by Shimada [143] is given as follows:

$$A(\lambda) = \sum_{i=1}^{m} A_i(\lambda) + G(\lambda)$$

$$A(\lambda) = \sum_{i=1}^{m} \varepsilon_i C_i \overline{l_i}(C_1,...,C_m,\lambda) + G(\lambda) \qquad (4.33)$$

where the subscript, i, refers to the ith chromophores and $\overline{l_i}(\lambda)$ is the path length in the area whereby the ith chromophore is dispensed. Path length, $\overline{l_i}(\lambda)$ rely not only on C_i but also C_1, K, C_m, though the effects of C_j ($j \neq i$) are small. The path length in the region where plural chromophores exist is regarded as the path length of both chromophores. $\bar{l_t}(\lambda)$ and $G(\lambda)$ vary with wavelength λ because the scattering coefficients are different at each λ.

Using the absorption properties of skin layers (blood, water, melanin and chromophores content), the following modified Beer–Lambert can be utilised to simulate the skin reflectance spectra:

$$
\begin{aligned}
A_{skin}(\lambda) = {} & \varepsilon_{eumelanin}C_{eumelanin}\bar{l}_{eumelanin}(\lambda) + \varepsilon_{pheomelanin}C_{pheomelanin}\bar{l}_{pheomelanin}(\lambda) \\
& + \varepsilon_{oxy-haemoglobin}C_{oxy-haemoglobin}\bar{l}_{oxy-haemoglobin}(\lambda) \\
& + \varepsilon_{deoxy-haemoglobin}C_{deoxy-haemoglobin}de\,\bar{l}_{oxy-haemoglobin}(\lambda) \\
& + \varepsilon_{beta-carotene}C_{beta-carotene}\bar{l}_{beta-carotene}(\lambda) + \varepsilon_{bilirubin}C_{bilirubin}\bar{l}_{bilirubin}(\lambda) + A_0
\end{aligned}
$$

$$(4.34)$$

with $A_0(\lambda) = \bar{A}_0(\lambda) + G(\lambda))$ where $A_0(\lambda)$ is the absorbance of skin base.

It is found that the drawback of modified Beer–Lambert law is that the formula is only based on absorption while scattering is not considered ($G(\lambda)$ is made constant) making the light reflectance estimation not accurate.

4.4.6 Monte Carlo

MC technique was developed by Metropolis and Ulamin in order to understand a number of physical processes using a stochastic model [145]. The objective of MC method is to understand a deterministic problem using probabilistic technique and huge numbers. It is a stochastic approach and favours the analogy with physical reality. In the model of the light–skin interaction, the method will consider light as a very large set of photons and it is possible to converge to the steady state of the energy distribution in space after a number of iterations related to the optical properties of the medium by randomly simulating the random free path of photons in skin. For skin tissue, this method allows the evaluation of the reflected light energy (reflectance), directly linked to light energy absorbed by the different skin layers. After a photon is injected into skin, it propagates in it based on the knowledge of skin parameters. MC model statistically computes the optical pathways of each photon in an iterative manner. For accurate results, the simulation needs to perform numerous computations of the photon projection, thus requiring many photon histories. It is a very time-consuming process and therefore is computationally expensive.

MC approach has been utilized to simulate biological tissue optics. On account of skin–light interaction, photon histories are trailed as they are diffused and absorbed in the skin. Prahl proposed an MC-based methodology to model light transport in tissue for laser radiation [87]. Wang expanded the simulation to model light transport in multi-layered tissue,

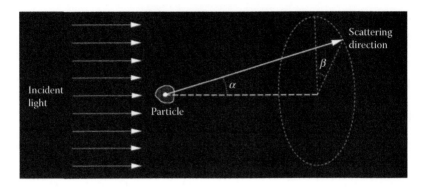

Figure 4.36 Scattering.

known as MCML (Monte Carlo simulation of light transport in multi-layered tissue) [146]. Besides MCML, Meglinski [55] and Krishnaswamy [80] have also developed a skin model based on MC approach.

The foundation of MC model is represented by the scattering profile of the particles, which can be depicted by a phase. When light hits a particle, it will be diffused. Figure 4.36 shows a diffusing process whereby the direction of diffusion is given by the polar angle α at which the light is bent and an azimuthal angle β is in a plane normal to the direction of incidence. A phase function denoted by $\Gamma(\theta, \beta)$ describes the amount of light diffused from the direction of incidence to the direction of scattering [147].

In astrophysics, a phase function is regarded as probability distribution, and its normalization desires that the integral over all angle be equal to the unity:

$$\int_{4\pi} \Gamma(\alpha, \beta) d\omega = 1 \qquad (4.35)$$

where $d\omega$ is the differential solid angle.

The average cosine of the phase function, asymmetry factor, is used to represent the degree of asymmetry of the phase function and it can be interpreted as

$$g = \int_{4\pi} \Gamma(\alpha, \beta) \cos \alpha \, d\omega \qquad (4.36)$$

The simplest phase function is when $g = 0$:

$$\Gamma(\alpha, \beta) = \frac{1}{4\pi} \qquad (4.37)$$

The term, phase function, is not related to the phase of light but originated from astronomy to study the lunar phase. One of the phase functions developed for astrophysical application is known as the Henyey–Greenstein Phase Function (HGPF), the most common phase function used in skin optics [148].

The HGPF was presented by Henyey and Greenstein to approximate the scattering of diffuse radiation in galaxies. The approximation of HGPF here can be formulated as

$$\Gamma_{HG}(g,\alpha) = \frac{1-g^2}{(1+g^2 - 2g\cos\alpha)^{3/2}} \tag{4.38}$$

where α is the angle when the light is bent and g is the asymmetry factor.

The HGPF actually is a function with three parameters. The approximation assumes that the azimuthal angle (β) is constant. In order to compute the trajectories of the scattered photons, Prahl [87] used a warping function to derive the HGPF.

$$\cos\alpha = \frac{1}{2g}\left[1+g^2 - \left(\frac{1-g^2}{(1-g+2g\xi)}\right)^2\right] \tag{4.39}$$

where ξ is an uniformly distributed random number on the interval [0,1]. For symmetric scattering ($g = 0$), the expression $\cos\alpha = 2\xi 1 - 1$ is used.

The azimuthal angle can be generated as

$$\beta = 2\pi\xi \tag{4.40}$$

where ξ is a random number uniformly distributed on the interval [0,1]. The drawback of MC method is that it requires a high computational power to conduct the simulation.

Table 4.5 summarises the pros and cons of the above-mentioned computational skin models.

Although it is known that the most precise skin model is referencing on MC method [33,39,52,80,89,92,115,116], the approach is computationally extensive. In order for the method to be applicable in clinical settings, the processing time of the simulation process must be significantly reduced. In this work, the proposed skin analysis uses the MC approach for accuracy and is implemented using NVIDIA graphics processing units (GPUs) to achieve simulation times appropriate for clinical applications.

Table 4.5 Comparison of computational skin models

Model	Advantages	Disadvantages
K–M	• Easy to implement • Suitable on multiple layer tissues	• Lacking details of the structure • Lacking details of optical properties
Adding-doubling method	• Easy to implement • Suitable on iterative problem	• Not accurate (assuming that skin layer is homogeneous) • Computationally extensive
Diffuse reflectance approximation	• Fast and easy to apply	• Not accurate (simplifying many factors) • Poor approximation when absorption coefficient is not significantly smaller than the scattering coefficient
Modified Beer–Lambert law	• Fast and easy to apply	• Not accurate (calculation is based only on the absorption of components)
MC-based method	• Most accurate skin simulation method	• Computationally extensive

4.5 Inverse MC analysis for determination of melanin types

4.5.1 Proposed inverse analysis of MC skin model method

Skin–light model provides an outcome of spectral distribution (reflectance and transmittance) of skin tissues. These skin and light models can be used in a few inversion techniques [114]. An inversion technique is an approach to determine the optical and biochemical properties from *in situ* and non-invasive surface acquisitions [80]. The expression "inversion" infers an inversion of the real procedure of computing reflectance and transmission, that is, using reflectance and transmission values as input to find out the absorption and scattering properties of the tissues (Figure 4.37).

In this section, the creation of an inverse analysis based on MC skin model for the determination of skin optical characteristics is presented. The MC approach itself is regarded as the most precise skin–light propagation model [33,38,92,150]. However, due to the high computational requirements of the inverse of MC method, it has not been attempted for skin analysis purposes.

By applying the inverse model analysis, skin optical characteristics or parameters, namely the relative concentrations of eumelanin and pheomelanin, volume fraction of melanosomes in epidermis and epidermal thickness from the reflectance spectrum of skin can be determined.

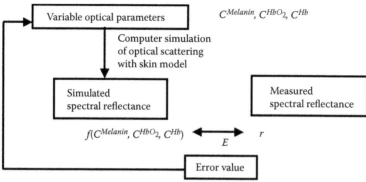

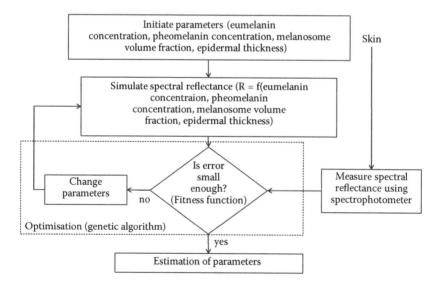

Figure 4.37 Inverse analysis reproduced from Tsumura [149]. (Reprinted with permission from IS&T: The Society for Imaging Science and Technology sole copyright owners of the *Journal of Imaging Science and Technology*.)

Figure 4.38 shows the flow chart of the proposed inverse model analysis to determine the above-mentioned skin optical parameters.

As depicted in the figure, preliminary values of the skin parameters are irregularly determined and referencing on these preliminary values, the reflectance (and transmission) is then simulated using the

Figure 4.38 Flow chart of the proposed inverse analysis.

forward model of optical scattering in human skin. Error is then computed between the simulated reflectance and acquired reflectance. The values of the parameters are revised, and reflectance spectrum is simulated again; this process is repeated until the error is minimised, that is, reduced to a given threshold. An optimisation methodology is utilized to find out new values for the skin parameters to further speed up the procedure.

Many researchers have used a number of different optimisation techniques. Tsumura et al. [149] used several linear optimisation techniques in their calculation. Ela Claridge et al. [133], Zhang et al. [92] and R. Jolivot [135] utilised Genetic Algorithms (GAs). Meanwhile, Choi et al. utilised a combination of Simplex Algorithm and Genetic Algorithm (GA) [151]. Aeda et al. furthermore, used a conventional optimisation technique [152]. Yudovsky and Pilon used Levenberg–Marquardt algorithm [72].

Generally, researchers choose the optimisation technique based on the skin and light model being used. For the MC model, most of the researchers [38,92,153] use GA due to the nature of the MC problem. Erik Alerstam has proposed a hardware optimisation for the usage of MC in GPUs [154] and found that while CPU and GPU codes produce similar results, GPU usage is 1080 times faster than traditional CPU.

This section discusses the MC approach, in particular the MC for multi-layered media. More importantly, the section presents the reflectance of skin used, the optimisation of the MC in multi-layered tissues using GAs and its implementation on GPUs for inverse modelling of skin properties.

4.5.2 MC modelling of light transport in multi-layered tissues

In 1993, Wang and Jacques wrote a standard C-code for MCML. Since then, many researchers have used the code. Generally, the MCML program constitutes following operations for photons: (1) launching of photon, (2) simulating propagation distance, (3) moving the photon, (4) internal reflection, (5) photon absorption, (6) changing photon direction by diffusing and (7) computing quantities (i.e., diffuse reflectance, specular reflectance, absorbance).

MCML simulates the path of a photon on a multi-layered tissue in which each layer of the tissue is infinitely wide and described by the following parameters: thickness, refractive index, absorption coefficient, μ_a, scattering coefficient, μ_s and anisotropy factor, g. The absorption coefficient, μ_a is defined as the probability of photon absorption per unit path length, and the scattering coefficient, μ_s is defined as the probability of photon scattering per unit path length. The total interaction of coefficient, μt refers to the sum of the absorption coefficient and the scattering coefficient. The interaction of coefficient refers to the probability of photon interaction per unit path length. Furthermore, the anisotropy, g represents the average of the cosine value of the deflection angle.

In MCML, photon absorption, fluencies, reflectance and transmittance are the physical quantities to be modelled. Two coordinate systems namely the Cartesian coordinate system (Figure 4.39) and cylindrical coordinate system, are simultaneously used in the MC simulation. Here, a Cartesian coordinate framework is utilized to follow photon packets. The source of the coordinate framework is the photon incident point on the tissue surface, and the z-axis is always the normal of the surface pointing towards the inner layer of the tissue. The xy-plane, in this manner, is on the tissue surface.

A cylindrical coordinate framework is utilized to record the internal photon absorption, $A(r, z)$ where r and z serve as the radial and z-axis coordinates of the cylindrical coordinate framework, respectively. The Cartesian coordinate framework and the cylindrical coordinate framework have the same source and the z-axis. The r coordinate of the cylindrical coordinate framework is also utilized for the diffuse reflectance and total transmittance.

Photon position are recorded on tissue surface as reflectance, $R(r, \alpha)$ or transmittance, $T(r, \alpha)$, respectively, where α represents an angle between the photon exiting direction and the normal (z-axis for reflectance and z-axis for transmittance) to the tissue surfaces. A moving spherical coordinate framework whose z-axis is aligned with the photon propagation direction dynamically is utilized for the sampling of the propagation direction change of a photon packet. In this spherical coordinate framework, the deflection angle, θ and the azimuthal angle, ψ are first sampled due to diffusion. The photon direction is then revised in terms of the directional cosines in the Cartesian coordinate framework.

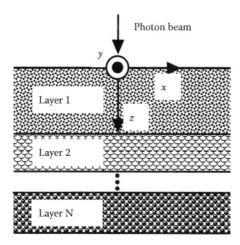

Figure 4.39 Cartesian coordinate of a photon in MCML.

4.5.2.1 Random variables

The MC method relies on the random sampling of variables from well-defined probability distributions [155]. A random variable is used for a variable step size for a photon to take between photon–tissue interaction sites or the angle of deflection of a scattered photon experience due to a scattering event.

For a random variable, χ, the probability density function that defines the distribution of χ over the interval (a, b) is formulated as

$$\int_{a}^{b} p(\chi)d\chi = 1 \tag{4.41}$$

Most of the MC-based works use the pseudorandom number generator algorithm – an algorithm for generating a sequence of numbers that approximates the properties of random numbers. The sequence is not truly random for being completely determined by a relatively small set of initial values, including a truly random seed.

The most well-known pseudorandom number generator used for MCML is Mersenne twister algorithm [154]. It is a pseudorandom number generator developed in 1997 by Makoto Matsumoto and Takuji Nishimura [156] and can provide fast generation of very high-quality pseudorandom numbers.

In MCML, a random number is denoted by ξ, which is consistently disseminated over the interval $(0, 1)$. The cumulative distribution function of this consistently disseminated random variable is

$$F_\xi(\xi) = \begin{cases} 0 & \text{if } \xi \leq 0 \\ \xi & \text{if } 0 < \xi \leq 1 \\ 1 & \text{if } \xi > 1 \end{cases} \tag{4.42}$$

4.5.2.2 Launching a photon

The method considers light as a very large set of photons. In the simulation, each photon packet is initially assigned a weight, W, equal to unity. Each photon packet is then injected into the skin tissue. The initial positions in the Cartesian coordinate are set to $(0, 0, 0,)$ and to $(0, 0, 1)$ in the directional cosines. The current position of the photon can be specified by the Cartesian coordinates (x, y, z) and can be equivalently described by the directional cosines (μ_x, μ_y, μ_z).

$$\begin{aligned} \mu_x &= r \cdot x \\ \mu_y &= r \cdot y \\ \mu_z &= r \cdot z \end{aligned} \tag{4.43}$$

where x, y, and z are unit vectors along each axis and r is a unit vector.

When the photon is launched, specular reflectance will occur if there is a mismatched boundary at the tissue surface. The specular reflectance is then computed by

$$R_{sp} = r_1 + \frac{(1-r_1)^2 r_2}{1-r_1 r_2} \qquad (4.44)$$

where r_1 and r_2 are the Fresnel reflectance on two boundaries of the glass layer.

$$r_1 = \frac{(n_1 - n_2)^2}{(n_1 + n_2)^2} \qquad (4.45)$$

$$r_2 = \frac{(n_3 - n_2)^2}{(n_3 + n_2)^2} \qquad (4.46)$$

The photon weight is decremented by R_{sp} and the specular reflectance R_{sp} is recorded in the output data file.

$$W = 1 - R_{sp} \qquad (4.47)$$

4.5.2.3 Moving a photon

In the tissue, photon is moved based on a step size, s in which the position of the photon packet is updated by

$$x \leftarrow x + \mu_x s$$
$$y \leftarrow y + \mu_y s \qquad (4.48)$$
$$z \leftarrow z + \mu_z s$$

The step size is calculated based on the sampling of the probability distribution for photon's free path $s \in [0,\infty]$. According to the definition of interaction coefficient, μ_t, the interaction coefficient refers to the probability of photon interaction per unit path length. Prahl formulated it in the interval $(s', s' + ds')$ as [87]

$$\mu_t = \frac{-dP\{s \geq s'\}}{P\{s \geq s'\}ds'} \qquad (4.49)$$

or

$$d(\ln(P\{s \geq s'\})) = \mu_t ds' \qquad (4.50)$$

The above equation can be integrated over s' in the range $(0, s_1)$ and leads to an exponential distribution where $P[157] = 1$ is used:

$$P\{s \geq s_1\} = \exp(-\mu_t s_1) \tag{4.51}$$

Equation 4.11 can be rearranged to yield the cumulative distribution function of free path s:

$$P\{s \geq s_1\} = 1 - \exp(-\mu_t s_1) \tag{4.52}$$

This cumulative distribution function can be assigned to the uniformly distributed random number ξ as discussed in the previous section. Considering this, the equation can be rearranged to provide a means of choosing step size:

$$s_1 = \frac{-\ln \xi}{\mu_t} \tag{4.53}$$

4.5.2.4 Energy absorption of photon

After a photon takes a step, a fraction of the photon's weight, W, will be deposited in a local grid element due to absorption. Here, the attenuation of photon weight must be calculated. The amount of deposited photon weight, ΔW, is calculated as

$$\Delta W = W \frac{\mu_a}{\mu_t} \tag{4.54}$$

The total accumulated photon weigh $A(r, z)$ deposited in the local grid element is updated by adding ΔW,

$$A(r,z) \leftarrow A(r,z) + \Delta W \tag{4.55}$$

The photon weight will be updated as

$$W \leftarrow W - \Delta W \tag{4.56}$$

4.5.2.5 Photon scattering

Once a photon packet has been moved and its weight has been decremented, the photon packet is scattered. There will be a deflection angle,

$\theta \in (0, \pi)$ and an azimuthal angle, $\psi \in (0, 2\pi)$ to be statistically sampled. The probability distribution for the cosine of the deflection angle, $\cos \theta$, is described by the scattering function as defined by Henyey and Greenstein [158] as follows:

$$p(\cos\theta) = \frac{1-g^2}{2(1+g^2 - 2\cos\theta)^{3/2}} \tag{4.57}$$

where the anisotropy, g, has a value between –1 and 1. Here, a value of –1 indicates complete back scattering while a value near 1, indicates a strong forward-directed scattering.

Jacques et al. (1987) experimentally determined that the Henyey–Greenstein function described single scattering in tissue very well. The values of g range between 0.3 and 0.98 for tissues, but quite often g is ~0.9 in the visible spectrum. The choice for $\cos \theta$ can be expressed as a function of the random number, ξ:

$$\cos\theta = \begin{cases} \dfrac{1}{2g}\left\{1+g^2 - \left[\dfrac{1-g^2}{1-g+2g\xi}\right]^2\right\} & \text{if } g>0 \\[2ex] 2\xi - 1 & \text{if } g=0 \end{cases} \tag{4.58}$$

Subsequently, the azimuthal angle, ψ, which is uniformly distributed over the interval 0 to 2π is sampled as

$$\psi = 2\pi\xi \tag{4.59}$$

Once the deflection angle and azimuthal angle are chosen, the new direction of the photon packet is calculated as follows:

$$\mu'_x = \frac{\sin\theta}{\sqrt{1-\mu_z^2}}(\mu_x\mu_z \cos\psi - \mu_y \sin\psi) + \mu_x \cos\theta$$

$$\mu'_y = \frac{\sin\theta}{\sqrt{1-\mu_z^2}}(\mu_y\mu_z \cos\psi + \mu_x \sin\psi) + \mu_y \cos\theta \tag{4.60}$$

$$\mu'_z = -\sin\theta\cos\psi\sqrt{1-\mu_z^2} + \mu_z \cos\theta$$

The current photon direction is updated as

$$\mu_x = \mu'_x, \mu_y = \mu'_y, \mu_z = \mu'_z \tag{4.61}$$

4.5.2.6 Photon termination

After a photon packet is launched, it can be naturally terminated using a reflection or a transmission out of the tissue. For a photon packet still propagating inside the tissue, if the photon weight, W, falls below a threshold value (e.g., $Wth = 0.0001$), further propagation of the photon will yield little information. A proper termination must be executed to ensure an energy conservation (or number of photons) without skewing the distribution of photon deposition. A technique called roulette is used to terminate the photon packet in a condition of $W \leq Wth$. The technique gives the photon packet one chance in m (e.g., $m = 10$) of surviving with a weight of mW. If the photon packet does not survive the roulette, the photon weight will be reduced to zero and the photon will be terminated.

$$W = \begin{cases} mW & \text{if } \xi \leq 1/m \\ 0 & \text{if } \xi > 1/m \end{cases} \tag{4.62}$$

where ξ is the uniformly distributed pseudo-random number. This method conserves energy, yet terminates photons in an unbiased manner [146].

4.5.2.7 Implementation of MCML on GPU using CUDA programming

MCML is currently considered as a gold standard tool for simulating light propagation in multi-layered turbid media – particularly in skin and light simulation [159,160]. MCML is used for the validation of photon modelling schemes as well as a starting point for custom-developed MC solutions [161,162]. However, its main drawback is that it requires high computational power. Thus, MCML simulations have been mainly used for forward modelling to calculate photon density distribution given skin tissue structures as well as their optical properties.

To enable the use of MCML simulations to solve inverse problems, GPU has recently emerged as a promising solution. Figure 4.40 shows the development of GPU technology and capability. Alerstam reported that the GPU implementation of MCML can achieve speedups of up to 3 orders of magnitude over CPU-based codes [154].

CUDA is a programming model and environment developed by NVIDIA, one of the graphic card companies producing GPU chips. In CUDA, NVIDIA includes a unified shared pipeline, allowing each of arithmetic logic unit (ALU) on the chip to be organised by a program for general-purpose computations. These ALUs are built to comply with IEEE requirements for single-precision floating-point arithmetic and designed to use an instruction set tailored for general computation [34,163].

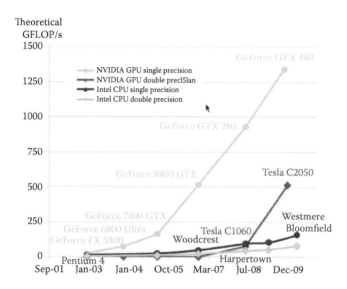

Figure 4.40 Emerging capability of GPU. (Reproduced from J. Sanders and E. Kandrot, *Cuda by Example: An Introduction to General Purpose GPU Programming.* Boston: Pearson Education, 2010.)

CUDA provides a C programming interface for NVIDIA GPUs known as CUDA C to facilitate a general-purpose computing on GPUs, as shown in Figure 4.41. In addition, to create a language to write code for the GPU, NVIDIA also provides a specialised hardware driver to exploit the CUDA computational power. Here, users are required neither to have any knowledge of the OpenGL nor DirectX graphics programming interfaces to force their problem to be solved as computer graphics task. However, the performance optimisation of a CUDA program requires the careful consideration of the GPU architecture. In CUDA, the host code and the device code are written in a single program. The host code is executed sequentially by the CPU, while the device code is executed in parallel by many threads on the GPU. Here, a thread is an independent execution context that, for example, can simulate an individual photon packet in the MCML algorithm. The device code is expressed in the form of a kernel function. It is similar to a regular C-language function, except that it specifies the work of each GPU thread, parameterised by a thread index variable. Correspondingly, a kernel invocation is similar to a function call. The difference is that the invocation must detail a grid of threads that will execute the kernel. A grid is composed of a number of thread blocks, each of which has a number of threads.

Table 4.6 presents a comparison about the CUDA implementation of MC simulation in terms of the folding factor, the system used and the availability of the codes.

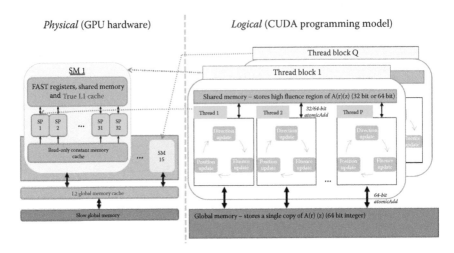

Figure 4.41 CUDA programming model. (Reproduced from E. Alerstam and S. Andersson-engels, *Monte Carlo Simulations of Light Transport in Tissue Computer Exercise.* Department of Physics, Lund, 2011, pp. 1–12.)

Table 4.6 CUDA-based MC simulation

Implementation	Folding factor	System	Code
Fang and Boas [37]	300x without atomic instruction 75x with atomic instruction	NVIDIA 8800 GT (112 processors)	None
Badal and Badano [164]	27x	NVIDIA 295 GTX (240 out of 480 processors)	http://code.google.com/p/mcgpu/.
Ren et al. [33].	10x	NVIDIA GTX 260 (192 processors)	None
Alerstam et al. [35].	600x	NVIDIA GTX 480 (480 processors)	http://code.google.com/p/gpumcm

From the table, it can be seen that work reported by Alerstam is by far the best in terms of speedup factor. To leverage on the speed and open source nature of the Alerstam's approach, the proposed inversion method implements the MCML based on GPU codes as developed by Alerstam. The codes are available at the end of this chapter.

For the proposed inversion method, the MCML is implemented on NVIDIA Quadro 2000 with 192 processors. Besides a CUDA-enabled GPU, the prerequisites of developing an application code in CUDA are a NVIDIA device driver, a CUDA development toolkit and a standard compiler [34]. For a NVIDIA device driver, NVIDIA provides system software that allows the code to communicate with the CUDA-enabled hardware. The NVIDIA GPU has to be installed perfectly for this software to be installed on our machine.

The second prerequisite is a CUDA development kit or known as CUDA toolkit. The CUDA toolkit provides a comprehensive development environment for C and C++ developers in building GPU-accelerated applications. The toolkit includes a compiler for NVIDIA GPUs, math libraries, data handlings and tools for debugging and optimising the performance of the GPU code. In the proposed method, the CUDA toolkit version 4.0.1.7 for Windows Operating System is installed and used (https://developer.nvidia.com/cuda-toolkit). The development kit is shared by NVIDIA for free.

For the standard compiler, NVIDIA recommends using the Microsoft Visual Studio compiler for Microsoft Windows [163]. NVIDIA currently supports the Visual Studi0 2005, the Visual Studio 2008 and Visual Studio 2010 families of products. Since we do not have access to a supported version of Visual Studio, a free version of Visual Studio is used instead. Microsoft provides free downloads of the Visual Studio Express edition on its website (http://www.visualstudio.com/downloads/download-visual-studio-vs). In the proposed method, Microsoft Visual Studio 2010 Express is used as the standard compiler.

The implementation is then tested and compared with the original MCLM codes which run on a normal CPU as shown in Table 4.7. The workstation used has a processor Intel Xeon E5645 (24 cores) and 24 GB memories. As shown in the table, the GPU enable a fast simulation of light–skin of MCML.

4.5.3 Skin reflectance

As seen from Table 4.4, the DRS is most appropriate for the work. The spectroscopy method measures the characteristic reflectance spectrum produced as light passes through a medium (Figure 3.9). The device called spectrophotometer measures a ratio value (between 0 and 1 or 0% and 100%) of reflectance from spectral bands 430 to 740 nm.

To investigate the characteristics of skin reflectance, analyses of skin reflectance were carried out. The reflectance spectrum data of 118 participants (22 females and 96 males) were obtained from their outer arm

Table 4.7 CPU versus GPU

Number of wavelength	Number of photons	System	Processing time
1	1,000,000	CPU	51 min
1	1,000,000	GPU	s

(facultative skin). The participants consist of 21 participants with skin photo type (SPT) III, 56 participants with SPT IV and 41 participants with SPT V. To understand the variability of skin reflectance at a particular wavelength, the standard deviation (SD) of reflectance data from all participants at a particular wavelength is plotted as well. In the graphs of Figure 4.42, the data points are the mean values of the skin reflectance with horizontal error bars indicating the corresponding SD ranges.

It is seen that the reflectance curves are not linear and thus, multiple linear regressions [165] may not give the best analysis. Nevertheless, it is hypothesized that the reflectance can be modelled by different linear regressions over different intervals of wavelength (piecewise linear regressions) [166,167]. A knot is a value at which the gradient in piecewise linear regression model changes. A knot is also defined as the *x*-value at which the two pieces of the linear model connect. Figure 4.43 depicts the second derivative of mean reflectance data of SPT V.

As seen from Figure 4.43, there are three knots in SPT V occurring in wavelength ranges of 500–530, 560–580 and 620–640 nm. Figure 4.44 shows the piecewise linear regression of SPT III, SPT IV and SPT V.

As seen from Figure 4.44, high correlations ($R^2 > 0.83$) between the piecewise linear regression reflectance models and the actual reflectance data have been achieved and thus, the piecewise linear regression can be used to model skin reflectance. Four linear regressions are identified for SPT III (Figure 4.44a), SPT IV (Figure 4.44b) and SPT V (Figure 4.44c). The spectral range for the first linear regression is from 430 to 510 nm, the second regression from 510 to 570 nm, the third regression from 570 to 630 nm and the fourth regression from 630 to 740 nm. In this work, data sampling for the analysis is performed on the spectral range of first linear regression because out of the four regressions, pigment melanin (eumelanin and pheomelanin) has the highest molar absorptivity in that range (430–510 nm), as shown in Figure 4.7. These nine spectral data from 430 to 510 nm with 10 nm difference are used as data samples. These sampling is necessary to ensure the convergence of the optimisation process.

4.5.4 Optimisation

The prerequisite to the MC simulation is that the skin optical parameters are known. Normally, the case is the opposite, the reflectance spectra are known, and the skin optical parameters need to be calculated. This inverse problem can be solved by tuning the parameters of the MC skin model until the simulated spectra match the measured spectra. Tuning the model manually is an overly tedious process. In order for the parameters of the MC skin model to be accurately tuned to the reflectance spectra, an error minimisation between simulated and acquired reflectance spectra is required. Error minimisation here is a subset of optimisation.

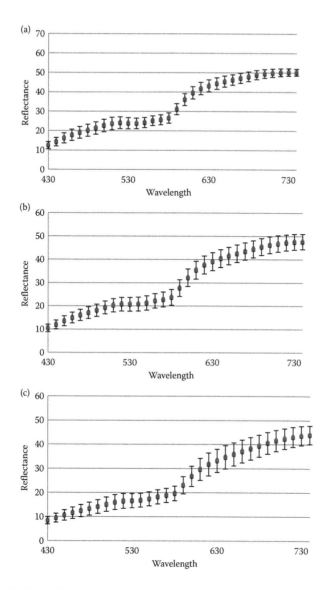

Figure 4.42 Mean skin reflectance of participants: (a) SPT III, (b) SPT IV and (c) SPT V.

Given an objective function f and a set of equality and inequality constraints, S, the main goal of optimisation is to determine a global minimum (or maximum) of the objective function, f, subject to the set of constraints, S [168]. Several general approaches to optimization are available as follows: (1) analytical methods, (2) graphical methods, (3) experimental methods and (4) numerical methods.

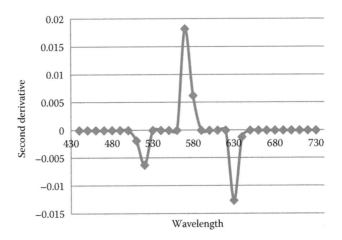

Figure 4.43 Second derivative analysis of SPT V.

Numerical methods such as GAs were invented by John Holland and developed in the 1960s and 1970s [169]. The algorithms start with an initial population of individuals generated at random. Each individual in the population represents a potential solution to the problem under consideration. The individuals evolve through successive iterations, called generations. During each generation, each individual in the population is evaluated using some measure of fitness. The population of the next generation is in turn created through genetic operators. The procedure continues until the termination condition is fulfilled.

The general framework of GAs is described as follows [169–172], where $P(t)$ denotes the population at generation.

$P(t)$ is a population that consists of t individuals representing a number of potential solutions to a problem. In GAs, an individual in a population is denoted by a string, i of length, n as follows:

$$i = i_1, i_2, \ldots, i_n \tag{4.63}$$

The string, i is regarded as a chromosome that consists of n genes. The character i_1 is a gene at the first locus and the different values of a gene are called alleles. The chromosome, i is called the genotype of an individual and a solution to the problem corresponding to string i is called the phenotype.

The mapping from phenotypes to genotypes is called a coding, and the mapping from genotypes to phenotypes is called a decoding. Both coding and encoding refer to encoding process in GA. As illustrated in Figure 4.45, after initiation, evaluation process is performed. Evaluation is a measurement of fitness value of every individual in a population using

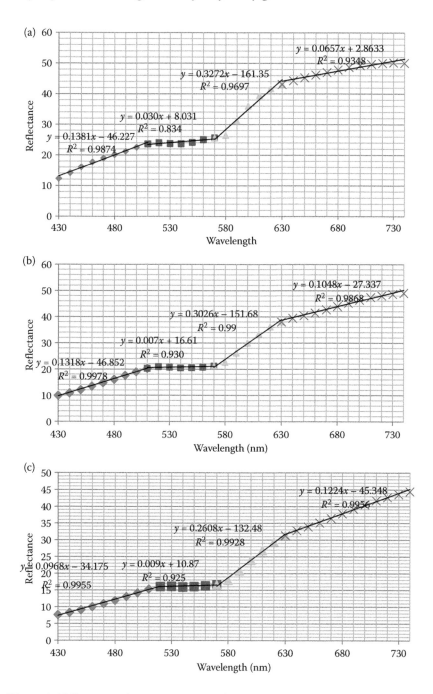

Figure 4.44 Piecewise linear regression of (a) SPT III, (b) SPT IV and (c) SPT V.

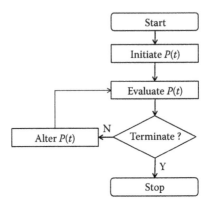

Figure 4.45 General framework of GA.

an objective function value, *f*. Termination is carried out if the requirement for termination is fulfilled. Otherwise, an alteration of population will be performed. There are three main genetic operators that are used in the alteration namely, reproduction, crossover and mutation to create the next generation.

4.5.4.1 Encoding

In encoding, candidate solutions (chromosomes) are encoded by a set of parameters [169]. Usually, a chromosome consists of several genes, each of which represents single variable/parameter of the model (Equation 4.63). Early GA applications used fixed-length, fixed-order bit strings to encode candidate solutions but nowadays several kinds of encoding such as binary encoding, real-value encoding and tree encoding are used. Table 4.8 presents the pros and cons among the three encoding methods.

In the proposed MC simulation, four parameters namely, concentration of eumelanin in epidermis, concentration of pheomelanin in epidermis, volume fraction of melanosome and epidermal thickness are used. As reported in the literature, the concentration of eumelanin approximately ranges from 0 to 122 g/L [75,86,173]. The concentration of pheomelanin, is reported to range from 0 to 18 g/L [14,173]. The volume fraction of melanosome is predicted to be from 0% to 43% [42,86] and the epidermal thickness ranges from 0.05 to 0.1 mm [174] (Table 4.9).

As seen in Table 4.8, the value ranges of the four parameters vary. Taking into account the pros and cons in Table 4.8, real-value encoding is chosen in the proposed method to ensure that all of the search space is explored with a high degree of resolution.

GA begins with the generation of a population *P* of *t* individuals. As illustrated in Figure 4.46, each individual is described by *n* genes containing the parameter model.

Table 4.8 Encoding type

Encoding type	Pro D	Con D
Binary	• Ease of implementation • Allowing higher degree of parallelism	• Limited space range • Problem in mapping from bits to real values
Real values	• Ease of implementation • Allowing higher degree of parallelism • Variable can be used directly for coding • Higher precision in comparison with binary encoding • Open search space	• Requiring high computational power
Tree	• Ease of implementation • Open search space	• Requiring high computational power • Possibility of uncontrolled solutions

Two important aspects of the population include the population sample size, (for example, Figure 4.47) and the number of generation. Both aspects depend on the problem but with a condition that the pool of individuals is able to cover and explore the whole search space.

A large population generally assures a higher probability that the search space will be more explored than that of a smaller population. However, convergence of algorithm will take longer time. The convergence time is related to both the population size (t) and the number of generation used (g). Larger t and g values will improve the likelihood of convergence but at the expense of longer computation times.

Many strategies are present in the evolution of population in a new generation. One strategy relies on several selected best individuals from an intermediate population composing children and parents to form a new generation. Another strategy is based on a new population totally consisting of children. This approach might lose the best individual from the previous generation. An alternative method is a compromise in which children replace the weakest individuals from the current generation. In

Table 4.9 Range of parameters

No	Skin optical characteristics	Range
1	Eumelanin concentration	0–122 g/L
2	Pheomelanin concentration	0–18 g/L
3	Volume fraction of melanosome	0–43%
4	Epidermal thickness	0.05–0.1 mm

Chromosome A
Gene 1A
Gene 2A
Gene 3A
Gene 4A
Eumelanin concentration
Pheomelanin concentration
Melanosome volume fraction
Epidermal thickness

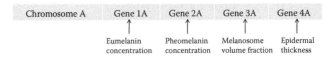

Figure 4.46 Individual and corresponding genes in a population.

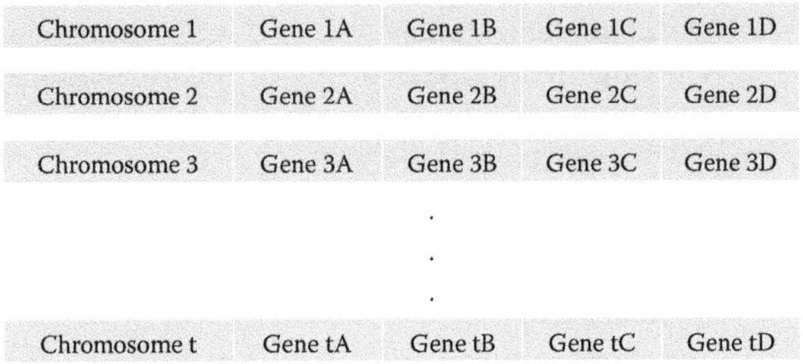

Chromosome 1
Gene 1A
Gene 1B
Gene 1C
Gene 1D
Chromosome 2
Gene 2A
Gene 2B
Gene 2C
Gene 2D
Chromosome 3
Gene 3A
Gene 3B
Gene 3C
Gene 3D
Chromosome t
Gene tA
Gene tB
Gene tC
Gene tD

Figure 4.47 Population sample.

this commonly used strategy, the best individual will preserve the best fitness of its generation and offers improvements to the next generation.

4.5.4.2 Fitness function

In GA, the population evolves through a number of selection and reproduction steps. The evolution leads to the creation of children from parents of the previous population. The population is iteratively evaluated by a fitness function, which selects the best individual in regard to the model [133,175,176].

In the study, the changing of parameters' values affect the entire spectra from 450 to 510 nm at 10 nm intervals. The fitness function is calculated over the entire spectra for all parameters. Note that fitness functions are problem-dependent, meaning that one fitness function may be useful in a particular problem but not necessarily others; it may not be generalized to other problems. Valisuo et al. compared several fitness functions such as mean square error (MSE), mean absolute error (MAE), relative MSE (rMSE) and relative MAE (rMAE). Although, rMSE was used in measuring the error data in their work, and as the fitness function for GA, the rMSE is not enough to reach the correct optimum point [153].

Data of 40 participants with similar skin tone are used to find the best-fitness function. Figure 4.48 shows the mean simulated and the measured reflectance using rMSE as the fitness function. The Euclidean distance, *Ed*, between the simulated and the measured reflectance are also calculated as follows:

$$Ed = \sqrt{\sum_{i=1}^{n} (Rs_i - Rm_i)^2} \tag{4.64}$$

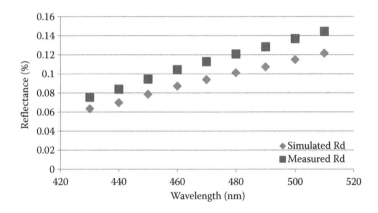

Figure 4.48 Simulated reflectance (mean) obtained with rMSE.

The Euclidean distance of the simulated and measured reflectance using rMSE is found to be 0.055. Figure 4.49 shows the error analysis between measured-simulated reflectance with the ideal.

To reduce the error and the Euclidean distance between the simulated reflectance and the measured reflectance, the gradient analysis is proposed for the fitness function. Hence, in this work, the rMSE is combined with the gradient error between the simulated reflectance and the measured reflectance.

The error data are calculated as follows:

$$Error\_data = 1 - rMSE = 1 - \frac{\sum\limits_{i=1}^{n} \sqrt{(Rs_i - Rm_i / Rm_i)^2}}{n} \quad (4.65)$$

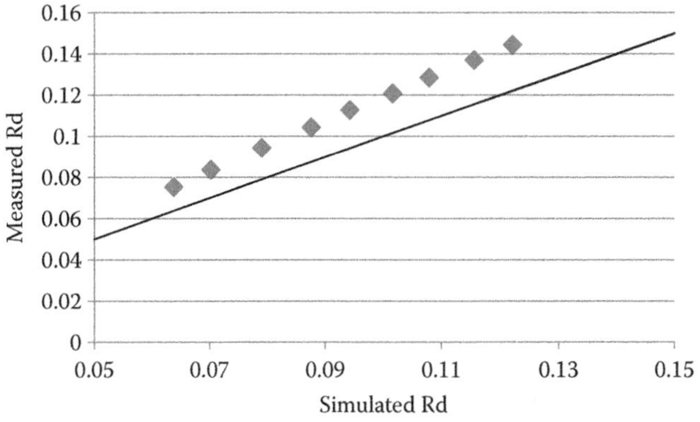

Figure 4.49 Error analysis of measured and simulated reflectance with rMSE.

The gradient error can be formulated as follows:

$$Error\_gradient = 1 - abs\left(\frac{G(Rm) - G(Rs)}{G(Rm)}\right)$$
(4.66)

The proposed fitness function used is as follows:

$$Fitness = Error\_data * Error\_gradient$$
(4.67)

where Rs is the simulated reflectance, Rm the measured reflectance, n the number of spectra, $G(Rm)$ the gradient of the simulated reflectance and $G(Rs)$ the gradient of the measured reflectance.

Figure 4.50 shows the mean simulated and the measured reflectance using our proposed fitness function and Figure 4.51 shows the error analysis. The Euclidean distance of the simulated and measured reflectance using the proposed method is 0.017. Comparing Figures 4.49 and 4.51, it can be seen that with the proposed fitness function, the simulated reflectance is closer to the measured reflectance.

4.5.4.3 Selection
Selection is based on the principal of adaptation of an individual from a population in its environment following the theory of natural selection. It is a technique to select chromosomes according to their fitness values. There are several strategies for the selection of the population as found in the literature [175].

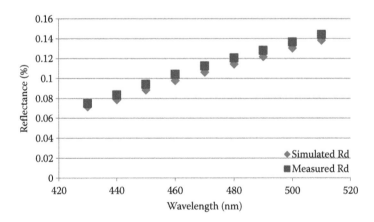

Figure 4.50 Simulated reflectance (mean) obtained with the proposed fitness function.

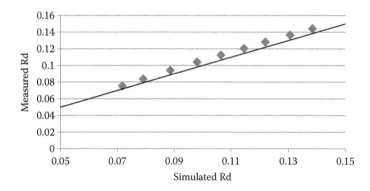

Figure 4.51 Error analysis of measured and simulated reflectance obtained with the proposed fitness function.

Generally, chromosomes with high fitness values will be selected. Following this concept, only fittest individuals to some criterion will survive and take part as parents in the generation of a new population. The type of selection pressure will then affect the convergence speed of the population. A high selection pressure leads to fast convergence rates. The selection process aims to apply selection pressure and to conserve population diversity. Several other techniques include roulette wheel, ranking, tournament and random selection to mention some. Table 4.10 presents a summary of the aforementioned selection methods.

Tournament and ranking methods can produce better generation. However, the methods can be trapped in local maxima or minima.

Table 4.10 Pros and cons of GA selection methods

Selection type	Pros	Cons
Roulette wheel	• Does not involve negative fitness value individual • Higher probability for better individual	• Discarding the least fit individual through after numerous spinning
Ranking	• Conserving the best individual of population • Creating a new generation based on the best parents of previous generation	• Probability of system to be trapped in local maxima/ minima
Tournament	• Creating new generation based on the best parents of previous generation	• Probability of system to be trapped in local maxima/ minima
Random	• Equal probability for all individuals	• Probability to have population with least fit individual

Nevertheless, this can be avoided by applying mutation as one of the GA operator. Among the different reproduction and evolution possibilities offered, Muhlebein stated that only mutation works well for evolution strategy [177]. To have a wider exploration of the search space, a crossover operation should also be applied [135].

In the proposed method, the ranking selection is chosen in which the population is ranked based on the fitness value. This is considered as an elitist selection. The best individuals are not only copied to the next generation but also kept in the current population. By so doing, they can still be selected by other genetic operators.

4.5.4.4 Alteration

Following the selection process, the population undergoes a reproduction to generate a new population. Two commonly used genetic operators are crossing and mutation. A crossing operation requires at least a pair of parents to generate two offspring/children. Alternatively, a mutation operation only necessitates one parent.

Crossover operation consists of swapping one randomly selected parameter between two randomly chosen parents to generate two offspring. It exchanges genetic information between parents and combines two parents to breed two children. The exchange of genetic information supposes that the children contain relevant information from their parents. The crossover operation is an important technique to increase the fitness of the population. Generally, the procedure of crossing are synthesised using four steps: selecting two individuals from the population by the crossing operator (single or multipoint crossing); selecting a random gene from the chromosome; interchanging the gene information between the two parents and generating two children. The crossing procedure interchanges the gene of two parents in one or several points. This operation can be applied to different types of coding (real-value and binary) for only involving a gene swapping.

The drawbacks of the crossing are related to that the product/children of one or two individuals with weak fitness is/are not alike. To avoid the effect of these numerous crossings, the operation can be directed towards the selection of individuals with good fitness to be parents. This process not only tends to limit the exploration of the search space but also may lead to premature convergence. The crossing of parents with close genes information rarely provides new information in the population, affecting the algorithm convergence speed. The crossing probability of an individual ranges from 0.6 to 0.95 [178,179]. Figure 4.52 shows the illustration of crossing operation between two parents.

Mutation on the other hand aims to maintain diversity in a population. It avoids the GA to be trapped into local minima by introducing randomness to the search and thereby increasing the probability that

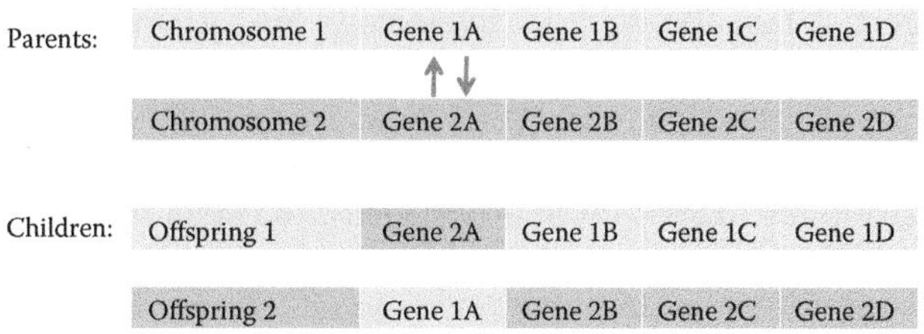

Parents:	Chromosome 1	Gene 1A	Gene 1B	Gene 1C	Gene 1D
		↑ ↓			
	Chromosome 2	Gene 2A	Gene 2B	Gene 2C	Gene 2D

Children:	Offspring 1	Gene 2A	Gene 1B	Gene 1C	Gene 1D
	Offspring 2	Gene 1A	Gene 2B	Gene 2C	Gene 2D

Figure 4.52 Sample of crossing operation.

all parts of the search space is explored. A number of individuals of the population will be selected for a mutation operation after the crossing process. The mutation operation randomly alters the genetic information of parameters/genes of individuals of the population.

For the binary coded solution, the mutation randomly selects and inverts a bit (named flipping). For real-value mutation, the gene is randomly selected and a new gene is randomly generated within its variation range. The mutation probability of an individual ranges from 0.02 to 0.3 [178,179].

Figure 4.53 illustrates the mutation operation.

These two processes (crossing and mutation) result in the generation of a new population with different chromosomes from the initial one. Genetic operators are not systematically applied to every individual from a generation. The most common scheme is to perform the crossing sequentially followed by the mutation operation on part of the population. However, there are an infinite number of possible combinations using multiple crossing and mutation operators in a single algorithm. If the fitness function is appropriately selected, this procedure, in turn, will increase the average fitness of the new population.

4.5.4.5 Termination

Generally, there are three ways for the GA to achieve the termination condition: by reaching a specific fitness value, by converging the population to an optimal solution, and by completing a predefined number of iteration. The random factors of GA operators produce the variety of solutions/chromosomes in the population. The diversity becomes null when the entire population is identical. It is then considered that the algorithm

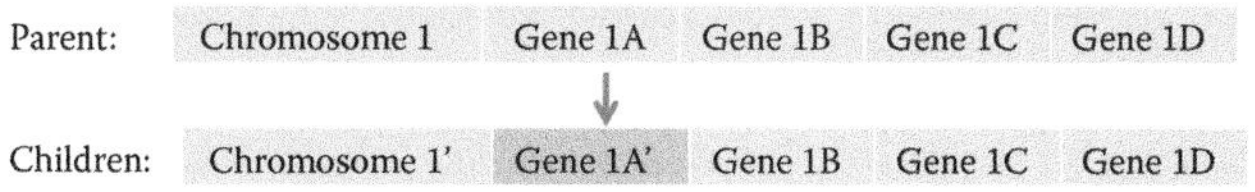

Parent:	Chromosome 1	Gene 1A	Gene 1B	Gene 1C	Gene 1D
		↓			
Children:	Chromosome 1'	Gene 1A'	Gene 1B	Gene 1C	Gene 1D

Figure 4.53 Sample of mutation operation.

has converged. When the genetic diversity is low, it is unlikely that the diversity will increase again. On the other hand, if the convergence happens early, it falls into local optima (premature convergence). Hence, it is important to preserve a genetic diversity without preventing convergence.

In designing the algorithm, it is necessary to find a trade-off between explorations of the search space (to avoid being trapped into a local optimum) and exploitation of the best individual. Too much exploitation, in turn, will lead to a convergence toward a local optimum whereas an over exploration will lead to the non-convergence of the algorithm. An exploitation step refers to a selection and crossing operation while exploration relates to the population initialisation and mutation. The effect of exploration and exploitation can be modified by the various algorithm parameters. However, the literature on GA does not provide a universal rule on how to tune the different parameters for a successful outcome. As a result, empirical testing and checking on the effects of the various algorithms are necessary.

In the selection of the termination, two major factors have to be considered: (1) defining a fitness value may lead to extensive computation time and (2) selecting a high fitness may trap the method into an infinite loop. Considering those factors, the termination operators must define an iteration number, which corresponds to the convergence of the population.

Using the previous set of data and parameters (the proposed fitness function), several iteration numbers ($N = 20, 50, 100, 150$) are applied.

Figure 4.54 show the number of iterations as a function of the fitness value. With 20 iterations, the algorithm does not have time to converge. For 20, 50 and 100 iterations, it is seen that after 70–80 iterations, the fitness value does not change significantly; the population is then considered to have converged. These values are the average convergences value obtained for the three spectra, which reflect the limit of the search space,

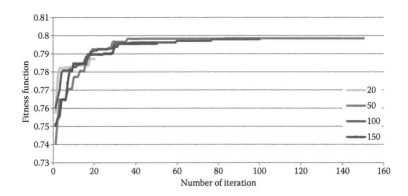

Figure 4.54 Number of iterations.

meaning that no drift has affected the test populations. Because of the convergence rate, the number of iterations selected is 100.

The convergence condition changes with the population size. A large population ensures the diversity over the search space and limits the risk of convergence towards local minima; a process was performed 10 times for each of the three spectra purposely to generalize the fitness value for different spectra. It means that the obtained spectra after the final iteration matches best the simulated one. However, a population with 20 individuals obtained similar fitness value with a population of 100 individual. A large population requires higher computational time and with precision only slightly better (0.2E-05) for a population of 300 than that of 100, the precision gained was not judged sufficient in comparison to the loss in computational time. Therefore, we select a population size of 20 individuals.

4.6 Non-invasive in vivo computerised pigmentation analysis

4.6.1 Computerised pigmentation analysis tool

With the developed system that analyses skin reflectance data, quantitative and objective assessment of skin pigmentation levels can be performed. The skin can then be categorised according to SPTs and the amount of different categories of melanin could be determined accurately in a non-invasive and *in vivo* manner. This analytical capability enables the assessment of treatment efficacy for skin disorders (by measuring the amount of repigmentation or depigmentation of the skin) and for cosmetic dermatology (by measuring the amount of melanin types before and after the treatment).

The computerised pigmentation analysis tool consists of a hand-held spectrophotometer and MCML skin analysis software running on GPU workstation, as shown in Figure 4.55. The spectrophotometer acquires multispectral skin reflectance data of pigmented lesion and the surrounding skin surface. The software analyses the skin reflectance data, that is, the different absorption spectra of pigments to distinguish melanin types from other pigments non-invasively. The GPU workstation is purposely set to achieve a fast computing time enabling skin analysis in clinical settings.

4.6.2 Validation of the pigmentation analysis and evaluation of the computerised pigmentation tool

The developed inverse analysis method of the skin pigmentation algorithm is validated with the RSM module of the ASAP software from BRO

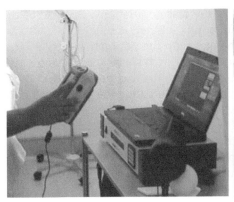
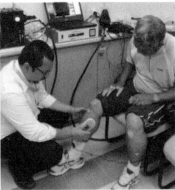

Figure 4.55 Spectrophotometer and GPU workstation.

and computerised pigmentation analysis tool is evaluated in two observational clinical studies.

The estimated epidermal optical parameters (namely the concentration of eumelanin and pheomelanin, the volume fraction of melanosome and the epidermal thickness) obtained using reflectance data of participants were inputted into the RSM module of the ASAP software from BRO, to model a computational simulated skin [180,181].

It is hypothesised that if the computational simulated skin produced by RSM results in similar reflectance data of the participants, the inverse analysis method is thus proven to be able to estimate correctly the epidermal skin optical parameters. As reported in the literature, the RSM can be modified to generate the reflectance data of skin and the reflectance data used as a ground truth for validating the analysis of skin optical parameters [41,42]. Figure 4.56 illustrates the skin model generated by RSM module of ASAP based on skin–light interactions.

Considering that skin is one of the complex and dynamic organs of the human body, many factors should be involved to model the skin accurately. RSM takes into account as many biologically relevant factors of the skin in its simulation. To model the scattering properties of the skin, the RSM uses a built-in volumetric scattering model in ASAP adopting the Henyey–Greenstein approximation for the angular distribution of scattered light. Four important parameters are required to create this model namely, anisotropy factor, scattering coefficient, absorption coefficient and fractional obscuration per unit area.

The Henyey–Greenstein scattering phase function is an approximate expression that accounts for the scattering of light in medium (Equation 4.57). The Henyey–Greenstein expression is a function of anisotropy factor (g values). Most biological tissues have g values in the range of 0.7–0.9. The scattering coefficient for tissue is a probability measurement towards

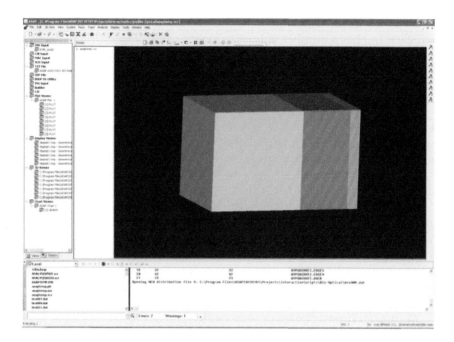

Figure 4.56 Skin modelling by RSM from ASAP software.

a scatter event. Scattering occurs when a photon interacts with a particle in the medium. The scattering of human skin is frequently modelled as a combination of Mie and Rayleigh scattering. The coefficient has a number of inverse length units as the scattering coefficient (μ_s) is the cross-sectional area per unit volume of medium.

$$\mu_s = \rho_s \sigma_s \tag{4.68}$$

For the simulation, the RSM assumed that each layer of skin tissues will have similar scattering coefficient. The scattering of human skin is frequently modelled as a combination of Mie and Rayleigh scattering as a function of wavelength [82] as follows:

$$\mu_s(\lambda) = \mu_{s.Mie}(\lambda) + \mu_{s.Rayleigh}(\lambda)$$
$$\mu_s(\lambda) = 2.10^5 . \lambda^{-1.5} + 2.10^{12} . \lambda^{-4.5} \tag{4.69}$$

Similar to the scattering coefficient, absorption coefficient defines the probability of a photon absorption event. The absorption coefficient in skin is mainly due to pigments deposited in epidermis or dissolved in blood located in the dermis. Similar with scattering coefficient, the absorption coefficient (μ_a) has a number of inverse length units.

$$\mu_a = \rho_a \sigma_a \qquad (4.70)$$

The fractional obscuration per unit area (f) is interpreted as the outcome of the particle number density (number of particles per unit volume) and the average particle cross-sectional area. The f value is roughly equivalent to the inverse mean free path length of the medium. In the RSM, the f value is set to 1 because RSM assumes that the absorption and scattering coefficients are similar for every region in one layer.

Using skin optical parameters, the RSM is used to generate the reflectance data of skin. These reflectance data are used to validate the inverse analysis of skin. BRO has developed a flexible and efficient optical system-modelling tool. It is able to simulate the interaction of light with optical and mechanical structures using MC ray-tracing techniques [182]. RSM uses the ray-tracing techniques to simulate the interaction of light with skin [181], as depicted in Figure 4.57.

All major chromophores of skin namely, melanin, haemoglobin and water are represented within the model along with lesser contributors

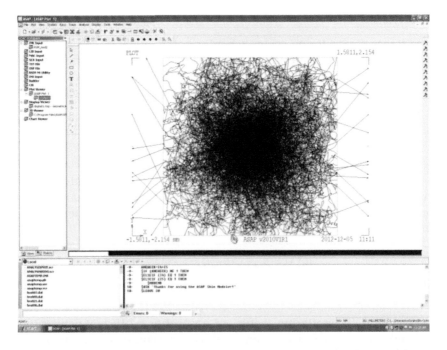

Figure 4.57 Screenshot of RSM showing the photon paths in the skin model.

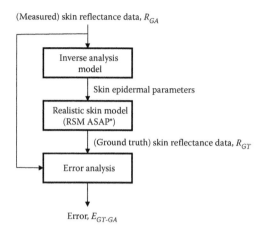

(Measured) skin reflectance data, R_{GA}

Inverse analysis
model

Skin epidermal parameters

Realistic skin model
(RSM ASAP*)

(Ground truth) skin reflectance data, R_{GT}

Error analysis

Error, $E_{GT\text{-}GA}$

Figure 4.58 Validation process.

such as bilirubin and beta-carotene. The flexibility of RSM to vary the concentrations for different chromophores has made it possible to model different skin conditions.

Figure 4.58 shows the validation process. First, based on the participants' skin reflectance spectral data according to SPTs, the skin optical parameters are determined using the developed inverse analysis algorithm (computerised pigmentation analysis system). The four parameters of skin epidermal attributes to be determined are eumelanin concentration, pheomelanin concentration, volume fraction of melanosome and skin epidermal thickness. After that, the determined skin parameters are being input to the RSM module of BRO ASAP software to regenerate the skin reflectance spectrum data to be compared with the measured data. To determine ground truth skin reflectance spectrum for the given epidermal parameters, the RSM module runs a simulation built based on optical parameters computed from the developed system.

In the RSM module, skin reflectance is computed as a cumulative energy of photon recorded upon contact with skin. To model closely the real world skin conditions, it is important to understand the amount of energy of light coming in contact with skin. The most important light source is the sun. The amount of energy from the sun that falls on Earth's surface is enormous. Outside Earth's atmosphere, the sun's energy contains about 1300 W/m². About one-third of this light is reflected back into space, and some are absorbed by the atmosphere (in part causing winds to blow). By the time it reaches the Earth's surface, the energy in sunlight would have fallen to about 1000 W/m² (0.001 W/mm²) at noon on a cloudless day [183].

The energy carried by an individual photon is given by the product of Planck's constant and the frequency of the radiation.

$$E = \frac{hc}{\lambda} \tag{4.71}$$

where E is the energy, h the Planck's constant (6.626×10^{-34} J s), c the speed of light (3×10^8 m/s) and λ the wavelength of light.

Sunlight is made up of a spectrum of colours with visible light wavelengths ranging from 340 to 760 nm. Taking a central wavelength of 550 nm as a sample, the energy of single photon of that particular spectrum is 3.61×10^{-19} W s. Using the above solar energy of 0.001 W/mm², this means that this represents about 2.77×10^{15} photons per second per square millimetres. Unfortunately, with the current computing technologies, it is impossible to run simulation with such numbers of photons. As reported in the literature, a simulation of a million photons should be adequate to produce a reliable result [35,112]. Therefore, the RSM module uses a million photons in the simulation.

The reflectance spectrum data obtained from the RSM module, R_{GT} is thus contrasted with the acquired reflectance utilized by the pigmentation analysis tool, R_{GA} to find out the error, E_{GT-GA}

$$E_{GT-GA} = \left| R_{GT} - R_{GA} \right| \tag{4.72}$$

There were 36 participants involved in the validation study and all are SPTs IV. Figure 4.59 shows the mean reflectance of the upper arm of all participants for the nine spectral bands. As explained in Section 4.5.3, only nine spectral bands are used in the analysis. The mean reflectance

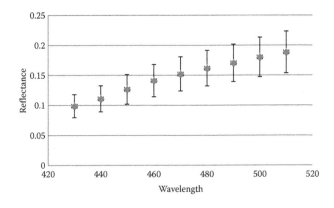

Figure 4.59 Mean reflectance of participants (SPT IV) upper arm.

Table 4.11 Statistical study of the system and the acquired reflectance

Items	Values
Measured reflectance (R_{GA})	0.148 ± 0.026
Pigmentation analysis system + RSM (R_{GT})	0.154 ± 0.028
Error between the measured reflectance data and reproduced reflectance ($E_{GT\text{-}GA}$)	0.0163 ± 0.009
Skewness	0.34
Kurtosis	−0.6

from the nine spectral bands is found to be 0.148 with an SD of 0.027 (the lower bound is 0.083 and the upper bound is 0.208).

The above measured mean reflectance spectra are then contrasted with the mean reflectance spectra computed from RSM, as shown in Figure 4.60.

As shown in Figure 4.60, the mean reflectance spectra attained from RSM falls within the error bar of the acquired reflectance. Table 4.11 depicts the statistical study of the error between the acquired reflectance information and reproduced reflectance due to pigmentation analysis methodology as set put by RSM ($E_{GT\text{-}GA}$).

The measured mean reflectance, RGA is 0.148 ± 0.026 and the mean reflectance attained from the RSM module, RGT is 0.154 ± 0.028. The absolute error is then calculated from the contrast of each spectrum between the acquired reflectance and the reflectance from the RSM module. The MAE is the mean of the error computed from each spectral band. From the 36 data, the MAE is found to be 0.0163 ± 0.009.

The MAE is 8.82%. Positive skewness shows that the distribution of error data is closer to the 0% error. A kurtosis of −0.6 portrays that the

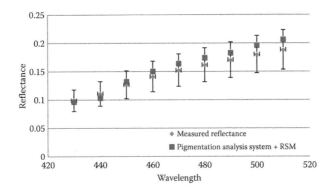

Figure 4.60 Plots of reflectance data between the acquired reflectance and the simulated reflectance obtained from the pigmentation analysis system.

error is nearly normally distributed, considering that a kurtosis of normal distribution is 0. It is also seen that the SD (0.009) was one order below the range of the reflectance data (0.036–0.0456) – indicating a satisfying precision. The relationship plots can be used to perform further study, as illustrated in Figure 4.61.

The graph demonstrated that the regression analysis line is close to the $X = Y$ line. The regression analysis of pigmentation analysis system error (EGT-GA) demonstrates that the system has a solid linear relationship measured data ($R^2 = 0.994$) showing a system with high accuracy and reliability.

4.6.3 Observational study I

Two observational studies have been conducted to evaluate the developed system. In these studies, the skin reflectance of participants and lesion reflectance data of patients have been obtained using spectrophotometer. The selected lesion and normal skin, in this case, must have an area with diameter not less than 7 mm.

For the scanning session, the room setting has been set as follows:

1. The room temperature must be set around 25°C to ascertain the effectiveness of the system
2. Distance: The spectrometer should be attached to the measured area

Figure 4.62 shows the data acquisition method for spectrophotometer assessment.

The sample size calculation method used in the studies [184] is as follows:

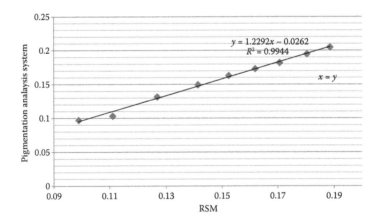

Figure 4.61 Regression study of the pigmentation study system.

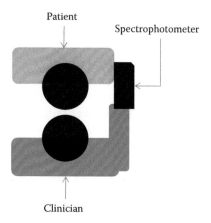

Figure 4.62 Assessment using spectrophotometer.

$$n = \frac{z_{1-\alpha/2}^2 p(1-p)}{d^2}$$

$$n = \frac{1.962 x 0.02 x (1-0.02)}{0.05^2} \tag{4.73}$$

$$n = 30 \pm 1.5$$

n = sample size to be determined
$z_{1-\alpha/2}^2$ = confidence level at 95% (standard value of 1.96)
p = estimated prevalence of vitiligo
d^2 = margin of error at 5% (standard value of 0.05)
p = assumed proportion of the parameter to the estimated population

The "p" value used is the prevalence of vitiligo cases in Dermatology Department of Hospital Kuala Lumpur as reported by Adawiyah et al. [185]. Between 2003 and 2007, there were 484 of new vitiligo cases in Hospital Kuala Lumpur. This represents 2% of all new cases referred to the Dermatology Department within the same period. The confidence level in this study is set to 95%. As shown above, the calculated sample size in this observational study is found to be 30 ± 1.5.

The observational study I was conducted at the two locations namely, Centre for Intelligent Signal and Imaging Research (CISIR), Universiti Teknologi PETRONAS, Malaysia, and University of Burgundy, France. The study aims to determine the baseline values for the various SPTs (normal skin with different skin tones based on Fitzpatrick classification). A number of undergraduate and postgraduate students from both institutions were employed as associates. In the analysis, the following inclusion requirements were set for the associates:-

1. Adults aged 18 years and above given written consent.
2. The absence of any dermatological diseases.

The exclusion requirements were set as follows:

1. Associates with jaundice or chronic medical disorders such as chronic renal failure and chronic liver failure.
2. The presence of dermatological diseases which could hamper the data analysis.

Figure 4.63 depicts the activities of the designed observational analysis.

First, all participants were given the study information sheet and were asked to approve on the consent form. In the following step, their skin reflectance data from different body areas, namely face, upper arm and lower back near buttock were obtained using a spectrophotometer. Here, the reflectance data of the face and the upper arm represented the reflectance of skin facultative data, while those of the lower back represented the reflectance of skin constitutive data. Facultative skin data can be obtained from skin areas that are affected by environment (sun or hormones). The environment impacts the original appearance of the

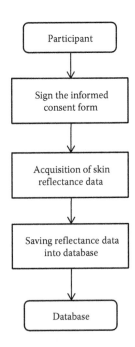

Figure 4.63 Study design of observational study I.

skin colour over time. Constitutive skin data, meanwhile, is determined by genetics [136,186]. The measured reflectance data were saved in a database. Overall, the process from participant's preparation to data acquisition took less than 7 min.

Overall, 110 participants were recruited in this study and divided based on their SPTs. Based on Fitzpatrick, SPT can be categorized into six types [11]. Generally, it is observed that

1. Caucasians have skin types I and II.
2. Asians and South Asians have skin types ranging from III, IV to V.
3. Africans have skin types VI.

Figure 4.64 shows the distribution of the participants based on their SPTs.

Figure 4.65 shows the mean reflectance spectrum of various SPTs obtained from 110 participants. It is shown that for a particular wavelength, participants with higher SPT generally will have smaller reflectance. This indicates that the skin of higher SPT absorb more energy as a result of a higher total absorption coefficient (μ_a). Assuming that the skin baseline absorption, the water spectral absorption and the dermis absorption are affected in a similar fashion, the occurrence of light photon absorption in skin is mainly caused by the pigments deposited in epidermis.

Generally, participants with higher SPT have higher concentration of pigments compared to participants with lower SPT. The graph also shows that the reflectance of skin is not linear. This is expected as the molar absorptivity of pigments has been found to be not linear. This has been shown in Figures 4.7 through 4.9, in which the respective molar absorptivity of pheomelanin, eumelanin and haemoglobin are not linear.

Figure 4.66 shows the relative concentration of eumelanin, volume fraction of melanosomes in epidermis and epidermal thickness obtained using the proposed inverse model. It was hypothesised that a higher SPT will have higher eumelanin (melanin) concentration and melanosome volume fraction; however, epidermal thickness of outer forearm will be similar.

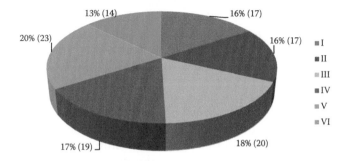

Figure 4.64 Participants distribution based on SPTs.

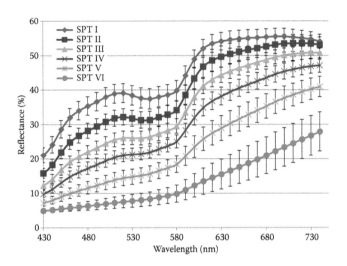

Figure 4.65 Reflectance of skin for different SPTs.

From Figure 4.66a, the concentrations of eumelanin (melanin) increased from white to dark skin (SPT I–VI) with 21.99 mg/ml for SPT I, 29.54 mg/mL for SPT II, 32.62 mg/mL for SPT III, 38.2 mg/mL for SPT IV, 51.56 mg/mL for SPT V and 57.26 mg/mL for SPT VI. These results are in concurrence with Jacques work reporting that the eumelanin concentration ranges from 0 to 100 mg/mL [47]. This confirms our hypothesis that eumelanin concentration corresponds to the SPT classification.

A different pigmentation level has different volume fraction of melanosome in epidermis. In Figure 4.66b, the proposed method estimated that SPT I has 0.039 volume fraction of melanosomes in epidermis, SPT II 0.07, SPT III 0.154, SPT IV 0.178, SPT V 0.29 and SPT VI 0.35. Jacques reported that light pigmented adults have 0.014–0.04 volume fraction of melanosome, 0.11–0.16 volume fraction for moderately pigmented adults and 0.18–0.43 volume fraction for darkly pigmented adults [86]. The results obtained in the present study are in line with those reported by Jacques [86].

As shown in Figure 4.66c, the estimated epidermal thickness of the outer forearm ranges from 0.079 to 0.084 mm. Lee and Hwang [187] performed biopsies on 452 healthy Korean volunteers and reported that the epidermal thickness on the outer forearm were 0.083 ± 0.036 mm. The values of epidermal thickness obtained by the system are within the ranges reported by Lee, indicating a correct estimation.

Figure 4.67 shows the ratios of relative pheomelanin to eumelanin concentration. It is estimated that the pheomelanin to eumelanin ratio of SPT IV is 0.05. The value is close to the value of 0.049 for SPT IV reported by Parsad [27].

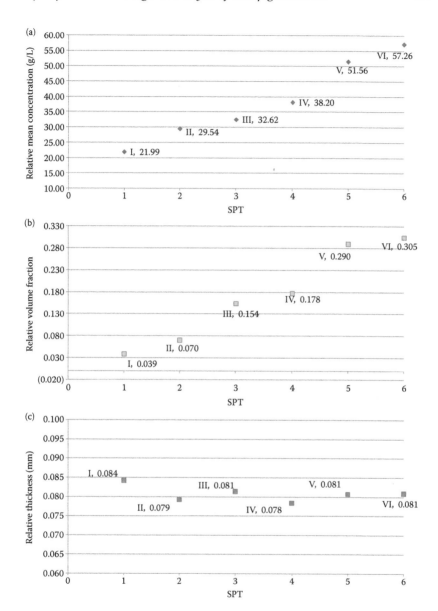

Figure 4.66 Epidermal skin parameters obtained from the proposed system: (a) relative eumelanin (melanin) concentration, (b) volume fraction of melanosomes in epidermis and (c) epidermal thickness.

To further evaluate the system, the above findings are compared with the results obtained from the analysis of skin reflectance with the modified Beer–Lambert law as discussed earlier.

Table 4.12 shows the comparison between ratios of relative pheomelanin to eumelanin concentration obtained by the modified Beer–Lambert law and the proposed system. It is shown that the value obtained by the system, especially for SPT IV, is in agreement with Parsad (0.049) in comparison with the value obtained by the modified Beer–Lambert law (0.49).

Table 4.13 summarises and compares parameters, that is, relative concentration of eumelanin, volume fraction of melanosomes in epidermis, epidermal thickness and ratio between pheomelanin and eumelanin, obtained using the system with those reported by other researchers. It is shown that the system is in good agreement. And as shown in Table 4.13, the system is superior to the other method (modified Beer–Lambert Law). It can be concluded, from the observational study I, that the system is potentially applicable in clinical conditions that require constant monitoring of changes in skin melanin pigments, volume fraction of melanosome in epidermis and epidermal thickness.

4.6.4 Observational study II

The observational study II was conducted at Hospital Kuala Lumpur and Hospital Serdang, Malaysia, by recruiting a number of patients suffering from melasma (hyper-pigmented disorder) and vitiligo (hypo-pigmented disorder). The study aims to evaluate the performance of the developed technique in analysing skin of vitiligo and melasma patients. The inclusion requirements were set as follows:

1. Adults aged 18 years and above given a written consent.
2. Clinically diagnosed to have either vitiligo or melasma.

The exclusion requirements were set as follows:

1. Associates with jaundice or chronic medical disorders such as chronic renal failure and chronic liver failure.
2. The presence of dermatological diseases other than vitiligo or melasma, which could hamper the analysis of the data.

Figure 4.68 depicts the activities of the designed observational analysis. All patients were given information sheet and required to sign the consent form. Next, dermatologist identified the areas of normal skin and lesion to be scanned. The reflectance data were then obtained using spectrophotometer and stored into a database. This

Table 4.12 Inverse analysis MCML system versus
modified Beer–Lambert law

SPT	Modified Beer–Lambert law	Inverse analysis MCML system
I	1.91	0.10
II	1.41	0.07
III	0.85	0.06
IV	0.49	0.05
V	0.26	0.04
VI	0.12	0.03

Table 4.13 Comparative results

Epidermal parameters	Inverse analysis MCML system	Jacques [47,86]	Lee [187]	Parsad [27]
Eumelanin	21.99–57.26 mg/mL	0–100 mg/mL	–	–
Vol. fraction of melanosome	0.039–0.35	0.014–0.43	–	–
Ratio pheomelanin to eumelanin	0.049	–	–	0.05
Thickness	0.079–0.084 mm	–	0.083 ± 0.036 mm	–

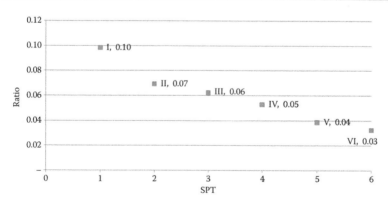

Figure 4.67 Ratio of relative pheomelanin to eumelanin concentration.

process typically takes less than 10 min from participant's preparation
to data acquisition.

In the observational study II, 43 patients were recruited (36% male,
64% female) and only patients suffering from vitiligo and melasma were
recruited. Figure 4.69 depicts the distribution of the data sets based on
lesion distribution.

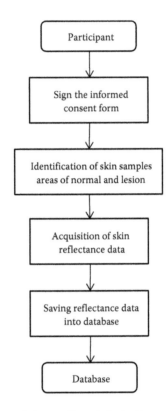

Figure 4.68 Study design of observational study II.

Figure 4.70 shows the skin reflectance data obtained from normal skin areas, melasma lesion and vitiligo lesion for various SPTs collected during the observational study. There are only three types of SPT collected during the second study. Melasma and vitiligo represent the different types of skin pigmentation disorders. In melasma, skin areas appear darker

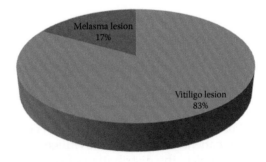

Figure 4.69 Lesion distribution.

than the surrounding skin due to the higher amount of pigment melanin. A higher production of melanin indicates that the light absorbance will be higher compared to the surrounding normal skin. Higher absorbance level will be reflected on the data of skin reflectance, which, in this case, will be lower than that of the normal skin, as shown in Figure 4.70.

Vitiligo lesion, however, is paler than the surrounding normal skin. Its lesion areas, in contrast with melasma, lack pigment melanin resulting in a lower light absorbance level. The reflectance of vitiligo lesion is slightly higher than the surrounding normal skin as shown in Figure 4.70.

The lesions are categorised based on the type of disease. Figure 4.71 shows the eumelanin concentration of vitiligo patients. Red squares represent the vitiligo lesion and blue dots represent the surrounding normal skin. It is found that the eumelanin concentrations of vitiligo lesions are lower (SPT III: 29.09 g/L, SPT IV: 27.85 g/L and SPT V: 41.56 g/L) than the surrounding normal skin (SPT III: 32.62 g/L, SPT IV: 38.2 g/L and SPT V: 50.56 g/L). This is because the melanocytes in vitiligo are not functioning normally; thus the production of the eumelanin and pheomelanin is affected.

Figure 4.72 shows the pheomelanin concentrations of the vitiligo lesion and the surrounding normal skin. Here, the pheomelanin concentrations of the vitiligo lesion (SPT III: 2.87 g/L, SPT IV: 4.26 g/L and SPT V: 5.82 g/L) are higher than the normal skin for all of the SPTs (SPT III: 0.97 g/L, SPT IV: 1.68 g/L and SPT V: 1.81 g/L). The higher pheomelanin results in paler skin tones.

The phenomena can also be observed in the ratio of pheomelanin to eumelanin. Figure 4.73 shows the ratios of pheomelanin to eumelanin of the vitiligo lesion for several SPTs (SPT III: 0.16, SPT IV: 0.21 and SPT V: 0.26) and the surrounding normal skin lesion (SPT III: 0.06, SPT IV: 0.05 and SPT V: 0.039). As the eumelanin concentration is lower, the pheomelanin concentration of vitiligo lesions tends to be higher than the surrounding normal skin.

Figure 4.74 shows the eumelanin concentrations of melasma lesion compared to normal skin. It is found that the eumelanin concentrations of melasma lesion (SPT III: 39.45 g/L, SPT IV: 44.93 g/L and SPT V: 60.06 g/L) are significantly higher than the surrounding normal skin (SPT III: 29.66 g/L, SPT IV: 37.86 g/L and SPT V: 51.39 g/L). The higher eumelanin concentration results in a darker skin tone compared to the surrounding normal skin.

Figure 4.75 shows the pheomelanin relative concentrations of melasma lesion and its surrounding normal skin. It is found that the pheomelanin concentrations (SPT III: 0.65 g/L, SPT IV: 1.16 g/L and SPT V: 1.28 g/L) are lower than the normal skin for all SPTs (SPT III: 0.79 g/L, SPT IV: 1.78 g/L and SPT V: 1.84 g/L) indicating that melasma disorder also affects the production of pheomelanin in skin.

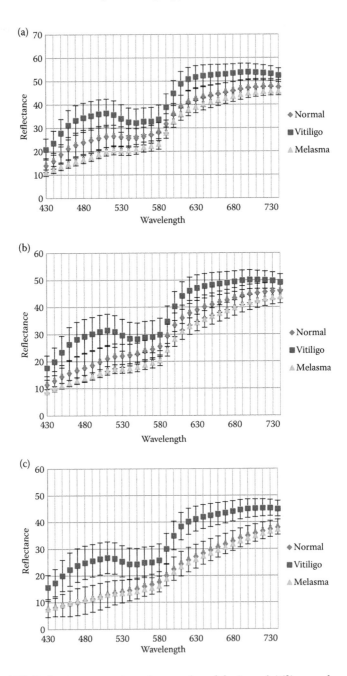

Figure 4.70 Reflectance spectra of normal and lesions (vitiligo and melasma) from (a) SPT III, (b) SPT IV and (c) SPT V.

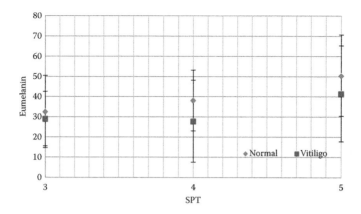

Figure 4.71 Eumelanin relative concentration of vitiligo patients.

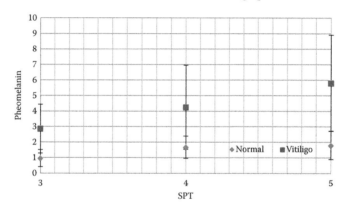

Figure 4.72 Pheomelanin relative concentration of vitiligo patients.

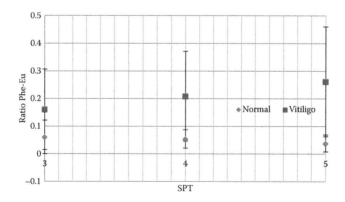

Figure 4.73 Ratio of pheomelanin to eumelanin of vitiligo patients.

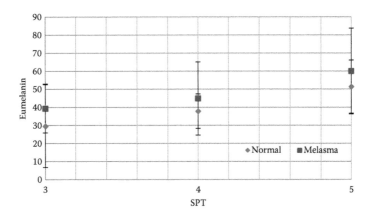

Figure 4.74 Eumelanin relative concentration of melasma patients.

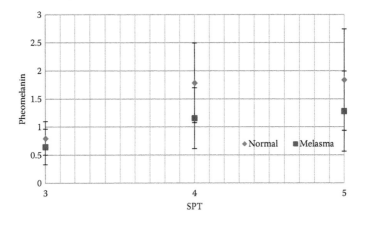

Figure 4.75 Pheomelanin relative concentration of melasma patients.

Figure 4.76 illustrates the ratios of pheomelanin to eumelanin of the melasma lesion and the surrounding normal skin. Here, the ratio of the melasma lesion (SPT III: 0.41, SPT IV: 0.33 and SPT V: 0.29) are significantly higher than the normal skin for all of the SPTs (SPT III: 0.067, SPT IV: 0.055 and SPT V: 0.0.365). The ratios of pheomelanin to eumelanin for melasma are around 6–7 times higher than that of the ratio of normal skin.

Results show that the concentrations of eumelanin of vitiligo are lower (Figure 4.72) and the concentration of pheomelanin of vitiligo are higher (Figure 4.73) than the concentration of eumelanin and pheomelanin of normal skin, resulting in lower light photon absorption. This observation corresponds to the reflectance spectrum data of vitiligo and normal skin, as shown in Figure 4.70.

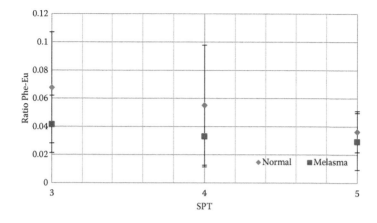

Figure 4.76 Ratio of pheomelanin to eumelanin of melasma patients.

It is also found that the concentrations of eumelanin (Figure 4.75) of all melasma are higher than that of eumelanin of normal skin but the concentrations of pheomelanin (Figure 5.23) are lower, resulting in higher light photon absorption. The result corresponds to the reflectance spectrum of melasma and normal skin in Figure 4.70.

4.7 Conclusion

In skin evaluation, visual cues play an important role. These cues are light reflectance which has been exposed to skin, scattered and re-emitted from the skin. According to the Dichromatic Reflection Model, the light reflectance can be identified as diffused reflectance, the light radiation which has entered the skin and absorbed or scattered within the skin layers. This re-emitted light or reflectance is a function of scattering and absorption of light within various skin layers. Current skin evaluation, however, has not able to use that information yet. The evaluation still depends on the judgement and the expertise of dermatologists. As a result, intra- and inter-observer variations may occur. Therefore, there is a growing need for an objective system which can assist dermatologist in the diagnostic process.

Pigmentation disorder is a condition that causes the skin to appear lighter or darker than normal skin. This condition is due to abnormal melanin production. Melanin is the main colour pigment. There are two categories of melanin, namely eumelanin and pheomelanin are synthesized. Eumelanin is the dark brown-black pigment, whereas pheomelanin is the light red-yellow pigment. It is important to determine the condition of skin pigments such as for assessing treatment efficacy of skin pigmentation disorders and effects of whitening cream. At present however, the assessment of melanin types is invasive; skin biopsy is conducted for chemical analysis of skin samples. Alternative methods that are non-invasive are required.

Moreover, the current evaluation depends on the human visual system and is based on the visual condition of skin surface and is not able to include the conditions of the underlying skin layers and pigments (melanin types and concentration). With the use of imaging technologies, better information of skin data can be obtained. The current skin imaging technologies can capture wider spectral information of skin. A wide spectral information of skin can provide valuable information to non-invasive *in vivo* approach in diagnosing various skin diseases [55]. Moreover, these imaging techniques are non-invasive and the recorded skin data (i.e., skin reflectance) that can be stored for future use. The analysis of the skin data, however, is not straightforward. A development of a system capable of analysing the skin data to obtain the information of the underlying skin layers, especially melanin types and concentrations is required.

Therefore, the objective is to develop such a system which is able of determining and quantifying the melanin types and concentration in a clinical setting based on a digital signal processing approach. The research work began by understanding the fundamental light–skin interaction and the models of light–skin interaction. These models, according to its similarities, can be grouped into five groups: K–M, adding-doubling method, diffuse reflectance, modified Beer–Lambert law and MC simulation. And, it is shown that the accurate model is the MC simulation [33,39,52,80,89,92,115,116]. However, it has not been implemented yet due to the long processing time required. In order for the method to be made available in clinical settings, the processing time of the simulation process must be shorter. In this study, the implementation of the MC simulation of multi-layered skin on a GPU workstation known as CUDA is proposed.

CUDA enables researchers to use the graphics hardware for common computational purpose and provide a better performance compared to the traditional central processing technologies application [34]. The previous work reported by Alerstam comes to be the best in terms of speedup factor. For this reason, the MC simulation on GPU developed by Alerstam is used. The GPU can run the simulation in 15 s only in comparison with 51 min using the traditional central processing unit (CPU).

Subsequently, the inverse process framework is developed. Here, the skin optical characteristics, namely the relative concentrations of eumelanin and pheomelanin and other optical parameters (volume fraction of melanosomes in epidermis and epidermal thickness) are determined from the reflectance spectrum obtained from a spectrophotometer. The inverse analysis uses the MC simulation of light transport in multi-layered tissue or known simply as MCML. MCML simulates the path of a light photon on multi-layered skin tissues. In the inverse procedure, the variable parameters of MCML are fine-tuned until the simulated reflectance and measured reflectance match. To ensure the convergence of this tuning process, an optimisation technique is used.

For MC-based approach, most researchers [38,92,153] propose the use of GA due to the nature of the MC problem. GAs start with an initial population of individuals randomly generated with each individual representing a potential solution. The individuals in GA evolve through successive iterations, called generations. During each generation, the population is evaluated by fitness function [133,175,176] and evolves through selection and reproductions. In our work we combine the rMSE with the gradient error between the simulated reflectance and the measured one as the fitness function. Selection refers to a GA operation to pick solution according to their fitness values.

To evaluate the system, the estimated parameters (namely the relative concentrations of eumelanin and pheomelanin, the volume fraction of melanosome and the epidermal thickness) obtained from the system using reflectance data of participants were inputted into the RSM module of the ASAP software from BRO, to model a computational simulated skin [180,181]. It is envisaged that if the computational simulated skin produced by RSM results in similar reflectance data of the participants, the inverse analysis method is proven to be correct. As reported in the literature, the RSM can be modified to generate the reflectance spectrum data of skin and thus, the reflectance spectrum data can be used for validating the analysis of skin optical parameters [41,42]. There were 36 participants involved in the validation study. From the statistical error analysis between the acquired reflectance spectrum information and reproduced reflectance spectrum due to pigmentation analysis system as determined by RSM, the MAE is only 8.82%, which is acceptable. It is found that the methodology has a solid linear relationship acquired data ($R^2 = 0.994$) showing a system with high accuracy and reliability.

The inverse MCML analysis method estimated that SPT I has 0.039 volume fraction of melanosomes in epidermis, SPT II 0.07, SPT III 0.154, SPT IV 0.178, SPT V 0.29 and SPT VI 0.35. Thus, different pigmentation levels have different volume fraction of melanosome in epidermis as reported by Jacques. Lightly pigmented adults have 0.014–0.04 volume fraction of melanosome, 0.11–0.16 volume fraction for moderately pigmented adults and 0.18–0.43 volume fraction for darkly pigmented adults [86].

The estimated epidermal thickness of the outer forearm ranges from 0.079 to 0.084 mm and these values are within the ranges reported by Lee, indicating a correct estimation. It is estimated that the ratio between pheomelanin and eumelanin of SPT IV is 0.05. The retrieved value is close to the value of 0.049 for SPT IV reported by Parsad [27]. The results obtained in the present study are in line with those reported in the literature indicating a correct estimation.

Observational study II aims to evaluate the performance of the system in analysing skin of vitiligo and melasma patients by recruiting a number of patients suffering from melasma (hyper-pigmented disorder) and vitiligo (hypo-pigmented disorder). Overall, 43 patients were involved in the study. For vitiligo, the method is able to point out the difference of eumelanin and pheomelanin, which resulted in a paler skin tone compared to the surrounding normal skin. It is found that the pheomelanin concentrations (SPT III: 0.65 g/L, SPT IV: 1.16 g/L and SPT V: 1.28 g/L) are lower than the normal skin for all SPTs (SPT III: 0.79 g/L, SPT IV: 1.78 g/L and SPT V: 1.84 g/L) indicating melasma disorder also affects the production of pheomelanin in skin. For melasma, the method is also able to determine the difference of the relative concentration of eumelanin and pheomelanin. It is found that for participants with melasma, their ratio of the melasma lesion (SPT III: 0.41, SPT IV: 0.33 and SPT V: 0.29) are significantly higher than the normal skin for all of the SPTs (SPT III: 0.067, SPT IV: 0.055 and SPT V: 0.0.365). These observations correspond to the reflectance spectrum data of vitiligo – normal skin and melasma – normal skin.

The computerised pigmentation analysis tool has shown the potential to assist dermatologists to monitor a pigmentation disorder and a skin-whitening treatment outcome objectively. It is able to analyse, determine and quantify *in situ* the melanin types and concentration in a non-invasive manner, as shown in the observational studies. It can also provide efficacy assessment to assist dermatologist in making an accurate diagnosis. The system is also able to provide information of eumelanin and pheomelanin concentrations, volume fraction of melanosome and epidermal thickness. With such capabilities, the system can establish a new non-invasive, simple and fast technique and can be performed in a healthcare setting.

In summary, this chapter presented the development of a non-invasive inverse skin analysis system to determine melanin types to solve the need of the objective evaluation of pigmented lesion and skin-whitening treatments. This innovative method will avoid the need of performing bio-chemical analysis, which is invasive, to determine melanin types and concentrations.

Second, the implementation of Monte Carlo for multi-layered skin tissues (MCML) in the system to analyse skin pigmentation is presented. MCML is the state-of-the-art of light–skin interaction simulation. However, it requires an extensive computational power. In the system, MCML is used in GPU settings which can significantly accelerate the skin-light simulations [154]. The GPU-accelerated MCML has a massive speedup factor in comparison with conventional CPU. This will enable the developed system to be run on clinics.

Finally, the development of the optimisation algorithm based on GA on the inverse analysis which enables detailed contribution of skin optical parameters is presented. In our system, the optimisation is used to determine melanin pigment types and concentrations. The determination of haemoglobin, for example, can be used in blood application.

4.8 MATLAB code: MCML

From the Table 4.1, it can be seen that the previous work reported by Alerstam is the best implementation of MCML using GPU [160]. The proposed method implements the MCML based on GPU codes as developed by Alerstam.

```
/*******************************************************************
***********
* Header file for common data structures and constants (CPU and GPU)
*******************************************************************
********
* This file is part of GPUMCML.

#ifndef _GPUMCML_H_
#define _GPUMCML_H_
#define SINGLE_PRECISION
////////////////////////////////////////////////////////////
////////////////////////////////////////////////////////////
// Various data types
typedef unsigned long long UINT64;
typedef unsigned int UINT32;
// MCML constants
#ifdef SINGLE_PRECISION
// NOTE: Single Precision
typedef float GFLOAT;
// Critical weight for roulette
#define WEIGHT 1E-4F
// scaling factor for photon weight, which is then converted to
integer
//
// This factor is preferred to be a power of 2, so that we can make
the
// following precision claim:
// If this factor is 2^N, we maintain N-bit binary digit precision.
//
// Using a power of 2 here can also make multiplication/division
faster.
//
#define WEIGHT_SCALE ((GFLOAT)(1<<24))
#define PI_const 3.1415926F
#define RPI 0.318309886F
#define COSNINETYDEG 1.0E-6F
#define COSZERO (1.0F - 1.0E-6F)
#define CHANCE 0.1F
#define MCML_FP_ZERO 0.0F
#define FP_ONE 1.0F
#define FP_TWO 2.0F
#else // SINGLE_PRECISION
// NOTE: Double Precision
```

```
typedef double GFLOAT;
// Critical weight for roulette
#define WEIGHT 1E-4
// scaling factor for photon weight, which is then converted to
integer
#define WEIGHT_SCALE ((GFLOAT)(1<<24))
#define PI_const 3.1415926
#define RPI 0.318309886
#define COSNINETYDEG 1.0E-6
#define COSZERO (1.0 - 1.0E-12)
#define CHANCE 0.1
#define MCML_FP_ZERO 0.0
#define FP_ONE 1.0
#define FP_TWO 2.0
#endif // SINGLE_PRECISION
#define STR_LEN 200
////////////////////////////////////////////////////////////
////////////////////////////////////////////////////////////
// Data structure for specifying each layer
typedef struct
{
 float z_min;    // Layer z_min [cm]
 float z_max;    // Layer z_max [cm]
 float mutr;          // Reciprocal mu_total [cm]
 float mua;           // Absorption coefficient [1/cm]
 float g;             // Anisotropy factor [-]
 float n;             // Refractive index [-]
} LayerStruct;
// Detection Grid specifications
typedef struct
{
 float dr;       // Detection grid resolution, r-direction [cm]
 float dz;       // Detection grid resolution, z-direction [cm]
 UINT32 na;      // Number of grid elements in angular-direction [-]
 UINT32 nr;      // Number of grid elements in r-direction
 UINT32 nz;      // Number of grid elements in z-direction
} DetStruct;
// Simulation input parameters
typedef struct
{
 char outp_filename[STR_LEN];
 char inp_filename[STR_LEN];
 // the starting and ending offset (in the input file) for this
simulation
 long begin, end;
 // ASCII or binary output
 char AorB;
 UINT32 number_of_photons;
 int ignoreAdetection;
 float start_weight;
 DetStruct det;
 UINT32 n_layers;
 LayerStruct* layers;
```

```
} SimulationStruct;
// Per-GPU simulation states
// One instance of this struct exists in the host memory, while the
other
// in the global memory.
typedef struct
{
// points to a scalar that stores the number of photons that are not
// completed (i.e., ,either on the fly or not yet started)
UINT32 *n_photons_left;
// per-thread seeds for random number generation
// arrays of length NUM_THREADS
// We put these arrays here as opposed to in GPUThreadStates
because
// they live across different simulation runs and must be copied back
// to the host.
UINT64 *x;
UINT32 *a;
// output data
UINT64* Rd_ra;
UINT64* A_rz;          // Pointer to a 2D absorption matrix!
UINT64* Tt_ra;
} SimState;
// Everything a host thread needs to know in order to run
simulation on
// one GPU (host-side only)
typedef struct
{
// GPU identifier
unsigned int dev_id;
// those states that will be updated
SimState host_sim_state;
// simulation input parameters
SimulationStruct *sim;

/* GPU-specific constant parameters */
// number of thread blocks launched
UINT32 n_tblks;
// the limit that indicates overflow of an element of A_rz
// in the shared memory
UINT32 A_rz_overflow;
} HostThreadState;

/////////////////////////////////////////////////////////////////
/////////////////////////////////////////////////////////////////
extern void usage(const char *prog_name);
// Parse the command-line arguments.
// Return 0 if successfull or a +ive error code.
extern int interpret_arg(int argc, char* argv[], char **fpath_p,
    unsigned long long* seed,
    int* ignoreAdetection, unsigned int *num_GPUs);
extern int read_simulation_data(char* filename,
    SimulationStruct** simulations, int ignoreAdetection);
```

```
extern int Write_Simulation_Results(SimState* HostMem,
   SimulationStruct* sim, float simulation_time);
extern void FreeSimulationStruct(SimulationStruct* sim, int
n_simulations);
#endif // _GPUMCML_H_
```

References

1. N. Shamsudin, *Efficacy and safety of tacrolimus ointment in vitiligo using a newly developed digital imaging analysis technique for evaluation of repigmentation progression*, Universiti Kebangsaan Malaysia, 2009.
2. K. Ongenae, L. Beelaert, N. Van Geel, and J.-M. Naeyaert, Psychosocial effects of vitiligo, *Journal of the European Academy of Dermatology and Venereology JEADV*, vol. 20, no. 1, pp. 1–8, 2006.
3. A. G. Smith and R. A. Sturm, Multiple genes and locus interactions in susceptibility to vitiligo, *Journal of Investigative Dermatology*, vol. 130, no. 3, pp. 643–645, 2010.
4. G. Laberge, C. M. Mailloux, K. Gowan, P. Holland, D. C. Bennett, P. R. Fain, and R. A. Spritz, Early disease onset and increased risk of other autoimmune diseases in familial generalized vitiligo, *Pigment Cell Research Sponsored by European Society for Pigment Cell Research and the International Pigment Cell Society*, vol. 18, no. 4, pp. 300–305, 2005.
5. R. J. Lutfi, M. Fridmanis, A. L. Misiunas, O. Pafume, E. A. Gonzalez, J. A. Villemur, M. A. Mazzini, and H. Niepomniszcze, Association of melasma with thyroid autoimmunity and other thyroidal abnormalities and their relationship to the origin of the melasma, *Journal of Clinical Endocrinology and Metabolism*, vol. 61, no. 1, pp. 28–31, 1985.
6. P. K. Buxton, *ABC of Dermatology*, 4th ed. London: BMJ Publishing Group, 2003.
7. S. Kingman, Growing awareness of skin disease starts flurry of initiatives, *Bulletin of the World Health Organization*, vol. 83, pp. 11–13, 2005.
8. J. Serup, G. Jemec, and G. Grove, *Handbook of Non-Invasive Methods and the Skin*. Boca Raton: CRC Press, 2006.
9. A. Abdul-Rahman and M. Chen, Spectral volume rendering based on the Kubelka-Munk Theory, *Eurographics*, vol. 24, no. 3, pp. 2005.
10. Z. U. Syed and I. H. Hamzavi, Photomedicine and phototherapy considerations for patients with skin of color, *Photodermatology, Photoimmunology and Photomedicine*, vol. 27, no. 1, pp. 10–16, 2011.
11. T. B. Fitzpatrick, The validity and practicality of sun-reactive skin types I through VI, *Archives of Dermatology*, vol. 124, no. 6, pp. 869–871, 1988.
12. Y. B. Choe, S. J. Jang, S. J. Jo, K. J. Ahn, and J. I. Youn, The difference between the constitutive and facultative skin color does not reflect skin phototype in Asian skin, *Skin Research and Technology Official Journal of International Society for Bioengineering and the Skin (ISBS) and International Society for Digital Imaging of Skin (ISDIS) and International Society for Skin Imaging (ISSI)*, vol. 12, no. 1, pp. 68–72, 2006.
13. I. Galván and J. J. Sanz, Brief report on Measuring plumage colour using different spectrophotometric techniques: A word of caution, *Ornis Fennica (Montgomerie)*, vol. 87, no. 2006, pp. 69–76, 2010.

14. A. Thody, E. Higgins, K. Wakamatsu, S. Ito, S. Burchill, and J. Marks, Pheomelanin as well as eumelanin is present in human epidermis, *Journal of Investigative Dermatology*, vol. 97, pp. 340–344, 1991.
15. J. M. Gillbro and M. J. Olsson, The melanogenesis and mechanisms of skin-lightening agents—Existing and new approaches, *International Journal of Cosmetic Science*, vol. 33, no. 3, pp. 210–221, Jun. 2011.
16. C. D. Villarama and H. I. Maibach, Glutathione as a depigmenting agent: An overview, *International Journal of Cosmetic Science*, vol. 27, pp. 147–153, 2005.
17. S. Zhong, Y. Wu, A. Soo-Mi, J. Zhao, K. Wang, S. Yang, Y. Jae-Ho, and X. Zhu, Depigmentation of melanocytes by the treatment of extracts from traditional Chinese herbs: A cell culture assay, *Biological and Pharmaceutical Bulletin*, vol. 29, no. 9, pp. 1947–1951, 2006.
18. K. D. Kim, M. H. Song, E. K. Yum, O. S. Jeon, Y. W. Ju, and M. S. Chang, 2,4-Dihydroxycinnamic esters as skin depigmenting agents, *Bulletin of Korean Chemical Society*, vol. 30, no. 7, pp. 1619–1621, 2009.
19. Global Industry Analysts, Skin lighteners: A global strategic business report, 2009.
20. C. M. Burgess, *Cosmetic Dermatology*, 1st ed. Berlin: Springer Verlag, 2005.
21. M. Storring, *Computer Vision and Human Skin Colour*, Aalborg University, Denmark, 2004.
22. V. Tuchin, Handbook of photonics for biomedical science, *Anticancer Research*, vol. 30, no. 8, pp. 3215–3216, 2010.
23. P. D. Burns and R. S. Berns, Color and Imaging Conference, 4th Color and Imaging Conference Final Program and Proceedings, Society for Imaging Science and Technology, vol. 4, pp. 19–22.
24. A. A. Christy, O. M. Kvalheim, and R. A. Velapoldi, Spectroscopy quantitative analysis in diffuse reflectance spectrometry: A modified Kubelka-Munk equation, *Vibrational Spectroscopy*, vol. 9, pp. 19–27, 1995.
25. S. Ito and K. Jimbow, Quantitative analysis of eumelanin and pheomelanin in hair and melanomas, *Journal of Investigative Dermatology*, vol. 80, no. 4, pp. 268–272, 1983.
26. K. Wakamatsu, S. Ito, and J. L. Rees, The usefulness of 4-amino-3-hydroxy-phenylalanine as a specific marker of pheomelanin, *Pigment Cell Research*, vol. 15, no. 3, pp. 225–232, 2002.
27. D. Parsad, K. Wakamatsu, A. J. Kanwar, B. Kumar, and S. Ito, Eumelanin and phaeomelanin contents of depigmented and repigmented skin in vitiligo patients, *British Journal of Dermatology*, vol. 149, no. 3, pp. 624–626, 2003.
28. A. Hennessy, C. Oh, B. Diffey, K. Wakamatsu, S. Ito, and J. Rees, Eumelanin and pheomelanin concentrations in human epidermis before and after UVB irradiation, *Pigment Cell Research*, vol. 18, no. 3, pp. 220–223, Jun. 2005.
29. R. Wolber, K. Schlenz, K. Wakamatsu, C. Smuda, Y. Nakanishi, V. Hearing, and S. Ito, Pigmentation effects of solar simulated radiation as compared with UVA and UVB radiation, *Pigment Cell & Melanoma Research*, vol. 21, no. 4, pp. 487–491, 2009.
30. D. G. Patil, Miles R Chedekel, and M. R. Chedekel, Sythesis and analysis of pheomelanin degradation products, *Journal of Organic Chemistry*, vol. 49, no. 10, pp. 997–1000, 1984.

31. L. Panzella, P. Manini, G. Monfrecola, M. d'Ischia, and A. Napolitano, An easy-to-run method for routine analysis of eumelanin and pheomelanin in pigmented tissues, *Pigment Cell Research*, vol. 20, no. 2, pp. 128–133, 2007.

32. B. Kongshoj, A. Thorleifsson, and H. C. Wulf, Pheomelanin and eumelanin in human skin determined by high-performance liquid chromatography and its relation to *in vivo* reflectance measurements, *Photodermatology, Photoimmunology and Photomedicine*, vol. 22, no. 3, pp. 141–147, 2006.

33. N. Ren, J. Liang, X. Qu, J. Li, B. Lu, and J. Tian, GPU-based Monte Carlo simulation for light propagation in complex heterogeneous tissues, *Optics Express*, vol. 18, no. 7, pp. 6811–6823, 2010.

34. J. Sanders and E. Kandrot, *Cuda by Example: An Introduction to General Purpose GPU Programming*. Boston: Pearson Education, 2010.

35. E. Alerstam, W. Chun, Y. Lo, T. D. Han, J. Rose, S. Andersson-engels, and L. Lilge, Next-generation acceleration and code optimization for light transport in turbid media using GPUs abstract, *Optics Express*, vol. 1, no. 2, pp. 658–675, 2010.

36. A. Doronin and I. Meglinski, Online Monte Carlo based calculator of human skin spectra and color, *Proceedings of SPIE*, vol. 8337, pp. 833702–833702-8, 2012.

37. Q. Fang and D. A. Boas, Monte Carlo simulation of photon migration in 3D turbid media accelerated by graphics processing units, *Optics Express*, vol. 17, no. 22, pp. 20178–20190, 2009.

38. P. Valisuo, *Photonics imulation and modelling of skin for design of spectrocutometer*, Universitas Wasaensis, 2011.

39. T. Lister, P. A. Wright, and P. H. Chappell, Optical properties of human skin, *Journal of Biomedical Optics*, vol. 17, no. 9, pp. 1–15, 2012.

40. A. E. Karsten and J. E. Smith, Modelling and verification of melanin concentration on human skin type, *Photochemistry and Photobiology*, vol. 88, no. 2, pp. 469–474, 2012.

41. R. R. Anderson and J. A. Parrish, The optics of human skin, *Journal of Investigative Dermatology*, vol. 77, no. 1, pp. 13–19, 198AD.

42. E. Angelopoulou, Understanding the color of human skin, Technical Report MS-CIS-99-29, Stevens Institute of Technology, 1999, pp. 1–14.

43. P.F. Millington and R. Wilkinson, *Skin (Biological Structure and Function)*. Cambridge University Press, 1983.

44. *Skin Anatomy* [Online]. Available: www.enchantedlearning.com. [Accessed 12 January 2014].

45. T. Igarashi, K. Nishino, and S. K. Nayar, The appearance of human skin: A survey, *Foundations and Trends® in Computer Graphics and Vision*, vol. 3, no. 1, pp. 1–95, 2007.

46. M. Doi and S. Tominaga, Spectral estimation of human skin color using The Kubelka-Munk Theory, *in SPIE-IS&T Electronic Imaging*, 2003, vol. 5008, no. May 2011, pp. 221–228.

47. S. L. Jacques, Origins of tissue optical properties in the UVA, visible and NIR region, in *Advances in Optical Imaging and Photon Migaration*. Optical Society of America, 1996, pp. 364–370.

48. S. Takatani and M. D. Graham, Theoretical analysis of diffuse reflectance from a two-layer tissue model, *IEEE Transactions on Biomedical Engineering*, vol. 26, pp. 656–664, 1987.

49. H. Du, R. A. Fuh, J. Li, A. Corkan, and J. S. Lindsey, PhotochemCAD: A computer-aided design and research tool in photochemistry, *Photochemistry and Photobiology*, vol. 68, pp. 141–142, 1998.

50. J. F. Blinn, Models of light reflection for computer synthesized pictures, in *ACM SIGGRAPH Computer Graphics*, 1977, pp. 192–198.

51. I. V Meglinski and S. J. Matcher, Modelling the sampling volume for skin blood oxygenation measurements, *Medical & Biological Engineering & Computing*, vol. 39, no. 1, pp. 44–50, 2001.

52. P. S. Holcomb, Under the skin, in *Optics Design: Virtual Prototyping*, 2006, pp. 56–58.

53. M. Storring, H. J. Andersen, and E. Granum, Estimation of the illuminant colour from human skin colour, in *Fourth IEEE International Conference on Automatic Face and Gesture Recognition*, 2000, no. March, pp. 64–69.

54. R. N. Clark, Reflectance spectra, in *Rock Physics and Phase Relations: A Handbook of Physical Constants*. American Geophysical Union, 1995, pp. 178–188.

55. I. V Meglinski and S. J. Matcher, Computer simulation of the skin reflectance spectra, *Computer Methods and Programs in Biomedicine*, vol. 70, no. 2, pp. 179–186, 2003.

56. A. Bhandari, B. Hamre, Ø. Frette, K. Stamnes, and J. J. Stamnes, Modeling optical properties of human skin using Mie theory for particles with different size distributions and refractive indices, *Optics Express*, vol. 19, no. 15, pp. 448–457, 2011.

57. D. Judd and G. Wyszecki, Color in Business, *Science and Industry*. New York: John Wiley & Sons, 1975.

58. E. Church and P. Takacs, Surface scattering, in *Handbook of Optics, Vol. I: Fundamentals, Techniques, & Design)*. New York: McGraw-Hill Inc., 1995, pp. 7.1–7.14.

59. McCartney, *Optics of the Atmosphere: Scattering by Molecules and Particles*. New York: John Wiley & Sons Inc., 1976.

60. M. Mishchenko, J. Hovenier, and L. Travis, *Light Scattering by Nonspherical Particles: Theory, Measurements, and Applications*. San Diego: Academic Press, 2000.

61. E. J. Parra, Human pigmentation variation: Evolution, genetic basis, and implications for public health, *Yearbook of Physical Anthropology*, vol. 50, pp. 85–105, 2007.

62. H. Zollinger, *Color: A Multidisciplinary Approach*, vol. 26, no. 3. New York: Wiley-VCH, 1999, pp. 1–258.

63. F. Träger, *Springer Handbook of Lasers and Optics*, vol. 72, no. 3. New York: Springer, 2007, p. 1332.

64. D. Eng and G. V. G. Baranoski, The application of photoacoustic absorption spectral data to the modeling of leaf optical properties in the visible range, vol. 45, no. 12, 2007, pp. 4077–4086.

65. J. van de Wijer and S. Beigpour, The dichromatic reflection model: Future research directions and applications, in *International Joint Conference on Computer Vision, Imaging and Computer Graphics Theory and Applications*, 2011.

66. K. P. Nielsen, L. Zhao, J. J. Stamnes, K. Stamnes, and J. Moan, The importance of the depth distribution of melanin in skin for DNA protection and other photobiological processes, *Journal of Photochemistry and Photobiology B*, vol. 82, no. 3, pp. 194–198, 2006.

67. M. Doi, N. Tanaka, and S. Tominaga, Reflectance spectrum estimation of human skin and its application to image rendering, *Journal of Imaging Science and Technology*, vol. 49, no. 6, 2005.

68. S. Tominaga and B. A. Wandell, Standard surface-reflectance model and illuminant estimation, *Journal of the Optical Society of America A*, vol. 6, no. 4, p. 576, 1989.

69. N. Tsumura, N. Ojima, K. Sato, M. Shiraishi, H. Shimizu, H. Nabeshima, S. Akazaki, K. Hori, and Y. Miyake, Image-based skin color and texture analysis/synthesis by extracting hemoglobin and melanin information in the skin, *Journal of the ACM Transactions on Graph*, vol. 22, no. 3, pp. 770–779, 2003.

70. S. A. Shafer, Using color to separate reflection components, *Color Research and Application*, vol. 10, no. 4, pp. 210–218, 1985.

71. G. Poirier, *Human Skin Modelling and Rendering*, University of Waterloo, 2003.

72. D. Yudovsky and L. Pilon, Retrieving skin properties from *in vivo* reflectance spectrum measurements, *Journal of Biophotonics*, vol. 4, no. 5, pp. 305–314, 2011.

73. J. A. D. Atencio, S. L. Jacques, and S. V. Montiel, Monte Carlo modeling of light propagation in neonatal skin, in *Applications of Monte Carlo Methods in Biology, Medicine and Other Fields of Science*, 1987.

74. B. C. Wilson and S. L. Jacques, Optical reflectance and transmittance of tissues: principles and applications, *IEEE J. Quantum Electron*, vol. 26, no. 12, pp. 2186–2199, 1990.

75. A. Krishnaswamy, *BioSpec: A biophysically-based spectral model of light interaction with human skin*, University of Waterloo, 2005.

76. J. Qin and R. Lu, Measurement of the optical properties of apples using hyperspectral diffuse reflectance imaging, in *ASABE Annual International Meeting*, 2006, vol. 0300, no. 06, pp. 2–16.

77. I. V Meglinski and S. J. Matcher, Quantitative assessment of skin layers absorption and skin reflectance spectra simulation in the visible and near-infrared spectral regions, *Physiological Measurement*, vol. 23, no. 4, pp. 741–753, 2002.

78. G. V. G. Baranoski, Biophysically-based appearance models: The bumpy road toward predictability, in *ACM Siggraph Asia*, 2009, no. December.

79. G. V. G. Baranoski and A. Krishnaswamy, Light interaction with human skin: From believable images to predictable models, in *SIGGRAPH ASIA*, 2008.

80. G. V. G. Baranoski and A. Krishnaswamy, *Light and Skin Interaction: Simulations for Computer Graphic Applications*. Burlington, MA: Elsevier, 2010.

81. Y. Yamaguchi, M. Brenner, and V. J. Hearing, The regulation of skin pigmentation, *Journal of Biological Chemistry*, vol. 282, no. 38, pp. 27557–27561, 2007.

82. A. N. Bashkatov, E. A. Genina, V. I. Kochubey, and V. V Tuchin, Optical properties of human skin, subcutaneous and mucous tissues in the wavelength range from 400 to 2000 nm, vol. 38, pp. 2543–2555, 2005.

83. E. Angelopoulou, The reflectance spectrum of human skin the reflectance spectrum of human skin (MS-CIS-99-29), 1999.

84. L. T. Norvang, T. E. Milner, J. S. Nelson, M. W. Berns, and L. O. Svaasand, Original articles skin pigmentation characterized by visible reflectance measurements, *Lasers in Medical Science*, vol. 12, pp. 99–112, 1997.

85. C. Donner, T. Weyrich, E. d'Eon, R. Ramamoorthi, and S. Rusinkiewicz, A layered heterogeneous reflectance model for acquiring and rendering human skin, *ACM Transactions on Graphics*, vol. 27, no. 5, p. 1, 2008.

86. S. L. Jacques, Laser-tissue interactions. Photochemical, photothermal, and photomechanical, Jun. 1992.

87. S. A. Prahl, M. Keijzer, S. L. Jacques, and A. J. Welch, A Monte Carlo model of light propagation in tissue, *Medicine (Baltimore)*, vol. I, no. 1989, pp. 102–1111, 1989.

88. V. Bartosova, *Skin effects and UV dosimetry of climate therapy in patients with psoriasis*, Norwegian University of Science and Technology, 2010.

89. T. Lister, P. Wright, and P. Chappell, Spectrophotometers for the clinical assessment of port-wine stain skin lesions: A review, *Lasers in Medical Science*, vol. 25, no. 3, pp. 449–457, 2010.

90. R. Lee, M. M. Mathews-Roth, M. A. Pathak, and J. A. Parrish, The detection of carotenoid pigments in human skin, *Journal of Investigative Dermatology*, vol. 64, no. 3, pp. 175–177, 1975.

91. T. Dwyer, H. K. Muller, L. Blizzard, R. Ashbolt, and G. Phillips, The use of spectrophotometry to estimate melanin density in Caucasians, *Cancer Epidemiology, Biomarkers & Prevention*, vol. 7, no. 3, pp. 203–206, 1998.

92. R. Zhang, W. Verkruysse, B. Choi, J. A Viator, B. Jung, L. O. Svaasand, G. Aguilar, and J. S. Nelson, Determination of human skin optical properties from spectrophotometric measurements based on optimization by genetic algorithms, *Journal of Biomedical Optics*, vol. 10, no. 2, pp. 1–11, 2005.

93. E. Claridge, S. Cotton, M. Moncrieff, and P. Hall, Spectrophotometric intracutaneous imaging (Siascopy): Method and clinical applications, in *Handbook of Non-Invasive Methods and the Skin*. 2006, pp. 315–325.

94. P. J. Matts, P. J. Dykes, and R. Marks, The distribution of melanin in skin determined *in vivo*, *British Journal of Dermatology*, vol. 156, no. 4, pp. 620–628, 2007.

95. J. K. Bowmaker and H. J. Dartnall, Visual pigments of rods and cones in a human retina, *Journal of Physiology*, vol. 298, no. 1, pp. 501–511, 1980.

96. B. Y. K. T. Mullen, Bornstein changes in brightness matches may have produced artifacts in previous isoluminant, pp. 381–400, 1985.

97. B. E. Bayer, *Color Imaging Array*, 555477, 1976.

98. M. H. Rowe, Trichromatic color vision in primates, *News in Physiological Sciences*, vol. 17, no. pp. 93–98, 2002.

99. T. Numahara, From the standpoint of dermatology,in *Digital Colour Imaging in Biomedicine*, pp. 67–72, 2001.

100. K. S. Nehal, S. A. Oliveria, A. A. Marghoob, P. J. Christos, S. Dusza, J. S. Tromberg, and A. C. Halpern, Use of and beliefs about baseline photography in the management of patients with pigmented lesions: A survey of dermatology residency programmes in the United States, *Melanoma Research*, vol. 12, no. 2, pp. 161–167, 2002.

101. J. L. Stone, R. L. Peterson, and J. E. W. Jr., Digital imaging techniques in dermatology, *Journal of the American Academy of Dermatology*, vol. 23, no. 5, pp. 913–917, 1990.

102. J. Yamamoto, A. Ikeda, T. Satow, M. Matsuhashi, K. Baba, F. Yamane, S. Miyamoto, T. Mihara, T. Hori, W. Taki, N. Hashimoto, and H. Shibasaki, Human eye fields in the frontal lobe as studied by epicortical recording of movement-related cortical potentials, *Brain*, vol. 127, no. Pt 4, pp. 873–887, 2004.

103. N. Smit, J. Vicanova, and S. Pavel, The hunt for natural skin whitening agents, *International Journal of Molecular Science*, vol. 10, no. 12, pp. 5326–5349, 2009.
104. K. Burton, J. Jeon, S. Wachsmann-Hogiu, and D. Farkas, Spectral optical imaging in biology and medicine, in *Biomedical Optical Imaging*. Oxford University Press, 2009, pp. 1–44.
105. M. Kalderon, Metamerism, constancy, and knowing which, *Mind*, vol. 117, no. 468, pp. 549–585, 2008.
106. J. Y. Hardeberg, F. Schmitt, and H. Brettel, Multispectral color image capture using a liquid crystal tunable filter, *Optical Engineering*, vol. 41, no. 10, pp. 2532–2548, 2002.
107. J. Brauers, N. Schulte, and T. Aach, Multispectral filter-wheel cameras: Geometric distortion model and compensation algorithms, *IEEE Transactions on Image Processing*, vol. 17, no. 12, pp. 2368–2380, 2008.
108. R. Liang, *Optical Design for Biomedical Imaging*. Washington: SPIE, 2010.
109. F. S. Azar and X. Intes, *Translational Multimodality Optical Imaging*. Norwood: Artech House, 2008.
110. M. G. Gore, *Spectrophotometry and Spectrofluorimetry: A Practical Approach*. New York: Oxford University Press, 2000, p. 368.
111. L. K. Pershing, V. P. Tirumala, J. L. Nelson, J. L. Corlett, A. G. Lin, L. J. Meyer, and S. A. Leachman, Reflectance spectrophotometer: The dermatologists' sphygmomanometer for skin phototyping? *Journal of Investigative Dermatology*, vol. 128, no. 7, pp. 1633–1640, 2008.
112. G. Zonios and A. Dimou, Modeling diffuse reflectance from homogeneous semi-infinite turbid media for biological tissue applications: A Monte Carlo study, *Biomedical Optics Express*, vol. 2, no. 12, pp. 3284–3294, 2011.
113. M. J. C. van Gemert, S. L. Jacques, H. J. Sterenborg, and W. M. Star, Skin optics, *IEEE Transactions on Biomedical Engineering*, vol. 36, no. 12, pp. 1146–1154, 1989.
114. G. Zonios, J. Bykowski, and N. Kollias, Skin melanin, hemoglobin, and light scattering properties can be quantitatively assessed *in vivo* using diffuse reflectance spectroscopy, *Journal of Investigative Dermatology*, vol. 117, no. 6, pp. 1452–1457, 2001.
115. D. Yudovsky and L. Pilon, Rapid and accurate estimation of blood saturation, melanin content, and epidermis thickness from spectral diffuse reflectance, *Applied Optics*, vol. 49, no. 10, pp. 1707–1719, 2010.
116. S. K. Alla, J. F. Clark, and F. R. Beyette, Signal processing system to extract serum bilirubin concentration from diffuse reflectance spectrum of human skin, *Conference Proceedings—IEEE Engineering in Medicine and Biology Society*, vol. 2009, pp. 1290–1293, 2009.
117. T. J. Farrell, M. S. Patterson, and B. Wilson, A diffusion theory model of spatially resolved, steady-state diffuse reflectance for the noninvasive determination of tissue optical properties *in vivo*, *Medical Physics*, vol. 19, no. 4, pp. 879–888, 1992.
118. R. M. Doornbos, R. Lang, M. C. Aalders, F. W. Cross, and H. J. Sterenborg, The determination of *in vivo* human tissue optical properties and absolute chromophore concentrations using spatially resolved steady-state diffuse reflectance spectroscopy, *Physics in Medicine and Biology*, vol. 44, no. 4, pp. 967–981, 1999.

119. N. T. Sumura, D. K. Awazoe, T. N. Akaguchi, N. O. Jima, and Y. M. Iyake, Regression-based model of skin diffuse reflectance for skin color analysis, *Optical Review*, vol. 15, no. 6, pp. 292–294, 2008.

120. C. Fan, A. Shuaib, and G. Yao, Path-length resolved reflectance in tendon and muscle, *Optics Express*, vol. 19, no. 9, pp. 8879–8887, 2011.

121. G. Zonios, A. Dimou, I. Bassukas, D. Galaris, A. Tsolakidis, and E. Kaxiras, Melanin absorption spectroscopy: New method for noninvasive skin investigation and melanoma detection. *Journal of Biomedical Optics*, vol. 13, no. 1, p. 014017, 2011.

122. H. Zeng, H. Lui, C. Macaulay, D. I. Mclean, and B. Palcic, Tissue optics: Optical spectroscopy for skin cancer diagnosis, *Cancer Imaging*, 2001.

123. N. Rajaram, J. S. Reichenberg, M. R. Migden, T. H. Nguyen, and J. W. Tunnell, Pilot clinical study for quantitative spectral diagnosis of non-melanoma skin cancer, *Lasers in Surgery and Medicine*, vol. 42, no. 10, pp. 716–727, 2010.

124. E. B. Smith, *Skin cancer detection by oblique-incidence diffuse reflectance spectroscopy*, Texas A&M University, 2006.

125. P. R. Bargo, S. A. Prahl, T. T. Goodell, R. A. Sleven, G. Koval, G. Blair, and S. L. Jacques, In vivo determination of optical properties of normal and tumor tissue with white light reflectance and an empirical light transport model during endoscopy, *Journal of Biomedical Optics*, vol. 10, no. 3, p. 034018, 2005.

126. C. Zhu and Q. Liu, Validity of the semi-infinite tumor model in diffuse reflectance spectroscopy for epithelial cancer diagnosis: A Monte Carlo study, *Optics Express*, vol. 19, no. 18, pp. 17799–17812, 2011.

127. P. Kubelka, New contributions to the optics of intensely light-scattering materials. Part I, *Journal of the Optical Society of America*, vol. 38, no. 5, pp. 448–457, 1948.

128. J. Saunderson, Calculation of the color of pigmented plastics, *JOSA*, vol. 32, no. 12, pp. 727–729, 1942.

129. P. Kubelka, New contributions to the optics of intensely light-scattering materials. Part II: Nonhomogeneous layers, *Journal of the Optical Society of America*, vol. 44, no. 4, p. 330, 1954.

130. A. Mandelis and J. P. Grossman, Perturbation theory approach to the generalized Kubelka–Munk problem in non-homogeneous optical media, *Applied Spectroscopy*, vol. 46, pp. 737–745, 1992.

131. S. Wan, R. R. Anderson, and J. A. Parrish, Analytical modeling for the optical properties of the skin with *in vitro* and *in vivo* applications, *Photochemistry and Photobiology*, vol. 34, no. 4, pp. 493–499, 1981.

132. S. Cotton, Developing a predictive model of human skin colouring, in *SPIE vol 2708, Medical Imaging*, vol. 2708, 1996, pp. 814–825.

133. E. Claridge and S. J. Preece, An inverse method for the recovery of tissue parameters from colour images, *Information Processing in Medical Imaging*, vol. 18, pp. 306–317, 2003.

134. M. Doi, R. Ohtsuki, and S. Tominaga, Spectral estimation of skin color with foundation makeup, *Image Analysis*, 2005, pp. 95–104.

135. R. Jolivot, *Development of an imaging system dedicated to the acquisition, analysis and multispectral characterisation of skin lesions*, University of Burgundy, 2011.

136. R. Jolivot, H. Nugroho, P. Vabres, M. H. A. Fadzil, and U. M. R. Cnrs, Validation of a 2D multispectral camera: Application to dermatology/cosmetology on a population covering five skin phototypes, in *European Conference on Biomedical Optics (ECBO)*, vol. 33, no. 0, Munich, Germany, 2011.

137. R. Jolivot, P. Vabres, and F. Marzani, Reconstruction of hyperspectral cutaneous data from an artificial neural network-based multispectral imaging system, *Computerized Medical Imaging and Graphics: Official Journal of the Computerized Medical Imaging Society*, vol. 35, no. 2, pp. 85–88, 2011.

138. H. C. Van De Hulst, *Light Scattering by Small Particles*, vol. 1, no. 275. Dover Publications, 1981, p. 470.

139. S. A. Prahl, M. J. C. Van Gemert, and A. J. Welch, Determining the optical properties of turbid media using the adding-doubling method, *Applied Optics*, vol. 32, pp. 559–568, 1996.

140. T. L. Troy and S. N. Thennadil, Optical properties of human skin in the near infrared wavelength range of 1000 to 2200 nm, *Journal of Biomedical Optics*, vol. 6, no. 2, pp. 167–176, 2001.

141. A. Ishimaru, *Wave Propagation and Scattering in Random Media*, vol. 2. New York: Academic Press, 1978, p. 600.

142. D. K. Sardar and L. B. Levy, Optical properties of whole blood, *Lasers in Medical Science*, vol. 13, pp. 106–111, 1998.

143. M. Shimada, Y. Masuda, Y. Yamada, M. Itoh, M. Takahash, and T. Yataga, Explanation of human skin color by multiple linear regression analysis based on the modified Lalnbert–Beer Law, *Optical Review*, vol. 7, no. 4, pp. 348–352, 2000.

144. A. F. M. Hani, H. Nugroho, N. M. Noor, K. F. Rahim, and R. Baba, A modified Beer–Lambert model of skin diffuse reflectance for the determination, in *IFMBE Proceedings* 35, 2011, pp. 393–397.

145. G. S. Fishman, Monte Carlo: Concepts, algorithms, and applications, *Nature Medicine (Springer)*, vol. 8, no. 6, p. 539, 1996.

146. L. Wang, S. L. Jacques, and L. Zheng, MCML—Monte Carlo modeling of light transport in multi-layered tissues, *Computer Methods and Programs in Biomedicine*, vol. 47, no. 2, pp. 131–146, 1995.

147. A. Krishnaswamy, G. V. G. Baranoski, N. Phenomena, and S. Group, *A Study on Skin Optics*, pp. 1–17, 2004.

148. A. N. Bashkatov, E. A. Genina, and V. V. Tuchin, Optical properties of skin, subcutaneous, and muscle tissues: A review, *Journal of Innovative Optical Health Sciences*, vol. 04, no. 01, p. 9, 2011.

149. N. Tsumura, M. Kawabuchi, H. Haneishi, and Y. Miyake, Mapping pigmentation in human skin by multi-visible-spectral imaging by inverse optical scattering technique, *Journal of Imaging Science and Technology*, vol. 45, no. 5, pp. 444–450, 2001.

150. B. T. Cox, S. R. Arridge, and P. C. Beard, Estimating chromophore distributions from multiwavelength photoacoustic images, *Journal of the Optical Society of America A. Optics Image Science and Vision*, vol. 26, no. 2, pp. 443–455, 2009.

151. S. H. Choi, Fast and robust extraction of optical and morphological properties of human skin using a hybrid stochastic-deterministic algorithm: Monte-Carlo simulation study, *Lasers in Medical Science*, vol. 25, no. 5, pp. 733–741, 2010.

152. T. M. Aeda, N. A. Rakawa, M. T. Akahashi, and Y. A. Izu, Monte Carlo simulation of reflectance spectrum using a multilayered skin tissue model, *Optical Review*, vol. 17, no. 3, pp. 223–229, 2010.

153. P. Välisuo, T. Mantere, and J. Alander, Solving optical skin simulation model parameters using genetic algorithm, in *2nd International Conference on Biomedical Engineering and Informatics*, 2009, pp. 1–5.
154. E. Alerstam, T. Svensson, and S. Andersson-Engels, Parallel computing with graphics processing units for high-speed Monte Carlo simulation of photon migration, *Journal of Biomedical Optics*, vol. 13, no. 6, p. 060504, 2008.
155. C. Andrieu, An introduction to MCMC for machine learning, *Science* no. 80, pp. 5–43, 2003.
156. M. Matsumoto and T. Nishimura, Mersenne Twister: A 623-dimensionally equidistributed uniform pseudorandom number generator, *ACM Transactions on Modelling and Computer Simulations: Special Issue on Uniform Random Number Generation*, 1998.
157. W. Sterry, R. Paus, and W. Burgdorf, *Thieme Clinical Companions: Dermatology*, 5th ed. Stuttgart, Gemany: Georg Thieme Verlag, 2006.
158. G. V. G. Baranoski, B. Kimmel, and M. Carlo, Revisiting the foundations of subsurface scattering, 2003.
159. S. Kumari and A. K. Nirala, Study of light propagation in human, rabbit and rat liver tissue by Monte Carlo simulation, *Optik—International Journal for Light and Electron Optics*, vol. 122, no. 9, pp. 807–810, 2010.
160. E. Alerstam and S. Andersson-engels, *Monte Carlo Simulations of Light Transport in Tissue Computer Exercise*. Department of Physics, Lund, 2011, pp. 1–12.
161. Q. Liu and N. Ramanujam, Sequential estimation of optical properties of a two-layered epithelial tissue model from depth-resolved ultraviolet-visible diffuse reflectance spectra, *Applied Optics*, vol. 45, no. 19, pp. 4776–4790, 2006.
162. G. M. Palmer and N. Ramanujam, Monte Carlo-based inverse model for calculating tissue optical properties. Part I: Theory and validation on synthetic phantoms, *Applied Optics*, vol. 45, no. 5, pp. 1062–1071, 2006.
163. NVIDIA, NVIDIA CUDA C Getting Started Guide For Microsoft Windows, *Development*, no. August. 2010.
164. A. Badal and A. Badano, Monte Carlo simulation of X-ray imaging using a graphics processing unit, *IEEE*, no. 3, pp. 4081–4084, 2009, DOI: 10.1109/NSSMIC.2009.5402382.
165. M. Shimada, Y. Yamada, M. Itoh, and T. Yatagai, Melanin and blood concentration in a human skin model studied by multiple regression analysis: Assessment by Monte Carlo simulation, *Physics in Medicine and Biology*, vol. 46, no. 9, pp. 2397–2406, 2001.
166. E. Vieth, Fitting piecewise linear regression functions to biological responses, *Journal of Applied Physiology*, vol. 67, no. 1, pp. 390–396, 1989.
167. G. F. Malash and M. I. El-Khaiary, Piecewise linear regression: A statistical method for the analysis of experimental adsorption data by the intraparticle-diffusion models, *Chemical Engineering Journal*, vol. 163, no. 3, pp. 256–263, 2010.
168. T. Weise, *Global Optimization Algorithms –Theory and Application*, 2nd ed. 2009.
169. M. Melanie, *An Introduction to Genetic Algorithms*, 5th ed. Cambridge, MA: MIT Press, 1999.
170. C. Reeves and J. Rowe, *Genetic Algorithms – Principles and Perspectives*. Dordrecht: Kluwer Academic Publishers, 2002.
171. R. L. Haupt, S. E. Haupt, and A. J. Wiley, *Practical Genetic Algorithms*. New Jersey: John Wiley & Sons, 2004.

172. D. A. Coley, *An Introduction to Genetic Algorithms for Scientists and Engineers.* Singapore: World Scientific Publishing, 1999.

173. N. Kollias and A. Baqer, On the assessment of melanin in human skin *in vivo*, *Photochemistry and Photobiology*, vol. 43, no. 1, pp. 49–54, 1986.

174. J. E. Calonje, T. Brenn, A. J. Lazar, and P. H. McKee, *McKee's Pathology of the Skin*, 4th ed. Philadelphia: Saunders, 2011, p. 1906.

175. S. N. Sivanandam and S. N. Deepa, *Introduction to Genetic Algorithms.* Berlin: Springer Verlag, 2008.

176. D. Yuret, From genetic algorithms to efficient optimization, *Massachusetts Institute of Technology*, 1994.

177. R. L. Haupt and S. E. Haupt, *Practical Genetic Algorithm.* New York: John Wiley & Sons, 2004.

178. G. Luque and E. Alba, *Parallel Genetic Algorithms: Theory and Real World Applications.* Springer Verlag, 2011.

179. P. C. P. Carvalho, L. H. de Figueiredo, J. Gomes, and L. Velho, *Mathematical Optimization in Computer Graphics and Vision.* Elsevier, 2008.

180. F. H. Mustafa, M. S. Jaafar, A. H. Ismail, A. F. Omar, Z. A. Timimi, and H. A. A. Houssein, *Red Diode Laser in the Treatment of Epidermal Diseases in PDT*, pp. 780–783, 2010.

181. Breault Research Organization, *Realistic Skin Model (RSM)*, no. 1. Breault Research Organization, 2012, pp. 1–60.

182. Breault Research Organization, *The ASAP Primer.* Breault Research Organization, 2012, pp. 1–560.

183. G. W. S. Institute, *How Much Solar Energy is Available?*, GW Solar Institute, 2009 [Online]. Available: http://solar.gwu.edu/FAQ/solar_potential.html.

184. J. E. Bartlett, J. W. Kotrlik, and C. C. Higgins, Organizational research: Determining appropriate sample size in survey research, *Information Technology, Learning and Performance*, vol. 19, no. 1, pp. 43–50, 2001.

185. J. Adauwiyah and H. H. Suraiya, Retrospective study of narrowband-UVB phototherapy for treatment of vitiligo in Malaysian Patients, *Medical Journal of Malaysia*, vol. 65, no. 4, pp. 299–301, 2011.

186. J. Y. Lin and D. E. Fisher, Melanocyte biology and skin pigmentation, *Nature*, vol. 445, no. 7130, pp. 843–850, 2007.

187. Y. Lee and K. Hwang, Skin thickness of Korean adults, *Surgical and Radiologic Anatomy*, vol. 24, no. 3–4, pp. 183–189, 2002.

188. T. S. Daily, Acute shortage of dermatologists in Malaysia, *Malaysian Medical News*, pp. 1–2, 2012. http://malaysianmedicine.blogspot.my/2012/06/acute-shortage-of-dermatologists-in.html.

189. P. Boyle and B. Levin, *World Cancer Report.* Lyon: World Health Organization, 2008, ISBN-13 9789283204237.

190. C. Turkington and J. Dover, *The Encyclopedia of Skin and Skin Disorders.* United States of America: Infobase Publishing, 2009.

191. Global Insight, *A Study of the European Cosmetics Industry.* European Commission Directorate General for Enterprise and Industry, 2007.

192. B. M. Yeomans, Global beauty market to reach $265 billion in 2017 due to an increase in GDP, pp. 11–14, 2013, www.cosmeticdesign.com.

193. D. Bird, H. Caldwell, and M. DeFanti, The quest for beauty: Asia's Fascination with Pale Skin, *Business Research Yearbook Global Business Perspectives International. Acad. Bus. Discip.*, vol. 12, no. 1, 2010.

194. M. Brenner and V. J. Hearing, Modifying skin pigmentation – Approaches through intrinsic biochemistry and exogenous agents, *Drug Discovery Today: Disease Mechanisms*, vol. 5, no. 2, pp. 189–199, 2009.

195. D. Scherer and R. Kumar, Genetics of pigmentation in skin cancer—A review, *Mutation Research*, vol. 705, no. 2, pp. 141–153, 2010.

196. A. Singh, A. E. Karsten, and J. S. Dam, Determination of optical properties of tissue and other bio-materials, vol. 1202, no. 2000, p. 6665, 2nd CSIR Biennial Conference, CSIR International Convention Centre Pretoria, 17 and 18 November 2008.

197. J. T. Whitton and J. D. Everall, The thickness of the epidermis, *British Journal of Dermatology*, vol. 89, no. 5, pp. 467–476, 1973.

198. G. Szabo, A. B. Gerald, M. A. Pathak, and T. B. Fitzpatrick, Racial differences in the fate of melanosomes in human epidermis, *Nature*, vol. 222, pp. 1081–1082, 1969.

199. G.A. Harrison, *Genetical Variation in Human Populations*. Pergamon, 1963.

200. Y. T. Jadotte and R. A. Schwartz, Melasma: Insights and perspectives, *Acta dermatovenerologica Croatica: ADC Hrvatsko dermatolosko Drustvo*, vol. 18, no. 2, pp. 124–129, 2010.

201. K. Maeda, Y. Yokokawa, M. Hatao, M. Naganuma, and Y. Tomita, Comparison of the melanogenesis in human black and light brown melanocytes, *Journal of Dermatological Science*, vol. 14, no. 3, pp. 199–206, 1997.

202. Papilary Layer of Dermis [Online]. Available: http://virtual.yosemite.cc.ca.us. [Accessed 12 January 2014].

203. P. Välisuo, I. Kaartinen, H. Kuokkanen, and J. Alander, The colour of blood in skin: A comparison of Allen's test and photonics simulations, *Skin Research and Technology*, vol. 16, no. 4, pp. 390–396, 2010.

204. J. K. Barton, S. Rollins, S. Yazdanfar, T. J. Pfefer, V. Westphal, and J. A. Izatt, Photothermal coagulation of blood vessels: A comparison of high-speed optical coherence tomography and numerical modelling, *Physics in Medicine and Biology*, vol. 46, no. 6, pp. 1665–1678, 2001.

205. S. K. Alla, A. Huddle, J. D. Butler, P. S. Bowman, J. F. Clark, and F. R. Beyette, Point-of-care device for quantification of bilirubin in skin tissue, *IEEE Transactions on Biomedical Engineering*, vol. 58, no. 3, pp. 777–780, 2011.

206. A. Krishnaswamy and G. V. G. Baranoski, A biophysically-based spectral model of light interaction with human skin, *Eurographics*, vol. 23, no. 3, 2004.

207. D. Parsad, R. Pandhi, S. Dogra, A. J. Kanwar, and B. Kumar, Dermatology Life Quality Index score in vitiligo and its impact on the treatment outcome, *Br J Dermatol*. vol. 148, no. 2, pp. 373–374, 2003.

208. G. Lewis, The conservation of photons, *Nature*, vol. 2981, no. 118, pp. 874–875, 1926.

209. G. Optics, Geometrical optics, *Nature*, vol. 199, no. 4895, pp. 753–753, 1963.

210. E. Hecht, *Optics*, 4th ed., vol. 1. New York: Addison-Wesley, 2001, p. 122.

211. P. Hanrahan and W. Krueger, Reflection from layered surfaces due to sub-surface scattering, in *the 20th Annual Conference on Computer Graphics and Interactive Techniques*, 1993, pp. 165–174.

212. M. A. Ansari and R. Massudi, Study of light propagation in Asian and Caucasian skins by means of the Boundary Element Method, *Optics and Lasers in Engineering*, vol. 47, no. 9, pp. 965–970, 2009.

213. T. Weyrich, H. W. Jensen, M. Gross, W. Matusik, H. Pfister, B. Bickel, C. Donner, C. Tu, J. McAndless, J. Lee, and A. Ngan, Analysis of human faces

using a measurement-based skin reflectance model, *ACM Transactions on Graphics*, vol. 25, no. 3, p. 1013, 2006.

214. M. Hammer and D. Schweitzer, Quantitative reflection spectroscopy at the human ocular fundus, *Physics in Medicine and Biology*, vol. 47, no. 2, pp. 179–191, 2002.

215. A. N. Bashkatov, E. A. Genina, V. I. Kochubey, A. A. Gavrilova, S. V. Kapralov, V. A. Grishaev, and V. V. Tuchin, Optical properties of human stomach mucosa in the spectral range from 400 to 2000 nm: Prognosis for gastroenterology, *Medical Laser Application*, vol. 22, no. 2, pp. 95–104, 2007.

216. B. G. Yust, L. C. Mimun, and D. K. Sardar, Optical absorption and scattering of bovine cornea, lens, and retina in the near-infrared region, *Lasers in Medical Science*, vol. 27, no. 2, pp. 413–422, 2012.

217. J. Qin and R. Lu, Measurement of the optical properties of fruits and vegetables using spatially resolved hyperspectral diffuse reflectance imaging technique, *Postharvest Biology and Technology*, vol. 49, no. 3, pp. 355–365, 2008.

218. M. L. Purschke, S. S. Southekal, and B. Ravindranath, Massively parallel image reconstruction for the BNL breast scanner PET tomograph using CUDA, in *IEEE Symposium on Nuclear Science*, 2009, pp. 2374–2375.

219. C.H. Huang, D. Racoceanu, L. Roux, and T. Putti, Bio-inspired computer visual system using GPU and visual pattern assessment language (ViPAL): Application on breast cancer prognosis, in *International Joint Conference on Neural Networks*, 2010.

220. T. S. Leung and S. Powell, Fast Monte Carlo simulations of ultrasound-modulated light using a graphics processing unit, *Journal of Biomedical Optics*, vol. 15, no. 5, p. 055007, 2010.

221. H. Scherl, B. Keck, M. Kowarschik, and J. Hornegger, Fast GPU-based CT reconstruction using the common unified device architecture (CUDA), in *IEEE Symposium on Nuclear Science*, 2007, pp. 4464–4466.

222. T. Reichl, J. Passenger, O. Acosta, and O. Salvado, Ultrasound goes GPU: Real-time simulation using CUDA, in *SPIE Proceedings 7261*, vol. 7261, 2009, pp. 1–10.

223. L. Pan, L. Gu, and J. Xu, Implementation of medical image segmentation in CUDA 1, in *5th Internation Conference on Information Technology and Application in Biomedicine*, 2008, pp. 82–85.

224. H. Shen and G. Wang, A tetrahedron-based inhomogeneous Monte Carlo optical simulator, *Physics in Medicine and Biology*, vol. 55, no. 4, pp. 947–962, 2010.

225. A. Badal and A. Badano, Accelerating Monte Carlo simulations of photon transport in a voxelized geometry using a massively parallel graphics processing unit, *Medical Physics*, vol. 36, no. 11, pp. 4878–4880, 2009.

226. W. C. Y. Lo, K. Redmond, J. Luu, P. Chow, J. Rose, and L. Lilge, Hardware acceleration of a Monte Carlo simulation for photodynamic therapy [corrected] treatment planning, *J. Biomed Journal of Biomedical Optics*, vol. 14, no. 1, p. 014019, 2009.

227. A. J. Chipperfield and P. J. Fleming, The MATLAB genetic algorithm toolbox, in *IEEE Collloquium on Applied Control Techniques using MATLAB*, 1995.

228. M. Affenzeller, S. Winkler, S. Wagner, and A. Beham, *Genetic Algorithms and Genetic Programming*. Boca Raton: Taylor & Francis, 2009.

229. L. Davis, *Handbook of Genetic Algorithms*. New York: Van Nostrand Reinhold, 1991.

230. D. Luebke, *CUDA: Scalable Parallel Programming for High-Performance Scientific Computing*, 2008, pp. 836–838.

chapter five

Retinal image enhancement and analysis for diabetic retinopathy assessment

Ahmad Fadzil Mohamad Hani, Hanung Nugroho,
Lila Iznita Izhar and Nor Fariza Ngah

Contents

5.1 Diabetic retinopathy

Diabetic retinopathy (DR), a complication threatening the sight due to diabetes mellitus affecting the retina, has become one of the leading causes of blindness in the world [1]. According to the National Eye Database 2007, of 10,856 cases with diabetes in Malaysia, 36.8% attains some forms of DR, 7.1% of them fall under proliferative diabetic retinopathy (PDR), severe non-PDR (NPDR), moderate NPDR and mild NPDR, as depicted in Figure 5.1 [2]. International Diabetes Federation (IDF) in 2009 reported that approximately 285 million people worldwide suffer from diabetes and predicted that the number would increase to 438 million within 20 years at the rate of 7 million people developing diabetes per year annually [3].

Determining DR severity is, therefore, essential in treating the disease. In grading DR, the International Clinical Diabetic Retinopathy Disease Severity Scale, shown in Table 5.1, is widely used [4]. An ophthalmologist using this scale needs to observe and determine DR-related abnormalities in the retinal fundus image. However, this pathology-based method for DR severity grading is time consuming, taking 20–30 min and often requires fundus fluorescein angiography (FFA) for an accurate diagnosis by highly trained and skilled clinicians. FFA refers to an invasive imaging procedure to highlight the retinal and choroidal circulation by injecting a contrasting agent (sodium fluorescein) into the blood vessels to obtain an angiogram of well-contrasted retinal blood vessels for diagnosis of retinal and choroidal pathologies [5]. Figure 5.2 illustrates DR severity with corresponding pathologies as observed in colour fundus images. Ophthalmologists and clinicians require extensive training to discern the pathologies. Figure 5.3 shows colour fundus and FFA retinal images of the

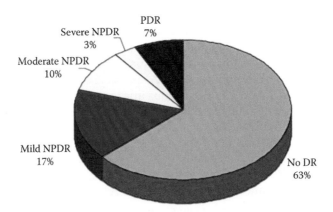

Figure 5.1 DR statistics of registered diabetic patients in Malaysia. (From P. P. Goh, 2007, *The Medical Journal of Malaysia*, vol. 63, pp. 24–28, 2008.)

Table 5.1 International clinical DR disease severity scale

Proposed disease severity level	Findings observable upon dilated ophthalmoscopy
No apparent retinopathy	No abnormalities
Mild NPDR	Micro-aneurysms only
Moderate NPDR	More than just micro-aneurysms but less than severe NPDR
Severe NPDR	Any of the following: 1. >20 intra-retinal haemorrhages in each of 4 quadrants 2. Definite venous beading in 2+ quadrants 3. Prominent intra-retinal microvascular abnormalities in 1 + quadrant 4. No signs of proliferative retinopathy
PDR	One or more of the following: 1. Neo-vascularisation 2. Vitreous/pre-retinal haemorrhage

Source: American Academy of Ophthalmology, *Preferred Practice Pattern* [Online].

same eye depicting pathologies such as micro-aneurysm. FFA enhances the pathologies for better visualisation of the pathologies.

5.2 Contrast problems in medical images

One of the most common problems for many medical-imaging modalities is varied contrast and low contrast of the produced images. Contrast

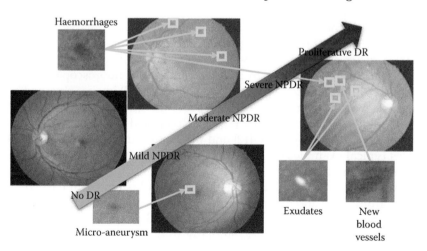

Figure 5.2 Colour fundus images of DR severity with corresponding retinal and choroidal pathologies.

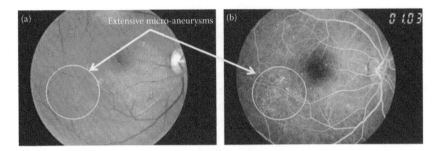

Figure 5.3 Extensive micro-aneurysms in retinal images: (a) colour fundus and (b) FFA. (From H. A. Nugroho et al. Fundus Image Database for Non Invasive Diabetic Retinopathy Monitoring and Grading System (FINDeRS). [Online].)

in an image refers to a measure of the magnitude of intensity differences between different regions or two adjacent pixels. Varied contrast is usually perceived as spurious smooth variation of image intensity and commonly referred to as uneven or non-uniform illumination, illumination variation, intensity inhomogeneity or non-uniformity, intensity variation, shading or bias artefact. Low contrast, however, appears when different objects in an image show similar intensity characteristics. Some of these problems are due to technical limitations of the medical-imaging devices and acquisition techniques while others correspond to the frequently unavoidable imaged objects. Some of these contributing factors include complexity of imaging situations, disease opacity, poor focus, variability of data among patients, inadequate illumination and imperfect image acquisition process, resulting in noise and artefacts [7].

The problems of small and diverse contrast that emerge in many medical images are due to image acquisition of the modalities used and characteristics of imaged organs. The problems, for instance, can be seen in retinal images obtained by fundus camera [8], fluoroscopic images obtained by fluoroscopy [9], magnetic resonance (MR) images obtained by magnetic resonance imaging (MRI) [10], mammography images obtained by digital x-ray mammography [11], CT (computed tomography) images obtained by CT angiography [12] and ultrasound images [13]. Figure 5.4 shows typical examples of medical images obtained from various medical-imaging modalities.

As seen from Figure 5.4a, retinal colour fundus image, in particular, suffers from small and diverse contrast problems due to the spherical surface of the retina, resulting in the reflection at the centre of the retina to be brighter than the periphery. Similarly in objects of interest in mammography and ultrasound images, malignant tissues usually appear in low contrast. In MR images, proper adjustment of T_1 and T_2 parameters is needed to obtain good quality images.

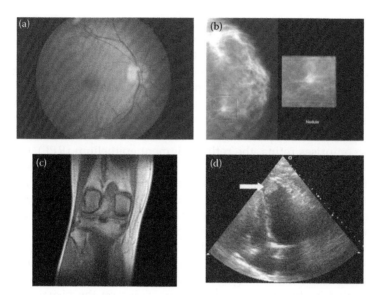

Figure 5.4 Examples of small and diverse contrast images obtained from different medical imaging modalities: (a) colour retinal fundus image (From A. Ciulla et al. *World Journal of Surgical Oncology,* vol. 6, p. 78, 2008.), (b) mammography image, (c) MR image (From T. Teng, M. Lefley and D. Claremont, *Medical and Biological Engineering and Computing,* vol. 40, pp. 2–13, 2002.) and (d) ultrasound image. (From S. Povoski, *World Journal of Surgical Oncology,* vol. 5, pp. 124, 2007.)

Accurate detection of pathologies in the early stages of diseases is important for treatment efficacy. In medical cases where images are required to monitor and grade the disease's severity level based on the pathological changes of the biological organs, accurate diagnosis may become difficult if the contrast between normal objects and abnormal ones (pathologies) is subtle. Noise and artefacts that make direct analysis of these images more difficult, often confound these low-contrast medical images.

Varied contrast in medical images similarly causes problems in a computer-aided diagnosis system especially for automated image analysis methods, such as segmentation [16,17], registration [18], feature extraction [19] and classification [20]. These problems do not merely degrade image quality but significantly hamper automated analysis [21]. This chapter investigates the problems in small and diverse contrast of colour retinal fundus pictures and develops a solution to overcome such problems.

5.2.1 Ocular fundus images

A digital fundus camera acquires retinal fundus images by registering the illumination reflected from the retina's spherical surface. During the acquisition process, (flash) light from the fundus camera illuminates various parts of the retina and the amount of illuminating light varies from eye to eye and depends on the direction of the illuminating flash.

Ocular fundus represents a structure of the back of the eyes and consists of multiple layers of tissue. Typically, the architecture of the eye can be characterized into two fundamental types: ocular media and ocular fundus [22]. Ocular media, which is situated between the ocular fundus and the observer, comprises cornea, lens and vitreous, while the ocular fundus comprises retina, the retinal pigment epithelium (RPE), the choroid and the sclera. Furthermore, the fundus layers beneath the retina consist of two pigments, namely melanin and haemoglobin, which dominate the overall appearance of the fundus. Referring to the cross section of the eye shown in Figure 5.5, the ocular fundus part is of importance since this part mainly affects the resulting colour fundus image.

The photoreceptor layer, which is also called the visual pigment, is composed of light-sensitive cells called rods and cones, characterized by different sensitivity to light. The cones are smaller and very highly concentrated in the fovea, the part of the retina on the visual axis and responsible for central vision. In addition, the layers of other cells and blood vessels covering the peripheral retina, thin out and disappear over the fovea, allowing uninterrupted exposure of the image. There are no rods in the fovea. However, rods dominate peripheral (non-central) vision. Under the photoreceptors is a dark layer known as RPE. The RPE contains melanin granules that absorb excess light and transport oxygen, nutrients and cellular wastes between the photoreceptors and the choroid.

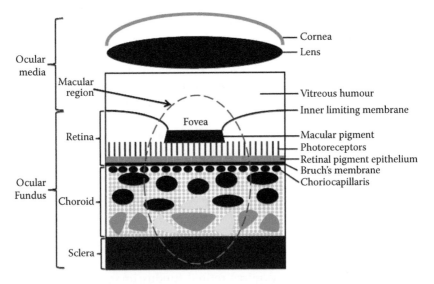

Figure 5.5 Cross section of the eye.

The choroid is a layer of blood vessels that supplies oxygen and nutrients to the outer layers of the retina. The innermost choroid, called the choriocapillaris, is a dense net of flattened capillaries that forms a blood-filled shell lying parallel to the basal side of the RPE. Bruch's membrane separates the blood vessels of the choroid from the RPE layer. The rest of the choroid is filled with larger blood vessels and melanin-containing melanocytes. The melanin content of the RPE varies among individuals. However, only the melanin content of the choroid depends on skin pigmentation. The final layer of significance is the sclera, the fibrous, thick, white outer covering of the eye. Therefore, a reflectance of the fundus can be understood as a ratio of a total amount of reflected light to the total incident light propagating through several fundus layers. Figure 5.6 depicts a model of ocular fundus showing possible pathways of the remitted light.

The slight changes of the biological structure and pigment construction lead to variation in colour of the retinal fundus. It is, therefore, necessary to understand the retinal fundus colour based on the structure and pigment construction to model fundus spectral absorbance image.

Despite the controlled acquisition process, retinal fundus images still suffer from varied contrast. Several factors that cause varied contrast are, for example, the curved surface of the retina, the presence of pathologies and pupil dilation, which vary highly among people. Some retinal pathologies, such as exudates and small blood leaks appear as bright spots due to the protein contents in these spots, which are more reflective than the retinal surface [23].

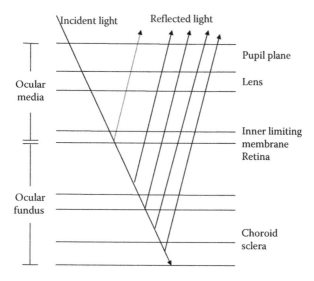

Figure 5.6 Model of ocular fundus showing pathways of remitted light.

The varied contrast prevents an absolute interpretation of the intensities in the image. For instance, the optic disc typically is the brightest object in the retinal image. The varied contrast often causes the area directly under the flash to appear the brightest. The curved retinal surface and the configuration of the light source and camera causes the peripheral part of the retina to appear darker than the central region. Figure 5.7 shows examples of contrast variations across colour retinal fundus images and within a colour retinal fundus image.

Instead of varied contrast, the contrast between retinal vessels and background is very low. Low contrast occurs particularly around retinal capillaries that are mostly located in the centre of the retina known as macular region. The retinal capillaries and vessels surrounding the macular region are of very low contrast since they are located in the choroidal layer underneath the macular pigment and the RPE, which contains melanin that absorbs light. Due to the small contrast between retinal blood vessels and the background in retinal fundus pictures, it is not easy to find out the retinal vasculature that can be utilized to identify macular region, foveal avascular zone (FAZ) and existence of pathology. Diverse and small contrast conditions in colour retinal fundus pictures generally reduces image quality and leads to inaccuracy of segmentation of retinal blood vessels and pathology detection; thus, leading to reduced accuracy, sensitivity and specificity in the diagnosis of the retinal-related diseases.

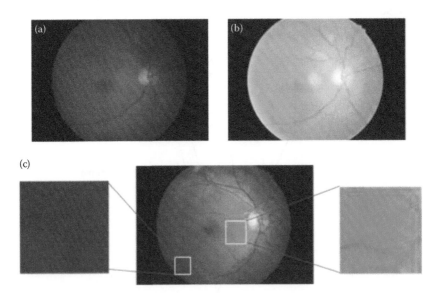

Figure 5.7 Uneven contrast occurs between images (a) and (b) and within an image (c).

5.2.2 Retinal image enhancement

Retinal image enhancement is an important pre-processing step to improve image quality for better visual perception and facilitate diagnosis of retinal-related diseases. In general, this can include transforming an image into a more suitable format for computer-aided image processing [24]. The quality of the enhanced image depends on five factors namely, spatial resolution, contrast resolution, temporal resolution, illumination and noise. Spatial resolution corresponds to image sharpness (edges) and features' fine detail, while contrast resolution – an ability to distinguish the intensity in an image represented into a grey scale quantisation – corresponds to discrimination of detail within and between objects. Noise consists of undesired objects that deteriorate the visibility of particular objects in an image. A good quality medical image is significantly important for both diagnosis process and subsequent computer-based automated image analysis.

Based on its invasiveness, there are two categorisation of image enhancement of medical images, that is, invasive and non-invasive enhancement. Invasive enhancement concerns exposing or injecting some contrasting agents into the human body. In radiography, for instance, the increase of the radiation dose to the patient results in better x-ray images. X-ray contrast media (e.g., barium, iodine) are often used in any x-ray related to medical-imaging modalities (e.g., angiography, CT, fluoroscopy and mammography) by injecting them into an artery or vein. Having absorbed x-radiation, x-ray contrast media thereby are able to increase the contrast between the organ of interest and the surrounding tissue. Injection of x-ray contrast media, however, may also result in death associated with nephropathy and allergic reactions, as reported in Reference 25.

In ophthalmology, fluorescein angiography could result in better contrast of retinal vasculatures; yet, due to its invasiveness by injecting contrasting agent (sodium fluorescein) within the blood vessels, this method can also cause physiological issues such as nausea, spewing and discombobulation [26]. The least unfavourable case of negative reactions after fluorescein injection, may be fatal anaphylactic shock, which can ultimately lead to death. It has been reported by Yannuzzi et al. that the frequency rate for death cases due to fluorescein injection is 1:222,000 [27]. Hence, even though fluorescein angiography can produce better contrast of retinal fundus images, it is not recommended for medical routine use [28].

In some cases related to the use of non-ionising imaging modalities for acquisition of medical images, injection of contrasting agent into the human body is not necessary to achieve better contrast of acquired images. Instead, patients must undergo an acquisition process with increasing power levels or a longer time exposure to obtain better contrast of images. For instance, the large power level of ultrasound may result in better ultrasound images. In the case of MRI, the longer the time of image acquisition, the better the MR images are. Even contrasting agents, for example, micro-bubble contrast agents [29] and gadolinium [30], are sometimes used in ultrasound and MRI, respectively, to enhance a specific tissue of interest. Nevertheless, the use of such contrast agents may result in adverse effects such as headache, nausea, vomiting and dizziness in the case of ultrasound [31] and in nephrogenic systemic fibrosis in MRI [32].

Implementation of these procedures is a compromise between technical evaluation and artistic appraisal. At this point, it must take account of the comfort and safety of the patients before acquiring medical images. Excessive radiation dose to obtain perfect images, is not acceptable. A suitable compromise between the power levels or the injection of contrasting agent and patient safety to achieve better image quality is sought. Alternatively, image quality can be improved by using non-invasive enhancement techniques.

Non-invasive image-enhancement techniques, also known as digital image-enhancement techniques, fundamentally, refer to mathematical techniques to improve the quality of a given image resulting in enhanced images that allow better visual perception and increase contrast of certain features than the original one for a specific problem-oriented application. Through digital image processing techniques, the implementation of non-invasive image enhancement is about manipulation of image intensities to improve image quality without any intervention into the human body. Most of the enhancement techniques focus on noise removal (smoothing), contrast enhancement (feature enhancement), contrast normalisation (illumination normalisation) and image sharpening to improve the visual perception of the image [33]. Other enhancement techniques provide better input for subsequent automated image processing algorithm in a computerised system such as edge detection and object segmentation [34].

In retinal images, it is important to enhance the low-contrast tiny objects of interest selectively. Yet, to distinguish low-contrast tiny objects and to increase their contrast without any distortions are complicated tasks. The major problem is how to discern the low-contrast tiny objects of interest and noise since most of the image-enhancement techniques tend to filter out the low-contrast tiny objects as noise. Moreover, fundus images suffer not only from low contrast, but also from varied contrast. For that reason, the main challenge in developing a non-invasive retinal image-enhancement technique is to determine significant image features and distinguish them from other objects, such as noise or artefacts to apply the enhancement process on image features only to obtain the best possible enhanced images.

Studies were conducted to correlate the achievement of several retinal image-enhancement techniques. Yousiff et al. [35] conducted a comparative study for performance evaluation of nine different techniques for contrast enhancement and illumination equalisation of retinal fundus image on two publicly available databases of a total of 60 images [36,37]. The eight different techniques are green band picture [38], histogram equalisation [39], adaptive histogram equalisation [40], adaptive local contrast enhancement [41], background subtraction of retinal blood vessels [42], division by an over-smoothed version [43], desired average intensity [44] and estimation of background luminosity and contrast variability [8]. The performance of each technique is evaluated by using a matched-filter vasculature segmentation algorithm [45]. The results show that adaptive histogram equalisation [40] is the most effective method, among others, for having the largest area of 0.874 under the receiving operating characteristics (ROC). It is then followed by the adaptive local contrast enhancement [41] with 0.833 and the histogram equalisation [39] with 0.787 at the second and the third, respectively [35], for improving the retinal vessels segmentation algorithm [41]. Youssif et al. [35] also applied hybrid method by combining Sinthanayothin's method on adaptive local contrast enhancement [41] with a method developed by Yang et al. on division by an over-smoothed image for contrast normalisation [43]. It is interesting to note that applying contrast enhancement techniques on varied contrast corrected image further, can enhance the image and in turn achieve better result in the segmentation process than just performing ordinary contrast enhancement techniques on the input image.

5.2.3 Challenges in retinal image enhancement

In the image formation model shown in Figure 5.8, image intensity I corresponding to a particular wavelength (λ) is a product of the illumination L and the reflectance R [46]. Varied contrast is defined as a smooth variation of image intensity that needs to be normalised as part of image enhancement. The varied contrast in the image occurs because of uneven illumination and or subtle difference in the reflectance. The latter is commonly due to the presence of objects in the image that have similar characteristics

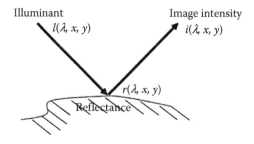

Figure 5.8 Image formation model.

or the presence of tiny objects, which also leads to the problem of low contrast.

Generally there are four main challenges in medical images. First, it is found that the contrast in medical images can vary due to geometrical surface of the objects and configuration of the acquisition system. In retinal fundus image, varied contrast occurs due to the spherical surface of the retina and the configuration of the light source in the camera.

Second, small objects of interest that are related to the biological structure or morphology often appear with low contrast in the acquired image as a consequence of the amount of light being absorbed or reflected by these particular objects. More often than not, these low-contrast objects need to be selectively enhanced and extracted (segmented) to facilitate diagnosis in direct observation or in automated image analysis. The challenge is significant when the diagnosis process involves the observation of these particularly low-contrast tiny objects to diagnose or to grade the severity level of a disease.

Third, the best-available method to enhance the low contrast is based on invasive method. In retinal imaging, FFA is used to enhance the retinal blood vessels and pathologies. Approaches involving invasive methods are, however, not preferable due to the side effects that may lead to physiological problems and in the worst case may cause death.

Fourth, noise in medical images if not handled properly can result in artefacts when images undergo enhancement. Image can be wrongly segmented resulting in errors (false positives) in diagnosis process.

Thus, it is important to develop a non-invasive digital imaging enhancement scheme that can enhance small and diverse contrast colour fundus images to be similar to, or better than the contrast produced by invasive method (FFA) without introducing noise or artefacts. Successful image enhancement of fundus images will enable direct observation and computer-based automated image analysis of the retina, which increase the accuracy, sensitivity and specificity of DR diagnosis and grading.

5.2.4 *Performance measures for retinal image enhancement by RETICA*

The performance of RETICA in normalising and enhancing the contrast of the retinal blood vessels in fundus images is investigated and this is conducted in three parts for: (1) contrast normalisation, (2) contrast enhancement and (3) contrast normalisation and enhancement. Three developed retinal fundus image models as described earlier are used.

Here, two problems are addressed: contrast normalisation and contrast enhancement. First, to measure the contrast normalisation, the kurtosis values of melanin, macular pigment and haemoglobin components are determined. As previously described, the kurtosis is used as a parameter to determine the optimum number of iteration of the Retinex. The highest kurtosis of the data corresponds to the optimum number of iteration of the Retinex and leads to the most homogenous intensity of the image. Second, to measure the contrast enhancement of the retinal blood vessels, contrast between the retinal blood vessels and the background needs to be determined. There are two kinds of background namely, melanin and macular pigment, in which the retinal blood vessels are fairly distributed.

Hence, to validate RETICA, four reference masks, as shown in Figure 5.9 are used to extract the region of interest (ROI) of a processed image. The mask is created in a binary form in which the value of 1 and 0 represent the ROI and the background, respectively. Hence, when the mask is multiplied with the enhanced image model, the result will be the extraction of ROI from the enhanced image model. From the extracted ROI, contrast normalisation and enhancement are validated.

The first mask (Figure 5.9a) shows the area of melanin and the second mask (Figure 5.9b) shows the area of macular pigment. The third

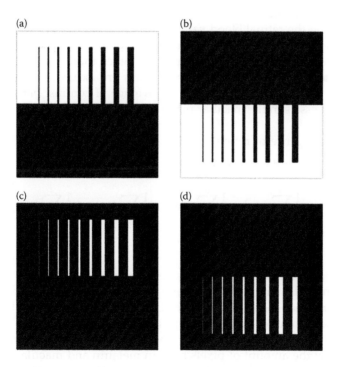

Figure 5.9 Reference masks for (a) melanin, (b) macular pigment, (c) haemoglobin (retinal blood vessels) on melanin and (d) haemoglobin (retinal blood vessels) on macular pigment.

(Figure 5.9c) and the fourth (Figure 5.9d) masks show the retinal blood vessels (haemoglobin) in the melanin and in the macular pigment, respectively.

After performing RETICA on the fundus image model, the masks are applied to the enhanced image to obtain the four areas of interest, that is, melanin, macular pigment, retinal blood vessels in melanin and retinal blood vessels in macular pigment. By identifying these areas, the contrast between the retinal blood vessels and each background can be determined.

The contrast between retinal blood vessels and the background $(C_{|bv-bg|})$ is interpreted as the absolute mean intensity gap between retinal blood vessels and the background and is calculated as

$$C_{|bv-bg|} = \left| \frac{1}{u} \sum_{i=1}^{u} Ibv_i - \frac{1}{v} \sum_{j=1}^{v} Ibg_j \right| \tag{5.1}$$

where Ibv is the intensities of the retinal blood vessels while Ibg is the background. The figures presented by u and v show the amount of pixels representing the retinal blood vessels and the background in the fundus picture model. The larger the figures presented by $C_{|bv-bg|}$, the higher the emergence of retinal veins in the picture. Since there are two kinds of background where the retinal blood vessels are located, the emergence of retinal veins is then defined as the average of contrast between retinal blood vessels in the macular pigment and retinal blood vessels in the melanin.

The emergence of retinal veins (C_{av}) in the fundus picture model is formulated as

$$C_{av} = \frac{\left| \frac{1}{a} \sum_{i=1}^{a} Ivml_i - \frac{1}{b} \sum_{j=1}^{b} Imel_j \right| + \left| \frac{1}{c} \sum_{k=1}^{c} Ivmc_k - \frac{1}{d} \sum_{l=1}^{d} Imac_l \right|}{2} \tag{5.2}$$

where $Ivml$ and $Ivmc$ are the intensities of retinal blood vessels in melanin and macular pigment, while $Imel$ and $Imac$ are intensities of melanin and macular pigment, respectively. The figures presented by a and c show the amount of pixels of the retinal blood vessels both in melanin and macular pigment correspondingly, while the figures presented by b and d show the amount of pixels both in melanin and macular pigment of the fundus image model. The higher the C_{av}, the better the emergence of retinal veins.

Three measures are used to evaluate the performance image-enhancement process. The first measure is image contrast, which is represented by the emergence of retinal veins (C_{av}), as expressed in Equation 5.2. The second measure is the image contrast normalisation (R_{sdc}), which is defined as the ratio between standard deviation, σ and the average contrast C_{av} of an image with the size of $m \times n$. The second measure is derived from the standard deviation that has been widely used to measure image contrast [47–51]. Rubin and Siegel showed that images with an equal standard deviation will have an equal contrast [48].

Theoretically, a standard deviation provides an indication of a sweep of data from its mean value in which a small standard deviation indicates that most of the data are focussed on their mean value and vice versa. In terms of image intensities, small standard deviation indicates that lion's share of the intensity values are near to the mean value. Whereas a high standard deviation indicates that the intensity values are spread out over a large range of values. Hence, the standard deviation can be used to indicate the homogeneity of intensity distribution. A low standard deviation obtained from an image area represents more homogeneous image intensities compared to the high one. This is in line with the objective of contrast normalisation in which the intensity distribution is made to be as homogeneous as possible. However, to use only one standard deviation is not sufficient if several objects in the image are present.

As the objective is also to enhance the contrast between an object and its background, in addition to standard deviation, σ, the average contrast, C_{av}, is used to measure contrast normalisation of the image since the average contrast shows the average of intensity difference between different objects. The fundus image model is the average of contrast between retinal blood vessels in the macular pigment and melanin. If the average contrast C_{av} is significantly high compared to the intensity variation indicated by its standard deviation σ, the image will be considered to have more homogeneous intensities. Conversely, if the average contrast C_{av} is significantly low compared to the intensity variation represented by its standard deviation σ, the image is considered to have more nonhomogeneous intensities. Hence, the lower the R_{sdc} is, the more superior the contrast normalisation of the picture will be.

By considering the standard deviation σ and average contrast C_{av} between objects in an image, the image contrast normalisation R_{sdc} actually measures not only pure contrast normalisation, but also contrast enhancement. However, both the aforementioned criteria can only be implemented in the image model where the objects have been predetermined. In the real image, the objects cannot be determined and separated from one and another before hand by such a system; hence, the average contrast that shows the average of intensity difference between different objects cannot be practically measured.

For the second measure, that is, image contrast normalisation, (R_{sdc}), is given by

$$R_{sdc} = \frac{\sigma}{C_{av}}, \quad \sigma = \frac{1}{mn} \sum_{i=1}^{(mn)} I_i - \bar{I} \qquad (5.3)$$

where I and $\bar{I}$ denote image intensity and its average correspondingly. The lower the R_{sdc} is, the more homogeneous the intensity and the more normalised the contrast is obtained. The task of measuring noise reduction can also use this principle because of operating a detailed picture improvement procedure. Noise can be characterised by the standard deviation of the image intensities. Ideally, the image without any noise will have one value of intensities or uniform intensity distribution, which is almost impossible to get from the real image. The idea of using R_{sdc} can be seen as being the value of R_{sdc} in direct proportion to the standard deviation. The standard deviation is also in direct proportion to the intensity variation. It also means that the more homogenous the intensity distribution will be.

The third measure is the contrast improvement factor (*CIF*) that is defined as a ratio between the emergence of retinal veins attained by a specific algorithm (C_{sp}) and reference (C_{ref}). In this case, C_{ref} uses the contrast of the retinal blood vessels in the green band picture. The *CIF* is therefore formulated as

$$CIF = \frac{C_{sp}}{C_{ref}} \qquad (5.4)$$

The higher the *CIF*, the better the performance of the algorithm.

5.3 Non-invasive image enhancement method for grading of DR severity

The developed colour fundus enhancement method addresses two main challenges – small and diverse contrast. First, in the image formation model, image intensity is a product of illumination and reflectance. The varied contrast due to illumination can be normalised by separating the illumination from the reflectance. The illumination varies slowly, leading its frequency spectrum assumedly to be distributed at low frequencies. If the varied contrast can be determined in a local neighbourhood, the contrast can then be normalised by specialised methods such as Retinex

[117–119]. Second, objects are related to the reflectance. By determining the actual sources from the observed (low contrast) RGB (red, green and blue) image using methods such as Independent Component Analysis (ICA), the objects or areas due to the source of interest can then be enhanced separately without introducing unwanted artefacts. If the varied contrast can be normalised (contrast normalisation) and low-contrast objects can be enhanced (contrast enhancement), the accuracy, sensitivity and specificity of the diagnosis through either direct observation or computer-assisted diagnosis system will increase. These two challenges, that is, varied contrast normalisation and low-contrast enhancement, are formulated and solved separately.

A non-invasive image-enhancement scheme based on Retinex and ICA called RETICA is proposed to overcome the problem of small and diverse contrast with application to medical images; particularly to colour retinal fundus images. A model of small and diverse contrast picture is formed to evaluate the achievement of RETICA. The model is based on data collected from two clinical studies conducted at Selayang Hospital, Malaysia, from July 2008 to March 2010. This database named Fundus Image for Non-invasive Diabetic Retinopathy System (FINDeRS) consists of 315 colour fundus images to be tested. Several parameters have been adopted to measure the performance of RETICA and to compare with other enhancement methods. The proposed method is also implemented as part of a computerised DR system to improve the quality of digital colour fundus image for classifying of DR severity levels. The problem in finding out the FAZ in digital colour retinal fundus images has become an initial motivation for this work. The FAZ is formed by connecting the endpoints of fine retinal vessels in the macular region. These fine retinal vessels, however, are of low contrast and present in varied contrast of colour fundus images. Even though the proposed method is mainly developed based on colour fundus images, it can also be implemented to other medical images, which have similar characteristics, that is, problem of small and diverse contrast objects.

5.3.1 Development of RETICA

RETICA is a non-invasive digital imaging enhancement method capable of enhancing small and diverse-contrast colour fundus images to be similar to, or better than the contrast produced by FFA without introducing noise or artefacts. However, the method does not address reducing or eliminating noise in fundus images. This will be covered in Chapter 6. In this section, the details of RETICA are discussed and applied to the small and diverse-contrast fundus images. It is validated using developed retinal fundus image models in which its performance is evaluated and compared against other selected non-invasive image-enhancement methods.

Image intensity, as previously discussed, is a product of illumination and reflectance. In the image, the varied contrast occurs due to slow varied illumination, whereas the low contrast in some objects of interest is related to the reflectance. If the varied contrast can be determined in a local neighbourhood, it is possible to normalise the contrast by some specialised methods such as Retinex. In addition, by determining the actual sources that resulted in the observed (low contrast) RGB image using methods such as ICA, the objects or areas due the source that is of interest, can then be enhanced separately without introducing unwanted artefacts. The advantage of contrast normalisation and enhancement is an increase in accuracy, sensitivity and specificity of the diagnosis through either a direct observation or a computer-assisted diagnosis system.

In principal, the proposed method called as RETICA enhances the diverse and small contrast colour retinal fundus pictures using two processes, that is, contrast normalisation referencing on Retinex and contrast enhancement based on ICA. The input of RETICA refers to colour image that has been separated into three channels, that is, red, green and blue channels. First, RETICA performs normalisation on the diverse contrast utilizing an improved iterative Retinex, a methodology to separate the part of picture with source of light from part of picture with the reflectance.

The improved iterative Retinex uses kurtosis to determine the optimum number of iteration and overcomes the problem of standard iterative Retinex in which the number of iteration is fixed and pre-determined. Normalisation of varied contrast is followed by separating the retinal pigments makeup, namely macular pigment, haemoglobin and melanin, using ICA. Independent component (IC) image due to haemoglobin exhibits higher contrast of retinal vessels. The use of ICA to improve the contrast of retinal vessels by revealing the underlying sources in colour retinal fundus images is another contribution of this work since most of the image-enhancement methods use pixel manipulation.

The block diagram of RETICA is depicted in Figure 5.10. As illustrated in Figure 5.10, the three channels of RGB are inputted to the first step of the RETICA implementation, which constitutes normalisation of the contrast in reference to Retinex. These images undergo the said process to become three contrast-normalised output pictures. Before these images are being used in the second step of the RETICA, it is necessary to

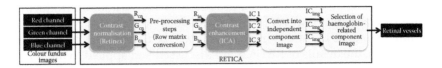

Figure 5.10 Proposed method (RETICA) for contrast normalisation and contrast enhancement of retinal blood vessels on colour fundus image.

perform a pre-processing task that is able to convert the picture matrix to row matrices so that the calculation at the second step can be accelerated.

At the second step, the ICA is being implemented to improve the contrast enhancement by separating the independent components (ICs) from their mixture. The ICs, resulting from the second step are eventually converted from row matrices back to image matrix. Further explanation on the processes involved in each step are available in the following sections.

5.3.2 Contrast normalisation: Retinex

The contrast normalisation stage is referenced on the Retinex methodology purposively to normalise the diverse contrast of the retinal fundus picture by estimating the sensory response of lightness in the picture. The contrast-normalised picture is advantageous for the subsequent image-processing techniques, for example, contrast enhancement, as it will enable an effective enhancement on the overall image. Among the Retinex algorithms, the iterative method based on McCann algorithm [52,53], which is an improvement of the random walks Retinex algorithm [54], is chosen. Unlike non-iterative methods in which several parameters, such as the weighted scale, must be pre-determined to obtain good dynamic range and tonal rendition, the iterative Retinex method only needs to determine the number of iterations. A typical number of iteration for natural image is 4 as suggested by Funt et al. [55]. However, in our developed algorithm, a parameter to measure contrast normalisation based on kurtosis is used to determine the optimum number of iteration for the Retinex rather than to use a fixed number of iteration. A flowchart showing the algorithm for contrast normalisation based on the iterative Retinex is given in Figure 5.11.

Referring to Figure 5.11, the RGB input picture is first divided into three channels, whereby all is applied with the Retinex methodology. For all the three colour channels, the input picture is converted from linear form to logarithmic form to streamline the calculation from multiplication to addition and from division to subtraction. In the iterative Retinex, the averaging process is performed on the fundus image in order to create a multiple resolution pyramid from the input. These iterative Retinex methods [52,53] work out the long-distance interactions initially before gradually moving to short-distance interactions between the pixels. The methodology thereafter correlates the highest averaged pixel or the top stage of the pyramid.

In each progression, the distance between the pixels being correlated decreases. The direction between pixels also changes at each progression in a clockwise order. In each progression, the correlation of pixels is done to predict the reflectance part using the ratio–product–reset–average process, which is iteratively calculated in a predetermined iteration. This

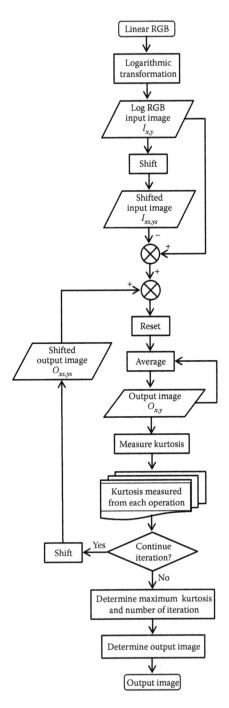

Figure 5.11 Flowchart for contrast normalisation based on Retinex algorithm.

amount of iteration appears to be an important picture-dependent criterion in the methodology. After estimating the reflectance part of the image at the longest distance, the resulting values are used as an initial estimation of reflectance for the next level of interaction. Subsequent correlations between pixels are continuously done to refine the predicted reflectance to a level whereby the distance reaches to only one pixel, finally obtaining the final product.

Ratio and product are operations of adding and comparing, creating a revised new product from each pixel correlation operation. Reset process is to standardize the revised new product surpassing the sustainable maximum. The goal of the averaging process is to predict and revise one pixel's luminance. The ratio–product–reset–average process is done by working out the ratio between pictures I (in a certain channel) and its spatially shifted version and displaced by certain lengths calculated as

$$\log O^*_{x,y} = \frac{Reset\left[(\log I_{x,y} - \log I_{xs,ys}) + \log O_{xs,ys}\right] + \log O_{x,y}}{2} \tag{5.5}$$

where $(\log I_{x,y} - \log I_{xs,ys})$ is the ratio and $[(\log I_{x,y} - \log I_{xs,ys}) + \log O_{xs,ys}]$ represents the product. Reset operation is performed to update the maximum intensity of the image scene L^{scene}_{max} if $[\log I_{x,y} - \log I_{xs,ys} + \log O_{xs,ys})] > \log L^{scene}_{max}$. The term $\log O^*_{x,y}$ is a result of averaging with $\log O_{x,y}$ and $O^*_{x,y}$ itself is an updated output produced iteratively that will be used as an input for the next iteration.

The kurtosis of the data, melanin, macular pigment and haemoglobin is measured and saved iteratively. After all iterations have been performed, the maximum kurtosis can be found and the related number of iterations is determined as the optimum number of iteration for the Retinex.

5.3.3 Contrast enhancement: ICA

For contrast enhancement, ICA is utilized to identify the original signals from blends of signals from a few independent sources [56,57]. ICA is a process that can improve the contrast of a certain item or component (used in this case for the emergence of retinal veins), by extracting each of the components (in this case macular pigment, haemoglobin and melanin) from their blends. In reference to the fundus spectral absorbance model that indicates spectral characteristics of the absorbance components in the ocular fundus, ICA is able to show helpful data to distinguish the absorbance components [58].

The linear consolidation of the absorption coefficients of melanin, haemoglobin and macular pigment is modelled from three absorbance $\mu_a(\lambda_1)$, $\mu_a(\lambda_2)$ and $\mu_a(\lambda_3)$ at three wavelengths λ_1, λ_2 and λ_3. These wavelengths

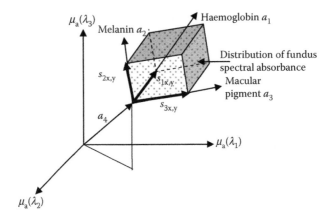

Figure 5.12 Model of spectral absorbance of the ocular fundus.

represent the red (R), green (G) and blue (B) channels. Figure 5.12 shows a model of spectral absorbance of the ocular fundus to highlight the concept of using ICA to separate the spatial distributions of melanin, haemoglobin and macular pigment in the ocular fundus.

According to the model of spectral absorbance of the ocular fundus, the colour density vector of the fundus can be stated as

$$v_{x,y} = A\tilde{s}_{x,y} + a_4 \tag{5.6}$$

$$\tilde{s}_{x,y} = [\tilde{s}_{1x,y}, \tilde{s}_{2x,y}, \tilde{s}_{3x,y}]^T \tag{5.7}$$

with mixing matrix $A = [a_1, a_2, a_3]$ and $\tilde{s}_{x,y}$ representing pure colour vectors of the three components (melanin, haemoglobin and macular pigment) per unit quantity. It is assumed that a linear consolidation of reciprocally independent pure colour vectors of $\tilde{s}_{1x,y}, \tilde{s}_{2x,y}$ and $\tilde{s}_{3x,y}$ with mixing matrix, A results in the composite colour vectors of $v_{1x,y}, v_{2x,y}$ and $v_{3x,y}$ on the image coordinate (x, y). The composite colour vector $v_{x,y}$ is obtained referencing on the outcome of the Retinex methodology whereby the input images to the ICA are contrast-normalised. The input for the ICA is determined as

$$[\mu_a(\lambda_1), \mu_a(\lambda_1), \mu_a(\lambda_1)] = [Rr_{x,y}, Rg_{x,y}, Rb_{x,y}] \tag{5.8}$$

Here, the values of $Rr_{x,y}, Rg_{x,y}$ and $Rb_{x,y}$ correspond to pixel intensity in the channels of red, green and blue, respectively, as the outputs of the Retinex for contrast normalisation. The composite colour vector is denoted as

$$v_{x,y} = [\mu_a(\lambda_1), \mu_a(\lambda_1), \mu_a(\lambda_1)] \tag{5.9}$$

By applying the ICA to the composite colour vectors in the image, the relative quantity and pure colour vectors of each IC are determined with no prior information on both the quantity and colour vector. The quantities of melanin, haemoglobin and macular pigment are assumed to be reciprocally independent for the picture coordinate. The separating matrix, W is used to separate vector, $\tilde{s}_{x,y}$ using the following equations:

$$\tilde{s}_{x,y} = W\tilde{v}_{x,y} \tag{5.10}$$

The estimated ICs, $\tilde{s}_{1x,y}$, $\tilde{s}_{2x,y}$ and $\tilde{s}_{3x,y}$ can be the same as $s_{1x,y}$, $s_{2x,y}$ and $s_{3x,y}$ respectively. A flowchart showing the ICA algorithm is depicted in Figure 5.13.

Vector v as the input for ICA consists of three colour channels that have been processed by Retinex to perform contrast normalisation. The output of the Retinex are three images from three different colour channels, that is, RGB. Each of these images is transformed from matrix of $m \times n$ into a row matrix, $1x(mn)$. Since there are three colour channels, v will be $3x(mn)$. v is initially centred and whitened prior to performing the ICA algorithm. The result of this process is zero-mean and whitened vector, $\tilde{v}$. Following this, $\tilde{v}$ undergoes the ICA algorithm. The algorithm uses the FastICA [59], which is based on a fixed-point iteration for maximisation of non-Gaussianity of $w\tilde{v}$ to obtain the estimated IC $\tilde{s}$, as indicated in Equation 5.10. Since FastICA uses approximation of negentropy, the maxima of the approximation of $w^T\tilde{v}$ are obtained at certain optima $E\{G(w^T\tilde{v})\}$.

For estimation of several ICs, a symmetrical orthogonalisation that obtains the ICs in a parallel process is used and the detailed steps are outlined as follows:

1. Choose h ICs and set iteration $i = 1$. In this study, number of ICs h is equal to 3, that is, melanin, macular pigment and haemoglobin.
2. Initialise random w_i, $i = 1, 2, 3$ to unit form and carry out orthogonalisation of the matrix w.
3. For each i: $w_i^+ = E\{\tilde{v}g(w_i^T\tilde{v})\} - E\{g'(w_i^T\tilde{v})\}w_i$ and update each column of the separating matrix w from the previous iteration.
4. Orthogonalisation of $w^+ = (ww^T)^{-1/2}w$.
5. Check the criteria for convergence. If $|w - w^+| \leq \varepsilon$ is not fulfilled, the process will be back to step 3. The convergence parameter ε is set to 0.0001.

The iteration process ends when the convergence is achieved or the iteration has reached its maximum number of iteration, which is 1000. Once the optimum separating matrix W is obtained, the estimated ICs can be determined.

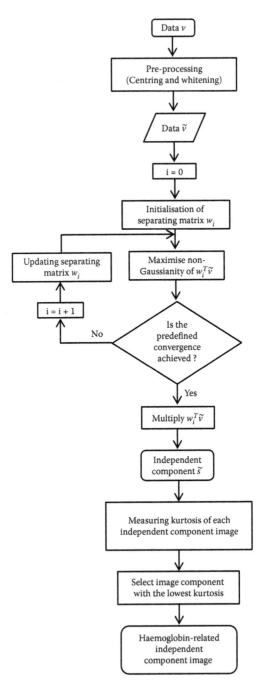

Figure 5.13 Flowchart of contrast enhancement of retinal vessels based on ICA.

However, since the order of the ICs cannot be determined, the haemoglobin-related IC cannot be automatically selected. Therefore, the fourth-order statistics, that is, kurtosis, is utilized to discriminate the haemoglobin-related IC from the other components. Kurtosis is a measure of how distributed the data are. Kurtosis is formulated as

$$kurtosis = \frac{\sum_{i=1}^{M}(I_i - \bar{I})^4}{(M-1)\sigma^4} \tag{5.11}$$

where I_i refers to the intensity value of data point, i from the total data point, M, $\bar{I}$ is the mean of the intensity and σ is the standard deviation of the data. For normal distribution, the kurtosis of the data equals to 3.

In both the melanin-related IC and the macular pigment-related IC images, the emergence of retinal veins is expected to be low for the intensity distribution dominated by the intensities of the melanin and that of the macular pigment, respectively, whereas in the haemoglobin-related IC image, the contrast of retinal vessels is significantly higher than that of the other two IC images. However, due to significantly smaller region of haemoglobin (retinal blood vessels) compared to that of macular pigment and melanin in the fundus image, the kurtosis measured from the haemoglobin-related IC is expected to be smaller than that of the other two ICs. The haemoglobin-related IC is, therefore, distinguished from the other two ICs since it has the least value of kurtosis. The use of kurtosis to discriminate the haemoglobin-related ICs from the two other ICs can be applied to fundus images in which both macular pigment and melanin are also significantly dominant compared to haemoglobin (retinal blood vessels).

5.3.4 Fundus image models

To model fundus images, 44 fundus images were randomly selected from FINDeRS database. As previously discussed, there are three components – macular pigment, melanin and haemoglobin – that significantly influence the appearance of colour retinal fundus images. For modelling, these three components are estimated from the real colour retinal fundus images. While the macular pigment is estimated from the centre area of the retina, the haemoglobin and the melanin are estimated from the sample of retinal blood vessels and the background, respectively. An example of colour retinal fundus images showing the selection of these three components is shown in Figure 5.14.

The statistics of macular pigment, haemoglobin and melanin from three channels, that is, RGB are shown in Table 5.2.

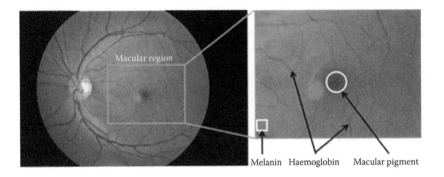

Figure 5.14 Colour retinal fundus image with enlarged macular region.

It can be seen from Table 5.2 that the intensity means of the three components are different in each colour channel. The macular pigment and melanin have the lowest and the highest means, respectively. The difference in intensity means of macular pigment, haemoglobin and melanin is expected due to different spectral absorbance of these three components. This characteristic is useful to separate these three components using ICA. Standard deviation and minimum–maximum intensities also vary among these three components. Standard deviations and intensity ranges shown in the table indicate the homogeneity of intensity distribution of each component in each channel. A small standard deviation indicates that intensity distribution tends to centre on the mean indicating a more homogeneous intensity distribution. Conversely, a high standard deviation implies that data intensities are spread out over a large range of values indicating a more inhomogeneous intensity distribution. The variation of standard deviation and intensity range is expected and implies that the contrast of the retinal fundus image is varied. Like standard deviation, the highest intensity range belongs to the red channel followed by

Table 5.2 Statistics of macular pigment, haemoglobin and melanin intensities in RGB channels

	Macular pigment			Haemoglobin			Melanin		
	R	G	B	R	G	B	R	G	B
Mean	93.40	46.21	7.77	120.88	62.21	15.64	158.16	95.93	35.29
Stdev	37.76	17.656	6.21	34.23	20.37	11.45	29.44	25.20	22.07
Min	0	0	0	18	0	0	35	0	0
Max	228	124	33	227	115	55	255	197	120
Skewness	0.048	0.0796	0.695	−0.036	−0.066	0.416	−0.045	−0.026	0.232
Kurtosis	−0.107	0.056	−0.016	−0.018	0.025	−0.363	0.022	0.167	−0.416

the green and the blue channel. It implies that intensity variation mostly occurs in the red channels rather than in the other two colour channels.

The minimum and maximum of intensity are important to set up the intensity range of the varied-contrast fundus image model that will be developed. Moreover, skewness and kurtosis of the components show that the intensities of the three components tend to have normal (Gaussian) distribution. This is expected since the data intensities of the three components are sampled from real colour fundus images. Probability density functions (pdfs) of the components are used to develop the low-contrast fundus image model. Statistics of the components shown in the table are important to characterise the intensity distribution of samples used in the development of varied contrast and low-contrast image models.

5.3.4.1 Varied-contrast fundus image model development

Varied contrast in an image is characterised by spurious smooth variation of image intensities. Variation of image intensities is mainly due to the effect of illumination. Illumination determines the lightness of an image. Land showed that the relationship between reflectance and lightness is not linear but, generally can be approximated with cube root, square root and logarithmic functions [60]. Here, smooth variation of image intensities is modelled using a mathematical function

$$Y = k \cdot X^{\alpha} \tag{5.12}$$

where k and α are constants. The above function is a general function in which cube root and square root are obtained for α equal to $(1/3)$ and $(1/2)$. A smooth image intensity variation $i(x)$ as a function of pixel's position x is mathematically formulated as

$$i(x) = k \cdot x^{\alpha} \tag{5.13}$$

Using the statistics of the samples as shown in Table 5.3, the mean $\bar{I}$ and the standard deviation σ of image intensities are used to model smooth variation of image intensity $i(x)$ so that $i_{\min} = \bar{I} - 2\sigma$ and $i_{\max} = \bar{I} + 2\sigma$. The value of $\bar{I} \pm 2\sigma$ is chosen for $i_{\min}$ and $i_{\max}$ instead of minimum and maximum intensity values due to the problem of extreme values (outliers) raised by the use of minimum and maximum intensity values. Moreover, the range $\bar{I} \pm 2\sigma$ covers 95% of all possible values [61]. While the value of x represents the position of specific pixel in the image, the value of i has the range as follow:

$$[i_{\min}, i_{\max}] = \left[k \cdot x_{\min}^{\alpha}, k \cdot x_{\max}^{\alpha} \right] \tag{5.14}$$

Table 5.3 Constants k and α obtained for macular pigment, haemoglobin and melanin in RGB channels

	Macular pigment		Haemoglobin		Melanin	
	k	α	k	α	K	α
Red	17	0.453	53	0.263	100	0.152
Green	10	0.415	22	0.3177	46	0.228
Blue	1	0.590	1	0.753	1	0.861

Having known i_{min}, i_{max}, x_{min} and x_{max}, the constants k and α can be obtained for the three components on each RGB channel based on the collected data from 44 retinal fundus images as shown in Table 5.3.

Applying the obtained constants on Equation 5.13, the function $i(x)$ showing variation of image intensities based on pixel's position, x for macular pigment, melanin and haemoglobin in each colour channel can be generated as shown in Figure 5.15.

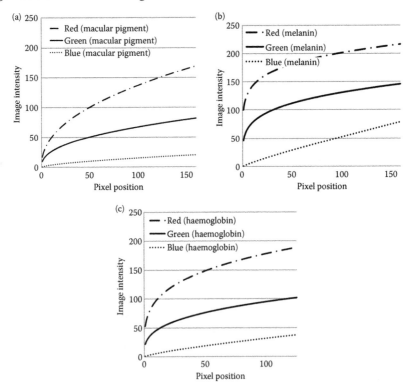

Figure 5.15 Image intensity variation $i(x)$ as a function of pixel's position x for (a) macular pigment, (b) haemoglobin and (c) melanin on each RGB channel.

As depicted in the graphs of Figure 5.15, image intensities increase as the pixel position increases. The increase in intensity variation is expected due to intensity ranges of the sample distribution and a result of applying Equation 5.13. The variation of image intensities occurs in a vertical profile line in the image model. In the image model, a pixel position is vertically set up from 0 started at the top of the image to 160 at the bottom of the image for macular pigment and melanin. For haemoglobin, the pixel position at the bottom of the image is set up to 125. The choice of these lengths is determined by the size of the related components, that is, macular pigment, melanin and haemoglobin in the developed fundus image model. Two fundus image models of 160 × 160 pixels showing the variations of image intensities for macular pigment and melanin and one fundus image model of 125 × 125 pixels showing the variations of image intensities for haemoglobin are depicted in Figure 5.16.

As shown in Figure 5.16, the image intensities increase as the pixel position increases vertically. In the image model, each vertical line shows an equal variation of intensities. Since the image model is square, for instance, in the image model of macular pigment, there are 160 equal vertical lines containing 160 pixels each used to form the image model. In other words, each horizontal profile line consists of 160 same pixel intensity values. The pixels positioned at the top of the image have the highest intensities while the pixels laid at the bottom of the image have the lowest intensity values. Therefore, the image models look darkest at the top and brightest at the bottom of the image. The image intensity variations of macular pigment, melanin and haemoglobin are then used to model the varied-contrast fundus image model where all of these components appear in one image.

The varied contrast image model of 320 × 320 pixels represents the macular region and its surrounding. The resolution for the fundus image model – 320 × 320 pixels – is determined based on the resolution of typical macular region in colour fundus image with resolution of 1936 × 1296 pixels. The image model consists of three components, that is, macular

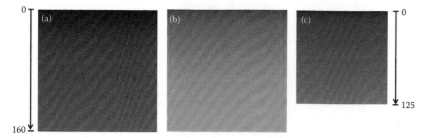

Figure 5.16 Variation of image intensities in fundus image models for (a) macular pigment, (b) melanin and (c) haemoglobin with the referred vertical pixel position.

pigment, haemoglobin and melanin. In the actual fundus picture, retinal blood vessels where the haemoglobin is fairly distributed exist in both the fovea, where the macular pigment are fairly distributed, and the background, where the melanin is fairly distributed.

The area of the fundus image model is divided into two: top half of the image model represents the fovea and bottom half represents the background. Retinal blood vessels are modelled in 9 straight lines, with the same height parallel to each other and the width ranging from 1 to 13 pixels, representing the width of retinal blood vessels from the real retinal fundus image. While the thin lines represent the retinal capillaries that mostly exists in the macular region, the wider lines represents wider blood vessels that mainly exist in the background. A varied-contrast fundus image model is shown in Figure 5.17.

The varied-contrast fundus image model, as illustrated in Figure 5.15, is developed by applying Equation 5.12 to generate the function of image intensity variation of macular pigment, haemoglobin and melanin. In the varied contrast image model, the melanin has the lowest intensity value at the top of the image. The melanin intensity increases as the pixel position moves down and reaches the highest value towards the middle of the image where the pixel position is 160.

5.3.4.2 Low-contrast fundus image model development

Based on the 44 collected image samples and the statistics shown in Table 5.2, normalised intensity distributions of the samples, that is, macular pigment, haemoglobin and melanin are shown in Figure 5.18.

These normalised intensity distributions are obtained from the estimated samples of macular pigment, haemoglobin and melanin in each colour channel. Based on these normalised intensity distributions, pixel values are generated to model the three related components

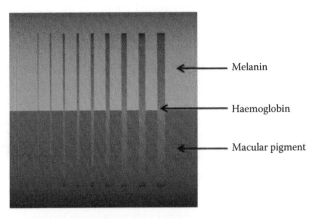

Figure 5.17 Varied-contrast fundus image model.

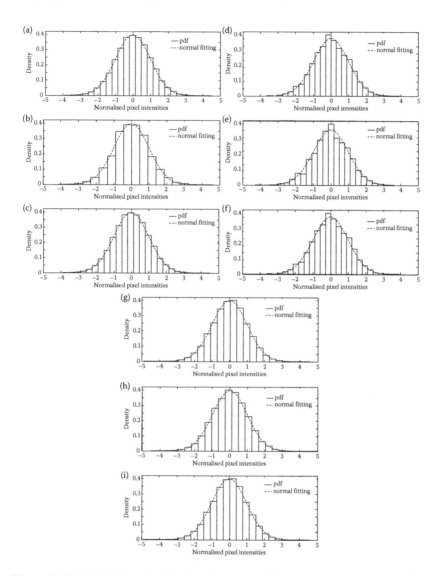

Figure 5.18 Probability distribution function of the normalised pixel intensities of macular pigment of (a) red channel, (b) green channel, (c) green channel. Haemoglobin of (d) red channel, (e) green channel, (f) green channel. Melanin of (g) red channel, (h) green channel, (i) green channel.

used in the low-contrast retinal fundus image model. A diagram of the development of low-contrast fundus image model is illustrated in Figure 5.19.

Based on the obtained pdfs and the mean of the components, colour distribution of each component is generated as shown in Figure 5.20.

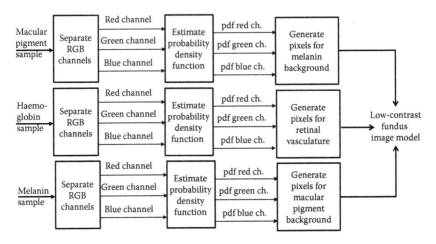

Figure 5.19 Development of low-contrast retinal fundus image model.

These three different colour distributions representing macular pigment, haemoglobin and melanin are used to develop the low-contrast retinal fundus image that contains these three components. Similar to the varied contrast image model, the low-contrast image model of 320 × 320 pixels, as depicted in Figure 5.21, represents the macular region and its surrounding.

In this image model, macular region containing the fovea is used to identify the improvement of retinal capillaries, which have a very small emergence of retinal veins – also known as the retinal vasculature. The area of the image model is divided into two, that is, top-half and bottom-half to represent the melanin and the macular pigment, respectively. Again, nine parallel straight lines with the width varied from 1 to 13 pixels are used to represent the retinal blood vessels. These three components are filled up by the generated pixels with the intensity values that are determined from the normalised pdfs obtained from the sample.

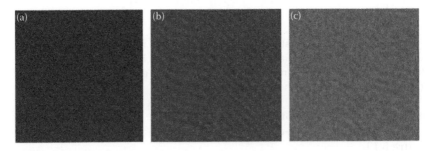

Figure 5.20 Colour distribution of (a) macular pigment, (b) haemoglobin and (c) melanin generated in an image model of 320 × 320 pixels.

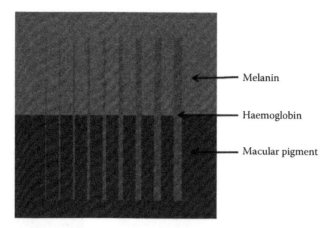

Figure 5.21 Low-contrast fundus image model.

5.3.4.3 *Small and diverse contrast fundus image model*

In physics of light, the brightness of a point (x, y), which in the image plane is also known as the image intensity and is independent for viewer direction, is defined as the amplitude of a function of illumination and surface properties at a particular wavelength λ [62–64]. In the image formation model, the function of $i(\lambda, x, y)$ is formed as a product of these two components – illumination (l) and reflectance (r) – that may form a formula as [46]

$$i(\lambda,x,y) = l(\lambda,x,y) \cdot r(\lambda,x,y) \tag{5.15}$$

Varied contrast in the images mostly occur because of uneven illumination and low contrast is due to the presence of the tiny objects or other objects in the image that have some similar characteristics resulting in a subtle difference in the reflectance. Responding to this, the small and diverse contrast image model is developed based on a combination of the two previous image models on varied contrast image model and low-contrast image model. At this point, the varied contrast image model represents an illumination part and the low-contrast one represents a reflectance part. Hence, the small and diverse contrast image model can be developed as a product of these two image models using Equation 5.15.

Since the small and diverse contrast image model is developed based on colour image, matrix element-by-element multiplication between illumination and reflectance parts – represented by the varied contrast and low-contrast image models – is conducted in each colour channel. As shown in Figure 5.22, outcomes from three multiplications between varied contrast image model and low-contrast image model in each channel are combined to obtain the small and diverse-contrast retinal fundus

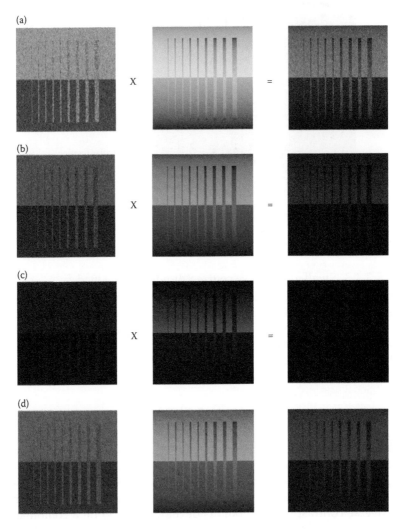

Figure 5.22 Small and diverse contrast fundus image model obtained from multiplication between low-contrast and varied-contrast image models: (a) red channel, (b) green channel (c) blue channel and (d) colour fundus image models for low contrast, varied contrast and small and diverse contrast.

image model. The resultant small and diverse-contrast image model is shown in Figure 5.23.

5.4 Results and analysis

Three fundus image models namely, varied-contrast image, low-contrast image and the small and diverse-contrast image models are used

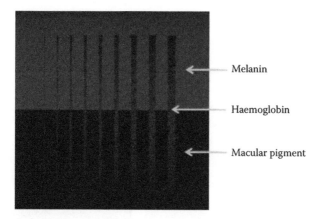

Figure 5.23 Small and diverse-contrast fundus image model.

to evaluate the performance of RETICA as well as comparing it against other image-enhancement algorithms. The improvement of retinal vasculature in the region around the macular area is investigated. Here, the contrast between the retinal vasculature and the macular background is usually small posing a challenge for image enhancement of small retinal capillaries.

As discussed earlier in Section 5.3.4, the area of the fundus image model is divided into two: the melanin and the macular pigment that are located at the top-half and the bottom-half of the image model, respectively. Retinal blood vessels are modelled in nine straight lines paralleling in height and ranging from 1 to 12 pixels in width, representing the width of retinal blood vessels from the real retinal fundus image. The thin lines are to represent the retinal capillaries that mostly exist in the macular region; while the wider lines are to represent wider retinal blood vessels that mainly exist in the background.

5.4.1 Contrast normalisation

The varied-contrast fundus image model as shown in Figure 5.24a is used to evaluate the contrast normalisation stage of RETICA.

As shown in Figure 5.24, the varied-contrast fundus image is separated into three channels, that is, red, green and blue channels that are inputted to the first stage of RETICA, which is based on the Retinex. Validation of the Retinex on the varied-contrast fundus image model is performed by observing the distribution of each component (melanin, macular pigment and haemoglobin) and determining the optimum iteration of the Retinex-based algorithm that results in the most homogenous pixel intensity distribution of each component.

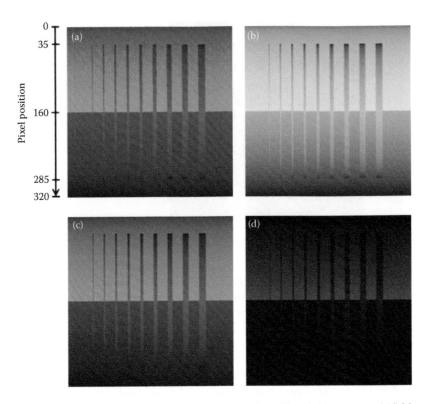

Figure 5.24 (a) Varied-contrast fundus image and its (b) red, (c) green and (d) blue channel images.

As shown in Figure 5.24, the varied-contrast fundus image is separated into three channels, that is, red, green and blue channel images that are applied to the first stage (Retinex) of RETICA. Validation of the Retinex on the varied-contrast fundus image model is performed by observing the distribution of each component (melanin, macular pigment and haemoglobin) and determining the optimum iteration of the Retinex-based algorithm that results in the most homogenous pixel intensity distribution of each component.

The varied-contrast fundus image model is developed by varying the intensity from low to high values as the position changes vertically. By performing the Retinex-based algorithm, the variation of intensities is reduced resulting in more homogeneous intensity distribution. Using the mask from Figure 5.9, each component of the fundus image model is separated.

A vertical line profile is then selected from the area of each component to show its homogeneity of the intensity variation. Referred to the pixel position in the varied-contrast image model shown in Figure 5.24, the original melanin intensity shows the lowest value at the top of the image and increases as the pixel position moves down and reaches the highest value towards the middle of the image where the pixel position is 160. Figures 5.25 through 5.27 depict the comparison of melanin's intensity variation on a vertical line profile taken from RGB channel images after performing Retinex algorithm with several different numbers of

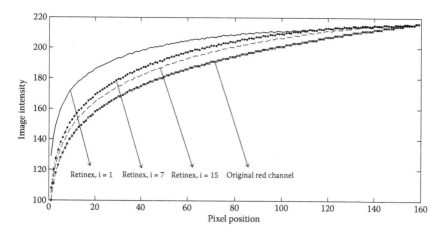

Figure 5.25 Comparison of melanin's intensity variation on an image profile between red channel image model and its Retinex output images with several iterations.

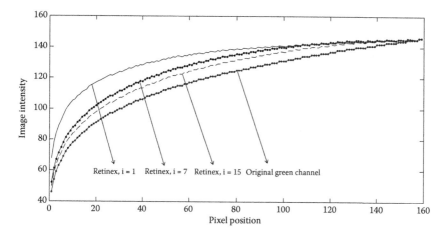

Figure 5.26 Comparison of melanin's intensity variation on an image profile between green channel image model and its Retinex output images with several iterations.

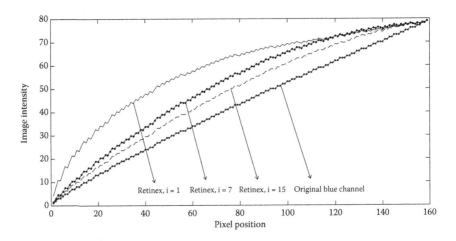

Figure 5.27 Comparison of melanin's intensity variation on an image profile between blue channel image model and its Retinex output images with several iterations.

iterations. The optimum number of iteration of the Retinex is determined when the most homogenous intensity distribution is achieved.

It can be seen from the graphs that the number of iterations results in different intensity variation for all components. Ideally, a homogenous intensity distribution is indicated by a completely flat line – meaning that all values of intensity are the same. However, it is difficult or even not possible to have a completely flat line in practice due to the presence of several different objects and varying illumination. From the above three graphs, the more homogeneous the intensity is, the flatter the line will be.

Qualitatively, all the three graphs show a similar pattern in which melanin has the highest intensity when the number of iterations of the Retinex equals to 1. This result is expected since the Retinex-based algorithm is applied on the varied-contrast fundus image model in which the intensity variation is regular and not random. The intensities of pixels in the operated image will be updated iteratively based on the ratio–product–reset–average operation of the Retinex. The more random the intensity variation is, the higher the optimum number of iterations of Retinex is. Performing Retinex on the varied-contrast fundus image model, as the number of iteration of the Retinex increases, the melanin's intensity values tend to decrease. It means that the most homogeneous melanin's intensity distribution is obtained when the number equals to 1 that makes this as the optimum number of iteration of the Retinex for the melanin in RGB channels.

The intensity of the pigment at the macular is highest at the middle of the image model (Figure 5.24). The intensity value decreases as the pixel position increases and reaches its minimum intensity value for the pixels located at the bottom of the image model where the position is 320, as shown in Figure 5.24. Similar results occur with the macular pigment's intensity variation for RGB channels in which the highest intensity is obtained by the Retinex with the number of iteration equal to 1, as shown in Figures 5.28 through 5.30.

In all cases, the macular pigment's intensity values tend to decrease as the number of iteration of the Retinex increases. These results similar

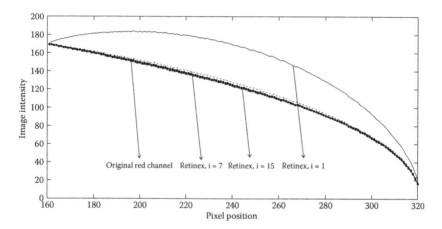

Figure 5.28 Comparison of macular pigment's intensity variation on an image profile between red channel image model and its Retinex output images with several iterations.

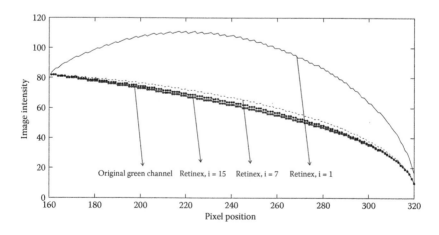

Figure 5.29 Comparison of macular pigment's intensity variation on an image profile between green channel image model and its Retinex output images with several iterations.

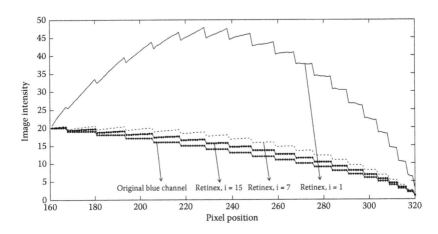

Figure 5.30 Comparison of macular pigment's intensity variation on an image profile between blue channel image model and its Retinex output images with several iterations.

to that of the melanin are expected since the Retinex-based proposed algorithm is applied on the varied-contrast fundus image model in which the intensity variation is regular (not random). Moreover, in the fundus image model, melanin and macular pigment have similar characteristics such as the size of area and regular intensity variation. The increase of the number of iterations of Retinex results in the change of intensities of the processed image according to the ratio–product–reset–average operation of the Retinex. Nevertheless, the objective is to get the most homogeneous intensity distribution. The more random the intensity variation is, the higher the optimum number of iteration of Retinex will be. Qualitatively, the image undergoing Retinex will look brighter indicated by the increase of intensity values. Quantitatively, the optimum number of iteration of Retinex is obtained when the operated image has the highest kurtosis measured from its intensity distribution. Quantitative results based on kurtosis will be further discussed in this section.

Moreover, similar to the melanin, the macular pigment obtained by the Retinex with the number of iteration equal to 1 has the most homogeneous melanin's intensity distribution and appears brighter than that of the Retinex with more numbers of iteration. Hence, the optimum number of iteration of the Retinex for the macular pigment in RGB channels is equal to 1. The increase of the number of iteration greater than the optimum one will result in more non-homogeneous intensity distributions. This is because the ratio between one image scene and the previous one used in the ratio operation is getting closer to one and the maximum intensity used in the reset operation is also getting smaller due to the regular intensity variation of the fundus image model. Hence, in the fundus image model, increasing the number of iteration of Retinex greater than 1 makes the image darker as indicated by the reduction of image intensity values.

A small difference in the optimum number of iteration of the Retinex is found in the case of the haemoglobin's intensity variation compared to that of the melanin and the macular pigment. Referring to the fundus image model shown in Figure 5.24, the haemoglobin is modelled by nine vertical straight lines of retinal blood vessel model parallel with varied width from 1 to 12 pixels and the same length that is, 250 pixels. The retinal blood vessel model has the highest intensity value at the middle of the image where the pixel position is 160 and its intensity values decrease as the pixel position vertically moves both up and down. The lowest intensity value meanwhile belongs to the pixels position at 35 as it moves up to position 285. Results for applying different number of iterations of the Retinex on the haemoglobin are shown in Figures 5.31 through 5.33.

Unlike that of melanin and macular pigment having the same optimum number of iteration for all channels, the optimum number of Retinex iterations for the haemoglobin is different in each channel. It is found that the optimum numbers of iteration of the Retinex in RGB channels are 2, 4 and 3, respectively. This is because the size and structure of the retinal blood vessel (haemoglobin) represented by nine vertical lines is different from that of melanin and macular pigment. However, since the intensity variation of the haemoglobin is regular (not being random), the optimum number of iteration of Retinex is relatively small.

Qualitatively, it is easy to determine the optimum number of iteration by observing the graphs in which the line showing the image intensity

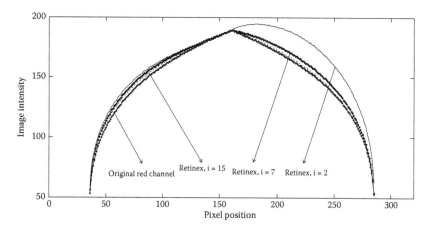

Figure 5.31 Comparison of haemoglobin's intensity variation on an image profile between red channel image model and its Retinex output images with several iterations.

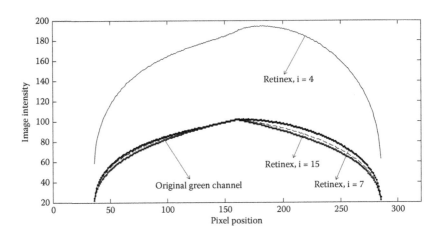

Figure 5.32 Comparison of haemoglobin's intensity changes on an image profile between green channel image model and its Retinex output images with several iterations.

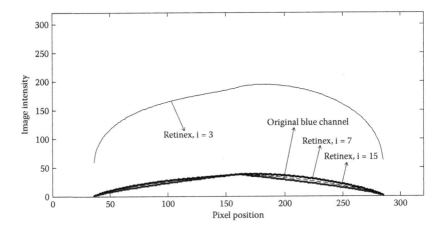

Figure 5.33 Comparison of haemoglobin's intensity changes on an image profile between blue channel image model and its Retinex output images with several iterations.

distribution tends to be flatter. However, in an automated algorithm, a specified parameter is needed to determine this optimum number of iteration. Since the optimum number of iteration of the Retinex is related to the homogeneity of the intensity distribution, kurtosis is then used as a parameter to determine this number. The higher the kurtosis is, the more homogenous the intensity will be. In other words, the highest kurtosis that can be obtained after performing several iterations corresponds to the most homogenous intensity distribution that can be achieved. Once the

Table 5.4 Kurtosis and related optimum number of iteration for Retinex algorithm for melanin, macular pigment and haemoglobin for each colour channel

	Melanin			Macular pigment			Haemoglobin		
	Red	Green	Blue	Red	Green	Blue	Red	Green	Blue
Kurtosis	7.76	8.26	7.75	6.98	8.06	8.20	6.25	6.58	7.23
Optimum number of iteration	1	1	1	1	1	1	2	4	3

highest kurtosis is determined, the related number of iteration is selected as the optimum number and its corresponding Retinex output image can be used as the best output images. Table 5.4 shows the highest kurtosis of melanin, macular pigment and haemoglobin data obtained from RGB channel in relation to the optimum number of iteration of Retinex.

As shown in Table 5.4, even though the optimum number of iterations of Retinex between the melanin and the macular pigment is the same, it does not occur for the haemoglobin. In the case of the fundus image model, even though these three components, that is, melanin, macular pigment and haemoglobin are present all together, it is easy to separate these components using the reference masks shown in Figure 5.9. Hence, it is possible to use different optimum number of iteration for each of the components in the fundus image model.

However, with real fundus images, there is no reference mask; thus, only one of the components is used as the reference in order to determine the optimum number of iteration. For real fundus images, the problem of varied contrast, particularly in the macular region, is due to the macular pigment. Therefore, the highest kurtosis obtained from the macular pigment data is used to determine the optimum number of iteration of the Retinex in each channel. These Retinex output images consisting of three colour channels are subsequently used as the input for the contrast enhancement process based on ICA.

Figure 5.34 shows the original RGB channels of the retinal fundus picture model and their corresponding Retinex output images in RGB channels based on the optimum number of iteration obtained from the macular pigment.

As depicted in Figure 5.34, the Retinex output images show better visualisation than that of the original images as the image intensity is more homogenous. The lower intensity values of the original input images that make the image seemingly darker have been brought up to higher intensity values in the output images that in turn make the output image seemingly to be brighter. As a result, the retinal blood vessel model in the output image is more visible than that of the input image.

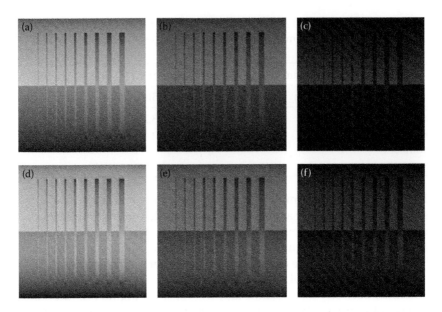

Figure 5.34 Retinal fundus image model in (a) red, (b) green and (c) blue channel images and their corresponding Retinex outputs in (d) red, (e) green and (f) blue channel images.

A significant improvement can be seen in the blue channel image of the Retinex (Figure 5.34f) with more homogeneous intensity than that of the original blue channel input image (Figure 5.34c). Retinal blood vessel model particularly at the macular pigment that cannot be clearly seen from the blue channel image is better visualised in the corresponding Retinex output image because of better homogeneity in the intensity of the macular pigment.

Obtaining more homogeneity in intensity implies that the varied contrast in the image model has been reduced. Retinex is able to make darker areas or sometimes referred as shadow areas into brighter appearance. With the objective of contrast normalisation, the dynamic contrast of the image has been significantly reduced by applying the Retinex algorithm.

In some cases, noise present in the image is represented as the standard deviation or the variance of image pixels. The more homogenous in intensity could lead to a lower standard deviation. This implies that the noise of the image is also reduced. Hence, the normalisation of the varied contrast significantly improves the quality of the image by reducing the intensity variation as well as the noise present in the image. With the normalised intensity and reduced noise, the contrast of image can be further enhanced without enhancing the noise (artefacts).

The result of more homogeneous intensity distribution is expected since the use of Retinex algorithm with its ratio–product–reset–average operation reduces the dynamic contrast of the image intensities. With the reference of the maximum intensity of the image scene, the lower intensities are brought up into higher values, which result in reduction of dynamic contrast. If a maximum intensity value is found in the iteration process, it will be used in the reset operation to update the reference. Therefore, not only is the dynamic range of intensity values reduced but also the lower intensities are raised resulting in brighter appearance of the image.

This contrast-normalised image is advantageous for the subsequent contrast-enhancement process to enhance image components since the intensity distribution of an image component is now more homogeneous and the noise present in the image has been somewhat reduced.

5.4.2 Contrast enhancement

The performance of the RETICA contrast-enhancement stage is evaluated using the low-contrast fundus image model (Figure 5.35).

As shown in Figure 5.35, the low-contrast fundus image model (a) is separated into RGB channels namely, red (b), green (c) and blue (d) channel images. The three channel images or RGB images are applied to the ICA stage of RETICA for contrast enhancement. Here, the capabilities of ICA to separate melanin, macular pigment and haemoglobin components from the mixing in RGB channel images and to determine the haemoglobin-related IC that gives the best contrast of the retinal blood vessels are evaluated.

The ICA algorithm works on an assumption that the components mixed in the RGB input images are independent. Since non-Gaussianity is related to independence, the separation of the ICs is achieved by maximising the non-Gaussianity of the components, as discussed in Section 5.3.3. Here, the objective is to enhance the contrast of the retinal blood vessels. Therefore, the haemoglobin-related IC is selected for the best emergence of retinal veins. Results of performing the ICA on the low-contrast fundus image model with the comparison to the green band picture are shown in Figure 5.36.

It can be seen from Figure 5.36 that the ICA algorithm successfully separates the components into three ICs. The first and second ICs are related to the pigment of the melanin and macular, respectively. The third IC is related to the haemoglobin. The order of the components is not unique meaning that if the fundus image model undergoes the ICA for the second, third and so forth, the order of the components might be different. However, this is not a problem since the ICs can be identified either qualitatively or quantitatively.

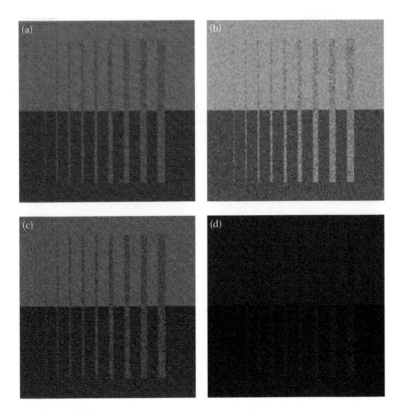

Figure 5.35 (a) Low-contrast fundus image model and its (b) red, (c) green and (d) blue channel images.

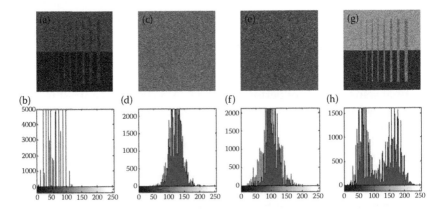

Figure 5.36 (a) Green band picture, (b) its corresponding histogram, (c) first IC image and (d) its corresponding histogram, (e) second IC image and (f) its corresponding histogram, (g) third IC image and (h) its corresponding histogram.

Qualitatively, the IC image is identified by visual inspection. Moreover, the histogram of the green band picture in Figure 5.36b has been shifted from lower to higher intensity values and more fairly distributed as shown by histograms of the IC images. In Figure 5.36d and f, the histograms tend to be normal having specific mean values. Nevertheless, unlike the previous two histograms of first and second IC images, the histogram of third IC shown in Figure 5.36h has two peaks and is fairly distributed in intensity ranging from 0 to around 250. These two peaks are related to the mean values of the intensity of the melanin and the macular pigment. Furthermore, the mean of haemoglobin's intensity is predicted to lie between these two peaks. The higher the difference between the mean of haemoglobin's intensity and that of the melanin is, the higher the emergence of retinal veins will be. This situation also occurs for haemoglobin and macular pigment in which the emergence of retinal veins increases with a higher difference between the mean of intensity of haemoglobin and macular pigment.

Quantitatively, the IC image is identified based on the statistics of intensity distribution of the related components as shown in Table 5.5. The parameter of emergence of retinal veins (C_{av}) as defined in Equation 5.2 is used to determine the haemoglobin-related IC image that has the highest C_{av}.

As can be seen from Table 5.5, the best emergence of retinal veins indicated by the highest C_{av} is the third IC image with C_{av} of 52.78. The third IC image which is also the haemoglobin-related IC image has significantly bigger emergence of retinal veins than that of the green band. Expectedly, the best emergence of retinal veins is found in the haemoglobin-related

Table 5.5 Statistics of green band of low-contrast image model and ICA component images

	Green band		ICA first component		ICA second component		ICA third component	
	Mean	SD	Mean	SD	Mean	SD	Mean	SD
Melanin (Mel)	78.84	13.14	134.23	18.73	99.04	27.53	168.18	22.38
Macular pigment (MP)	35.18	9.73	133.73	16.11	98.58	12.82	63.21	15.67
Haemoglobin (BV)	62.13	20.17	128.50	30.62	99.91	36.16	133.70	32.35
|BV–Mel|	16.71	7.02	5.73	11.89	0.86	8.62	34.48	9.97
|BV–MP|	26.95	10.43	5.23	14.51	1.33	23.34	70.49	16.68
Emergence of retinal veins (C_{av})	21.83		5.48		1.10		52.78	

IC image since the haemoglobin, which is related to retinal blood vessels, is extracted from its mixture with pigment of melanin and macular and results in the contrast enhancement of retinal blood vessels. With the extraction of the retinal blood vessels, the emergence of retinal veins with two kinds of background, namely the melanin and the macular pigment, is also enhanced. Using the emergence of retinal veins in the green band as the reference, the haemoglobin-related IC image achieves *CIF* of 2.42. This haemoglobin-related IC image is advantageous for showing the most-contrasted retinal blood vessels.

For contrast enhancement, the ICA successfully separates the ICs, that is, the melanin, the macular pigment and the haemoglobin. The haemoglobin-related IC image shows higher emergence of retinal veins than that of the green band picture with *CIF* of 2.42 for the low-contrast fundus image model.

5.4.3 RETICA for image enhancement

The performance evaluation of RETICA for both contrast normalisation and contrast enhancement is performed on the small and diverse-contrast fundus image model, as shown in Figure 5.37a. As seen in Figure 5.37, the small and diverse-contrast fundus image model is separated into three channel images, that is, red (b), green (c) and blue (d) channel images. These channel images are applied to RETICA.

In RETICA, the first stage is for contrast normalisation based on the Retinex and followed by the second stage that is, contrast enhancement based on the ICA. The same technique for contrast normalisation, as previously explained, is applied for this small and diverse-contrast image model. Maximum kurtosis and its related optimum number of iteration obtained from the macular pigment are shown in Table 5.6.

The Retinex output images are shown in Figure 5.38. The output images as shown in Figure 5.38d through f is obtained based on the above optimum number of Retinex iterations. The images are subsequently applied to the ICA stage of RETICA for contrast enhancement. As previously explained, the same technique for contrast enhancement is applied to separate the components (melanin, macular pigment and haemoglobin) that are mixed in the contrast-normalised RGB channel images. The haemoglobin-related IC that gives the best contrast of the retinal blood vessels is then determined. Images from Figure 5.38g through i shows the output images of contrast enhancement based on the ICA.

RETICA successfully separates the components into three ICs. It was mentioned earlier that the order of the components is not unique; the order of the components for this reason might be different if the related input image undergoes RETICA for the second, third and so forth. Referring to the results obtained, the haemoglobin is shown by the second IC, while

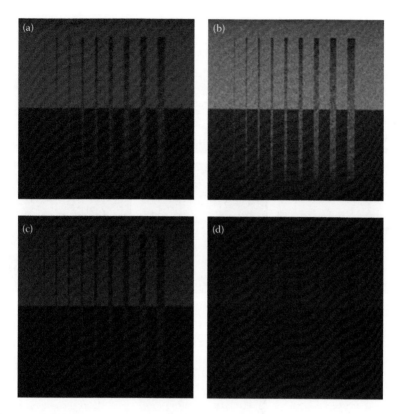

Figure 5.37 (a) Small and diverse-contrast fundus image model and its (b) red, (c) green and (d) blue channel images.

the first and third ICs are related to the melanin and the macular pigment, respectively.

Even though the haemoglobin-related IC can be qualitatively determined by visual inspection, quantitative results are required so that RETICA can be applied in a computerised medical diagnosis system. RETICA determines the haemoglobin-related IC by measuring the

Table 5.6 Kurtosis and related optimum number of iteration of RETICA for melanin, macular pigment and haemoglobin in each colour channel of the small and diverse-contrast image model

	Melanin			Macular pigment			Haemoglobin		
	Red	Green	Blue	Red	Green	Blue	Red	Green	Blue
Kurtosis	6.30	5.76	5.36	5.06	4.23	3.66	5.60	7.14	2.38
Optimum iterations	1	1	1	1	2	29	1	7	1

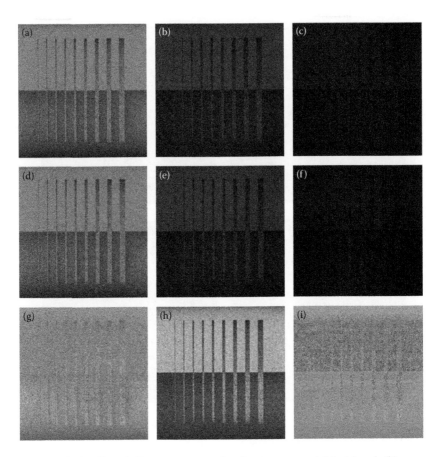

Figure 5.38 Small and diverse-contrast fundus image model in (a) red, (b) green and (c) blue channel images and their corresponding contrast normalisation outputs in (d) red, (e) green and (f) blue channel images and contrast enhancement outputs showing (g) first IC image, (h) second IC image and (i) third IC image.

kurtosis of each IC and determining the least value of kurtosis among the related ICs. Table 5.7 shows the statistics of the green band of the small and diverse-contrast fundus image model with its corresponding ICA images. The intensity I is measured in two forms, that is, I_{norm} and I, in which I_{norm} shows normalisation of I. I_{norm} ranges from 0 to 1, while I ranges from 0 to 255.

As shown in Table 5.7, the highest C_{av} belongs to the second IC image, which is also the haemoglobin-related IC image with C_{av} of 76.83. Moreover, the second IC image has R_{sdc} of 0.753, which is the lowest among the IC images. It means that the second IC has the best emergence of retinal veins as well as the least varied contrast among the IC images. As expected, the contrast of the retinal blood vessel is enhanced since the haemoglobin IC,

Table 5.7 Statistics of green band of small and diverse-contrast image model and ICA images

	Green band (Intensity I)		ICA first comp. (Intensity I)		ICA second comp. (Intensity I)		ICA third comp. (Intensity I)	
	I_{norm}	I	I_{norm}	I	I_{norm}	I	I_{norm}	I
Melanin (Mel)	0.14	36.40	0.63	159.51	0.72	183.78	0.61	154.45
Macular pigment (MP)	0.03	7.87	0.59	149.93	0.32	80.70	0.64	163.66
BV (Mel)	0.07	18.95	0.62	157.09	0.40	101.43	0.62	157.38
BV (MP)	0.07	18.94	0.64	164.04	0.60	152.01	0.64	163.04
Contrast of BV, C_{av}	0.06	14.26	0.03	8.27	0.30	76.83	0.01	1.77
Standard deviation, σ	0.06	15.11	0.11	28.12	0.23	57.86	0.11	27.48
Contrast norm, R_{sdc}	1.060		3.403		0.753		15.486	

which is related to retinal blood vessels, can be extracted from its mixture with the melanin and the macular pigment. This contrast normalised and enhanced image is advantageous as a pre-processed image to be further segmented and analysed in a computerised medical diagnosis system.

5.4.4 Performance evaluation of RETICA

The following performance measures as defined in Section 5.3.6 namely, average emergence of retinal veins, (C_{av}), image contrast normalisation measured, (R_{sdc}), as the ratio between standard deviation and average contrast and *CIF*, are used to evaluate the performance of RETICA. The performance of RETICA is also compared with the performance of six selected image-enhancement algorithms namely, contrast stretching (CS) [46], histogram equalisation (HE) [39], adaptive histogram equalisation (AHE) [40], adaptive contrast enhancement (ACE) [41], contrast limited adaptive histogram equalisation (CLAHE) [65] and homomorphic filtering (HF) [46].

Since the six selected algorithms work only on one channel out of three channels, the channel giving the best image quality in terms of optimum emergence of retinal veins and lowest noise present is selected based on three parameters – C_{av}, standard deviation, σ and R_{sdc}. A comparison of emergence of retinal veins among three channels of the small and diverse-contrast fundus image model is shown in Table 5.8.

According to the statistics shown in Table 5.8, the highest C_{av} belongs to the red channel image with C_{av} of 34.35 followed by the green channel image with C_{av} of 14.26. However, the red channel has a significantly

Table 5.8 Statistics of red, green and blue channels of the small and diverse-contrast fundus image model

	Red channel (Intensity I)		Green channel (Intensity I)		Blue channel (Intensity I)	
	I_{norm}	I	I_{norm}	I	I_{norm}	I
Melanin (mean)	0.40	100.63	0.14	36.40	0.015	3.77
Macular pigment (mean)	0.13	32.07	0.03	7.87	0.004	1
BV in melanin (mean)	0.28	71.03	0.07	18.95	0.007	1.89
BV in macular pigment (mean)	0.28	71.16	0.07	18.94	0.007	1.87
Contrast of retinal vessels, C_{av}	0.14	34.35	0.06	14.26	0.005	1.38
Standard deviation, σ	0.15	37.04	0.06	15.11	0.009	2.32
Contrast normalisation, R_{sdc}	1.078		1.060		1.686	

higher σ than that of the other two channels. The lowest σ, which is 2.32, belongs to the blue channel; yet the emergence of retinal veins of the blue channel is significantly low with C_{av} of only 1.38. Ideally, the image will be selected for that which the standard deviation σ is as low as possible and the emergence of retinal veins C_{av} is as high as possible. Nevertheless, those two conditions are not agreeable in this situation. Thus, the ratio R_{sdc} is used to further determine the best-enhanced image.

As previously discussed in Section 5.3.5, instead of specifically measuring contrast normalisation of the image, the ratio R_{sdc} also indirectly measures image contrast enhancement since it incorporates both σ and C_{av}. The ratio R_{sdc} is derived from the standard deviation σ, which measures the variation of data from its mean value and thus, specifically indicating the homogeneity of image intensity variation. The more homogeneous the intensities is, the more normalised the image contrast will be. Standard deviation σ is only suitable to measure the homogeneity of one object or an area in the image. If there are more than one object, each of which has a different intensity variation, measuring contrast normalisation based on standard deviation σ is no longer appropriate.

Therefore, the average contrast, C_{av}, which measures the average of intensity difference between different objects, is incorporated in the ratio R_{sdc} that specifically measures the contrast normalisation of the image and indirectly measures the contrast enhancement of the image. Moreover, the ratio R_{sdc} of the green channel is the lowest among the others. The lower the ratio R_{sdc} is, the better the contrast normalisation will be as well as the contrast enhancement. Therefore, the green channel with lowest R_{sdc} is selected to undergo the algorithms for comparative study. In real applications, the green channel is usually selected for enhancement of retinal blood vessels. Here, it is proven from fundus image model that the emergence of retinal veins in the green channel is actually lower than that of the red one. The green channel image undergoes six selected algorithms, that is, CS, HE, AHE, ACE, CLAHE and HF and the results are shown in Figure 5.39.

As depicted in Figure 5.39, the green band picture suffers from both small and diverse-contrast. The contrast of the retinal blood vessel model in the macular pigment, especially at the bottom of the image, is very low. Its histogram (Figure 5.39e) also shows that the intensity distribution is

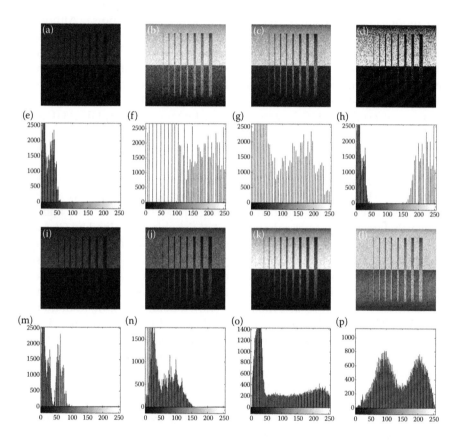

Figure 5.39 (a) Green band picture with (e) its corresponding histogram, (b) green band picture after HE with (f) its corresponding histogram, (c) green band picture after CS with (g) its corresponding histogram, (d) green band picture after AHE with (h) its corresponding histogram, (i) green band picture after ACE with (m) its corresponding histogram, (j) green band picture after CLAHE with (n) its corresponding histogram, (k) green band picture after HF with (o) its corresponding histogram and (l) haemoglobin-related component image with (p) its corresponding histogram.

concentrated at the low intensities values, meaning that the contrast of the image is low.

Applying different image-enhancement methods on the small and diverse image model changes the histogram of the image model. Enhanced images obtained by HE (Figure 5.39b) and CS (Figure 5.39c) have similar pattern of histograms (Figure 5.39f and g). These histograms show moderately and the equalised intensity distribution from 0 to 255 results in better contrast of retinal blood vessel model.

Unlike CS or HE methods, AHE does not qualitatively produce better enhanced image (Figure 5.39d) even though the contrast of retinal vessel model is further enhanced due to amplification of noise. Although the contrast of retinal vessels model in the melanin background is significantly enhanced, AHE fails to enhance the low contrast of retinal vessels in the macular pigment due to low and varied contrast of the image model. Furthermore, ACE produces slightly better contrast of retinal vessels model (as shown in Figure 5.39i) with no significant noise amplification as suffered by AHE. In general, these techniques – CS, HE, AHE and ACE – effectively enhance the contrast of the objects in the image model, but they do not overcome the problem of varied contrast occurred in the image model.

Unlike the aforementioned comparative selected algorithms, CLAHE and HF are better in solving the problem of varied contrast since it does not cause over-enhancement in the image models (Figure 5.39j and k). Nevertheless, the contrast enhancement of the object obtained by CLAHE is not as good as CS and HE as seen from the histogram of the image model by CLAHE (Figure 5.39n). However, CLAHE successfully increases its dynamic contrast resulting in better contrast of retinal blood vessel model than that of the green band picture. Qualitatively, HF produces better contrast of retinal vessels model (as shown in Figure 5.39k) than that of CLAHE. This result is further confirmed by its histogram (Figure 5.39o) showing more normalised intensity distribution than that of CLAHE. Nevertheless, it fails to overcome the problem of over-enhancement resulting in the 'washed-out' appearance of the image model.

RETICA overcomes both the problems of small and diverse-contrast of the image model as in the haemoglobin-related IC image (Figure 5.39). The haemoglobin-related IC image qualitatively shows a better contrast of retinal blood vessel model than that of the enhanced images produced by other selected enhancement methods.

Moreover, the histogram of the haemoglobin-related IC image (Figure 5.39p) shows better dynamic range than that of the green band and the CLAHE due to its more equalised histogram; yet, the histogram of the haemoglobin-related IC image is more concentrated than that of other comparative selected algorithms resulting in higher contrast of retinal blood vessel model.

Histogram of an image with better contrast will normally have a non-Gaussian distribution. Ideally, if there are two or more objects appearing in the image, the histogram will have the number of peaks that correspond to the number of objects. Each peak relates to the mean intensity value of the corresponding object that is represented by some specific intensity distribution. The further apart the peaks, the better the contrast, and the more non-Gaussian distribution the intensity of the object, the less varied contrast the image is.

In the case of the haemoglobin-related IC image, the histogram of third IC as previously explained has two peaks that are related to the mean values of the melanin's and the macular pigment's intensity. A higher difference between the mean of haemoglobin's intensity that is predictably located between these two peaks and that of the melanin or the macular pigment, will result in a larger emergence of retinal veins. Quantitative results represented by three parameters, that is, emergence of retinal veins, (C_{av}), standard deviation, σ and contrast normalisation, R_{sdc} are used to measure the quality of the enhanced image as shown in Table 5.9.

Table 5.9 Comparative results of several image enhancement algorithms on the small and diverse-contrast fundus image model

		Melanin	Macular Pigment	BV (mel)	BV (mac)	C_{av}	σ	R_{sdc}
Green band	I_{norm}	0.143	0.031	0.074	0.074	0.056	0.059	1.060
(Intensity I)	I	36.40	7.87	18.95	18.94	14.26	15.11	
HE	I_{norm}	0.777	0.237	0.499	0.499	0.270	0.293	1.086
(Intensity I)	I	198.16	60.50	127.28	127.24	68.81	74.71	
CS	I_{norm}	0.660	0.119	0.329	0.329	0.271	0.289	1.067
(Intensity I)	I	168.37	30.24	83.83	83.83	69.11	73.73	
AHE	I_{norm}	0.599	0.031	0.092	0.093	0.285	0.368	1.292
(Intensity I)	I	152.73	7.87	23.49	23.95	72.66	93.86	
ACE	I_{norm}	0.196	0.031	0.076	0.076	0.083	0.93	1.127
(Intensity I)	I	50.00	7.87	19.46	19.50	21.08	23.77	
CLAHE	I_{norm}	0.357	0.095	0.151	0.225	0.168	0.147	0.876
(Intensity I)	I	91.02	24.16	38.62	57.39	42.81	37.51	
HF	I_{norm}	0.720	0.097	0.349	0.253	0.264	0.329	1.248
(Intensity I)	I	183.59	24.80	88.87	64.63	67.27	83.97	
ICA	I_{norm}	0.577	0.177	0.388	0.388	0.200	0.210	1.051
(Intensity I)	I	147.23	45.15	98.84	98.98	51.11	53.67	
RETICA	I_{norm}	0.721	0.316	0.398	0.596	0.301	0.227	0.753
(Intensity I)	I	183.78	80.70	101.43	152.01	76.83	57.86	

As shown in Table 5.9, RETICA achieves the best contrast of retinal blood vessel model with the highest C_{av} of 76.83 among the selected image-enhancement methods followed by AHE and CS. However, to determine the quality of the enhanced image needs not only the contrast of the retinal blood vessels but also the contrast normalisation of the image represented by the reduction of the varied contrast including noise that results from the enhancement process. Hence, σ and R_{sdc} are used to measure the contrast normalisation of the image.

The green band picture has the value of σ which is 15.11 and after performing several enhancement methods, the minimum value of σ belongs to the enhanced image after ACE followed by CLAHE. Even though the enhanced images obtained by AHE, CS, HE and HF show better emergence of retinal veins model than that of CLAHE and ACE, they have significantly higher value of σ than that of CLAHE and RETICA. It means that the varied contrast and noise are more in AHE, CS and HE than that in CLAHE and RETICA. This is due to the nature of the AHE, CS and HE in which they enhance not only specific objects, but also noise that presents in the image. It can be seen from their histograms in which the distribution is made more equalised and spread out. Therefore, not only objects of interest, but also noise and the varied contrast are being enhanced resulting in the over-enhanced image.

Parameter R_{sdc} as previously explained is used to measure image quality in terms of contrast normalisation and enhancement by considering the ratio between σ and C_{av}. Moreover, as shown in Table 5.9, ICA with C_{av} of 51.11 produces higher contrast of retinal vessels model than that of CLAHE with C_{av} of 42.81; however, σ of CLAHE is less than that of ICA. Thus, applying ICA to the green band picture can produce better contrast of retinal vessels model in the enhanced image and can also enhance noise.

RETICA achieves the lowest R_{sdc} of 0.753 compared to the selected image-enhancement methods and the green band picture. RETICA enhances image optimally through contrast normalisation and enhancement. Moreover, using the green band picture as the reference, a contrast improvement achieved from the selected image-enhancement methods can be measured. Figure 5.40 depicts CIF and ratio R_{sdc} for images for comparison.

Figure 5.40 shows that among the selected non-invasive digital imaging enhancement methods, RETICA achieves the highest contrast of the retinal blood vessels in the small and diverse-contrast fundus image model with CIF of 5.389, which is slightly lower than that of the FFA with CIF of 5.796. The highest contrast improvement obtained by RETICA compared to other non-invasive image-enhancement methods is AHE with 5.097, CS with 4.848, HE with 4.826, HF with 4.719, followed by ICA with 3.595 and CLAHE with 3.003.

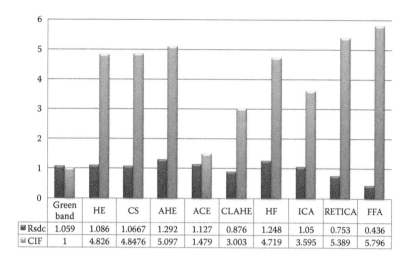

	Green band	HE	CS	AHE	ACE	CLAHE	HF	ICA	RETICA	FFA
■ Rsdc	1.059	1.086	1.0667	1.292	1.127	0.876	1.248	1.05	0.753	0.436
■ CIF	1	4.826	4.8476	5.097	1.479	3.003	4.719	3.595	5.389	5.796

Figure 5.40 CIF and ratio (R_{sdc}) between standard deviation and average contrast of the small and diverse fundus image model after performing seven different algorithms.

Since the fundus picture model is small and diverse in contrast, RETICA first addresses the problem of varied contrast using the contrast normalisation based on the Retinex and is followed by contrast enhancement based on the ICA. Contrast normalisation significantly reduces the intensity variation and minimises the noise present in the image so that the image can be further enhanced without enhancing the noise. Noise in the image is represented as a standard deviation or a variance of image intensities, which moreover can also be used to compare the contrast of two different images [47,48].

The two common problems, that is, varied contrast and low contrast have been addressed by RETICA, and expectedly, the result of image enhancement is better than that of the other selected non-invasive image-enhancement methods that address mostly only the problem of low contrast. The common image-enhancement methods such as AHE, CS and HE fail to produce better-enhanced images in that they do not specifically address the problem of noise present in the image. They are mainly focused on enhancing the contrast of the image. For this reason, if the image being enhanced contains noise, it will also result in an enhancement of the noise during the process.

The enhancement of contrast succeeded by RETICA is of great importance to minimize the utilization of invasive operations such as the FFA that has the best emergence of retinal veins. Nevertheless, due to its invasiveness by injecting contrasting agent into the veins, this method can also cause physiological issues such as nausea, spewing and discombobulation [26]. The least favourable case of negative reactions after fluorescein injection may be fatal anaphylactic shock, which can ultimately lead to death [66]. Furthermore, RETICA can be implemented as part of computerised medical diagnosis system to process the image prior to segmenting and analysing the results. The use of RETICA as an image-enhancement method is advantageous to increase sensitivity, specificity and accuracy of the system in diagnosing retina-related eye sicknesses, for example, DR.

5.5 Concluding remarks

A non-invasive picture-improvement scheme named RETICA is developed. RETICA addresses the issue of small and diverse contrast image, accommodated by using the Retinex for contrast normalisation and ICA for contrast enhancement. The three developed fundus image models are used to validate RETICA. The achievement of RETICA is assessed and compared to three common image-enhancement methods.

The first stage of RETICA is to normalise the varied contrast and to be developed based on the Retinex. Among the various Retinex algorithms, the iterative Retinex method is selected since only one parameter needs to be determined, that is, the number of iteration. The existing iterative Retinex method uses a predetermined number of iteration, which does not always yield the optimum results. Since the optimum number of iteration of the Retinex is related to the homogeneity of the intensity distribution, an iterative Retinex based on the kurtosis is developed to normalise the varied contrast by determining an optimum number of iteration. The higher the kurtosis is, the more homogenous the intensity will be. The contrast-normalised images are subsequently inputted to the second stage of RETICA.

The second stage of RETICA is to enhance the low contrast and to be developed based on the ICA, which in turn enhances the contrast of a specific object or component by separating each of the components that are mixed in the input images. The Fast ICA methodology with symmetrical orthogonalisation is utilized to obtain the predicted ICs due to its high accuracy and high calculation speed. One of the problems in the ICA is that the order of the components is not unique. In the case of fundus image model in which the related ICs are the melanin, the macular pigment and the haemoglobin, the fourth-order statistics, that is, kurtosis, is utilized to discriminate the haemoglobin-related IC from the other components. The haemoglobin-related IC image gives the best emergence of retinal veins among the IC images and higher emergence of retinal veins than that of the green band picture.

Three fundus image models, that is, varied contrast image model, low-contrast image model and small and diverse-contrast image models are developed to validate RETICA. Validation is performed in each stage of RETICA, that is, contrast normalisation and contrast enhancement and RETICA as an entire process. Three parameters, namely emergence of retinal veins (C_{av}), image contrast normalisation (R_{sdc}) and CIF are set up to measure quality of the contrast-enhanced image. Furthermore, the small and diverse-contrast fundus image model undergoes RETICA and six selected image-enhancement methods, that is, CS, HE, AHE, ACE, CLAHE and HF to evaluate the performance of RETICA.

Results of validation study for contrast normalisation show that the Retinex successfully normalises the varied contrast of fundus image model. Different numbers of iteration yield different results of contrast normalisation. Since three components are involved; the use of kurtosis may result in different number of iteration of the Retinex in each component. However, only one optimum number of iteration needs to be used. The optimum number of iteration obtained from the macular pigment is used in that the macular region in the application of RETICA for computerised DR system is selected for determination of FAZ and the varied contrast mainly occurs in the macular pigment. For contrast enhancement, the ICA is able to divide the components into three ICs, that is, melanin, macular pigment and haemoglobin. Even though the order of the component is not unique, the use of kurtosis is able to determine the haemoglobin-related IC that gives the best emergence of retinal veins among the IC images.

Results of comparative study indicate that RETICA is able to normalise the diverse contrast with R_{sdc} of 0.756 better than that of the other selected non-invasive image-enhancement methods. RETICA outperforms other enhancement methods in producing higher emergence of retinal veins with C_{av} of 76.83 followed by AHE, CS, HE, HF, CLAHE and ACE with C_{av} of 72.66, 69.11, 68.81, 67.27, 42.81 and 21.08, respectively. Using C_{av} of the green band picture (i.e., 14.25) as the reference, RETICA achieves CIF of 5.389 that is, slightly lower than that of the invasive FFA with CIFof 5.796. It means that without doing invasively, the emergence of retinal veins can be enhanced at similar level to that obtained by the invasive procedure, which possibly causes some physiological side effects.

In summary, RETICA successfully reduces the diverse contrast and significantly improves the small contrast of the small and diverse-contrast fundus image model. The contrast normalised and improved picture produces a larger emergence of retinal veins and is beneficial for the assessment of the retina-related eye diseases, such as DR through a direct observation or computerised medical diagnosis system. RETICA may be advantageous for retinal vasculature segmentation and determination of FAZ for grading of DR. This enhancement in contrast avoids the necessity of injecting contrasting agent into patients.

5.6 RETICA algorithm (MATLAB code)

```
% RETICA
% Input image is RGB and is processed to Retinex and followed by
% ICA to get the results in which one of them is the haemoglobin-
% related component image.

% LOAD IMAGE
[FileName,PathName] = uigetfile('*.*','Select any RGB image');
y = [PathName,FileName];
I = imread(y);

imgr = I(:,:,1);
imgg = I(:,:,2);
imgb = I(:,:,3);
[M2 N2] = size(imgg);
ratio = 0.4;

% Automatic cropping by selecting centre of the macular region
rectOri=[(x-0.5*ratio*M2) (y-0.5*ratio*M2) (round(ratio*M2))
(round(ratio*M2))];
Icr = imcrop(I,rectOri);
[xx yy] = size(Icr(:,:,2));
Icr = Icr(1:xx-mod(xx,2),1:yy-mod(yy,2),:);
figure(10), imshow(Icr)

% to substitute variable Icr dengan I and transform into log
Ircr = log(double(Icr(:,:,1)+1))/log(255);
Igcr = log(double(Icr(:,:,2)+1))/log(255);
Ibcr = log(double(Icr(:,:,3)+1))/log(255);

maximuter = 10;
dd = 2;
for muter =1:maximuter

    IrcrR2 = my3retinex_mccann99(Ircr, muter);
    IgcrR2 = my3retinex_mccann99(Igcr, muter);
    IbcrR2 = my3retinex_mccann99(Ibcr, muter);

    % Kurtosis Cropped Area
    kur_IrcrR2 = kurtosis(nonzeros(IrcrR2(:)));
    kur_IgcrR2 = kurtosis(nonzeros(IgcrR2(:)));
    kur_IbcrR2 = kurtosis(nonzeros(IbcrR2(:)));

    kur_IcrR2(dd,1) = kur_IrcrR2;
    kur_IcrR2(dd,2) = kur_IgcrR2;
    kur_IcrR2(dd,3) = kur_IbcrR2;

    dd = dd+1

end

% Select Component
kur_IcrR2_r = kur_IcrR2(:,1);
kur_IcrR2_g = kur_IcrR2(:,2);
kur_IcrR2_b = kur_IcrR2(:,3);
kur_IcrR2_max_r = find(kur_IcrR2_r==max(kur_IcrR2_r));
```

```
kur_IcrR2_max_g = find(kur_IcrR2_g==max(kur_IcrR2_g));
kur_IcrR2_max_b = find(kur_IcrR2_b==max(kur_IcrR2_b));

IrRkma = exp(my3retinex_mccann99(Ircr, kur_IcrR2_max_r)*log(255));
IgRkma = exp(my3retinex_mccann99(Igcr, kur_IcrR2_max_g)*log(255));
IbRkma = exp(my3retinex_mccann99(Ibcr, kur_IcrR2_max_b)*log(255));

% Output of Part 1 RETICA
imVCr = uint8(IrRkma);
imVCg = uint8(IgRkma);

imVCb = uint8(IbRkma);
imgrl2 = im2double(imVCr);
imggl2 = im2double(imVCg);
imgbl2 = im2double(imVCb);

% Input for PCA ICA
img_in2 = [imgrl2(:) imggl2(:) imgbl2(:)]';

% the next process is using the FastICA
[img_est2, A_est2, W2]=fastica(img_in2, 'approach', 'symm', 'g',
'tanh','stabilization','on');

Rout2 = img_est2(1,:);Gout2 = img_est2(2,:);Bout2 = img_est2(3,:);

% Rescale the image intensity value from min and max log into
0 to 255
Romax2 = max(Rout2);
Romin2 = min(Rout2);
Ro2 = round((255*(Rout2 - Romin2)/(Romax2-Romin2))); % With log
Gomax2 = max(Gout2);
Gomin2 = min(Gout2);
Go2 = round((255*(Gout2 - Gomin2)/(Gomax2-Gomin2))); % With log
Bomax2 = max(Bout2);
Bomin2 = min(Bout2);
Bo2 = round((255*(Bout2 - Bomin2)/(Bomax2-Bomin2))); % With log

ROim2 = uint8(reshape(Ro2,M2,N2));GOim2 =
uint8(reshape(Go2,M2,N2));BOim2 = uint8(reshape(Bo2,M2,N2));

% Find kurtosis for each of the components
kur(1)=kurtosis(double(ROim2(:)));
kur(2)=kurtosis(double(GOim2(:)));

kur(3)=kurtosis(double(BOim2(:)));

%% Find haemoglobin-related image component
[mkur pkur]=min(kur);
if pkur==1
    A20=ROim2;
end
if pkur==2
    A20=GOim2;
end
if pkur==3
    A20=BOim2;
end
```

```
A21=imcomplement(uint8(A20));
if mean2(A20)>mean2(A21)
    A1=A20;
else
    A1=A21;
end

imgica = A1;

figure(20), imshow(imgica)
```

References

1. D. S. Fong, L. Aiello, T. W. Gardner, G. L. King, G. Blankenship, J. D. Cavallerano, F. L. Ferris and R. Klein, Diabetic retinopathy, *Diabetes Care*, vol. 26, pp. s99–s102, 2003.
2. P. P. Goh, Status of diabetic retinopathy among diabetics registered to the diabetic eye registry, national eye database, 2007, *The Medical Journal of Malaysia*, vol. 63, pp. 24–28, 2008.
3. N. Unwin, D. Gan and D. Whiting, The IDF Diabetes Atlas: Providing evidence, raising awareness and promoting action, *Diabetes Research and Clinical Practice* vol. 87, pp. 2–3, 2010.
4. American Academy of Ophthalmology, *Preferred Practice Pattern* [Online].
5. G. Richard, G. Soubrane and L. Yanuzzi, *Fluorescein and ICG Angiography: Textbook and Atlas*, New York: Thieme; 2 Rev Exp edition, 23 April 1998.
6. H. A. Nugroho, M. H. Ahmad Fadzil, H. Nugroho and L. I. Izhar. Fundus Image Database for Non Invasive Diabetic Retinopathy Monitoring and Grading System (FINDeRS). [Online].
7. T. Teng, M. Lefley and D. Claremont, Progress towards automated diabetic ocular screening: A review of image analysis and intelligent systems for diabetic retinopathy, *Medical and Biological Engineering and Computing*, vol. 40, pp. 2–13, 2002.
8. M. Foracchia, E. Grisan and A. Ruggeri, Luminosity and contrast normalization in retinal images, *Medical Image Analysis*, vol. 9, pp. 179–190, 2005.
9. T. O. Ozanian and R. Phillips, Enhancement of fluoroscopic images with varying contrast, *Computer Methods and Programs in Biomedicine*, vol. 65, pp. 1–16, 2001.
10. A. A. Bhugaloo, B. J. J. Abdullah, Y. S. Siow and K. H. Ng, Diffusion weighted MR imaging in acute vertebral compression fractures: Differentiation between malignant and benign causes, *Biomedical Imaging and Intervention Journal*, vol. 2, p. e12, 2006.
11. V. Spyropoulou, N. Kalyvas, A. Gaitanis, C. Michail, G. Panayiotakis and I. Kandarakis, Modelling the imaging performance and low contrast detectability in digital mammography, *Journal of Instrumentation*, vol. 4, pp. 1–5, 2009.
12. S. Makrogiannis, R. Bhotika, J. Miller, J. Skinner and M. Vass, Nonparametric intensity priors for level set segmentation of low contrast structures, in *Medical Image Computing and Computer-Assisted Intervention—MICCAI 2009*, vol. 5761, G.-Z. Yang, D. Hawkes, D. Rueckert, A. Noble and C. Taylor, Eds. Berlin: Springer, 2009, pp. 239–246.

13. S. W. Smith, R. F. Wagner, J. M. Sandrik and H. Lopez, Low contrast detectability and contrast/detail analysis in medical ultrasound, *Sonics and Ultrasonics, IEEE Transactions on*, vol. 30, pp. 164–173, 1983.

14. A. Ciulla, G. Castronovo, G. Tomasello, A. Maiorana, L. Russo, E. Daniele and G. Genova, Gastric metastases originating from occult breast lobular carcinoma: Diagnostic and therapeutic problems, *World Journal of Surgical Oncology*, vol. 6, p. 78, 2008.

15. S. Povoski, The utilization of an ultrasound-guided 8-gauge vacuum-assisted breast biopsy system as an innovative approach to accomplishing complete eradication of multiple bilateral breast fibroadenomas, *World Journal of Surgical Oncology*, vol. 5, pp. 124, 2007.

16. A. A. H. A.-R. Youssif, A. Z. Ghalwash and A. A. S. A.-R. Ghoneim, Optic disc detection from normalized digital fundus images by means of a vessels' direction matched filter, *Medical Imaging, IEEE Transactions on*, vol. 27, pp. 11–18, 2008.

17. A. A. A. Youssif, A. Z. Ghalwash and A. S. Ghoneim, A comparative evaluation of preprocessing methods for automatic detection of retinal anatomy, in *Proceedings of the Fifth International Conference on Informatics & Systems (INFOS'07)*. Cairo, Egypt, 2007, pp. 24–30.

18. M. Ebrahimi and A. Martel, Image registration under varying illumination: Hyper-demons algorithm, in *Energy Minimization Methods in Computer Vision and Pattern Recognition*, vol. 5681, D. Cremers, Y. Boykov, A. Blake and F. Schmidt, Eds. Berlin: Springer, 2009, pp. 303–316.

19. W.-C. Kao, M.-C. Hsu and Y.-Y. Yang, Local contrast enhancement and adaptive feature extraction for illumination-invariant face recognition, *Pattern Recognition*, vol. 43, pp. 1736–1747, 2010.

20. J. Meier, R. Bock, G. Michelson, L. Nyúl and J. Hornegger, Effects of preprocessing eye fundus images on appearance based glaucoma classification, in *Computer Analysis of Images and Patterns*. W. G. Kropatsch, M. Kampel and A. Hanbury, Eds. Berlin: Springer 2007, pp. 165–172.

21. A. D. Fleming, S. Philip, K. A. Goatman, J. A. Olson and P. F. Sharp, Automated microaneurysm detection using local contrast normalization and local vessel detection, *Medical Imaging, IEEE Transactions on*, vol. 25, pp. 1223–1232, 2006.

22. R. W. Knighton, Quantitative reflectometry of the ocular fundus, *Engineering in Medicine and Biology Magazine, IEEE*, vol. 14, pp. 43–51, 1995.

23. A. Salvatelli et al., A comparative analysis of pre-processing techniques in colour retinal images, *Journal of Physics: Conference Series*, vol. 90, pp. 012069, 2007.

24. W. K. Pratt, *Digital Image Processing*, 2nd ed. New York: Wiley, 1991.

25. D. K. Wysowski and P. Nourjah, Deaths attributed to x-ray contrast media on U.S. death certificates, *American Journal of Roentgenology*, vol. 186, pp. 613–615, 2006.

26. S. Dithmar and F. G. Holz, *Fluorescence Angiography in Ophthalmology*, Heidelberg: Springer, 15 May 2016.

27. L. A. Yannuzzi, K. T. Rohrer, L. J. Tindel, R. S. Sobel, M. A. Costanza, W. Shields and E. Zang, Fluorescein angiography complication survey, *Ophthalmology*, vol. 93, pp. 611–617, 1986.

28. T. A. Ciulla, A. G. Amador and B. Zinman, Diabetic retinopathy and diabetic macular edema, *Diabetes Care*, vol. 26, pp. 2653–2664, 2003.

29. J. R. Lindner, Microbubbles in medical imaging: Current applications and future directions, *Nature Reviews Drug Discovery*, vol. 3, pp. 527–533, 2004.

30. C. Burtea, S. Laurent, L. Elst and R. N. Muller, Contrast agents: Magnetic resonance, in *Molecular Imaging I*, vol. 185/1, W. Semmler and M. Schwaiger, Eds. Berlin: Springer, 2008, pp. 135–165.

31. R. Senior, H. Becher, M. Monaghan, L. Agati, J. Zamorano, J. Louis Vanoverschelde and P. Nihoyannopoulos, Contrast echocardiography: Evidence-based recommendations by European Association of Echocardiography, *European Journal of Echocardiography*, vol. 10, pp. 194–212, 2009.

32. P. Marckmann, L. Skov, K. Rossen, A. Dupont, M. B. Damholt, J. G. Heaf and H. S. Thomsen, Nephrogenic systemic fibrosis: Suspected causative role of gadodiamide used for contrast-enhanced magnetic resonance imaging, *Journal of the American Society of Nephrology*, vol. 17, pp. 2359–2362, 1, 2006.

33. R. C. Gonzalez and R. E. Woods, *Digital Image Processing*. Upper Saddle River, NJ: Prentice-Hall, 2007.

34. J. C. Russ, *The Image Processing Handbook*. Boca Raton, FL: CRC/Taylor & Francis, 2007.

35. A. A. A. Youssif, A. Z. Ghalwash and A. S. Ghoneim, Comparative study of contrast enhancement and illumination equalization methods for retinal vasculature segmentation, in *Proceedings of the Third Cairo International Biomedical Engineering Conference*, Cairo, Egypt, 2006.

36. Clemson University, Clemson, SC, STARE project website [Online]. Available: http://www.ces.clemson.edu/~ahoover/stare

37. University Medical Center Utrecht, Image Sciences Institute, Research Section, Digital Retinal Image for Vessel Extraction (DRIVE) database [Online]. Available: http://www.isi.uu.nl/Research/Databases/DRIVE

38. D. J. Cornforth, H. J. Jelinek, J. J. G. Leandro, J. V. B. Soares, Jr. R. M. Cesar, M. J. Cree, P. Mitchell and T. Bossomaier, Development of retinal blood vessel segmentation methodology using wavelet transforms for assessment of diabetic retinopathy, *Complexity International*, vol. 11, pp. 50–61, 2005.

39. R. C. Gonzalez, R. E. Woods and S. L. Eddins, *Digital Image Processing Using MATLAB*. Berkeley: Gatesmark Publishing, 2004.

40. D. Wu, M. Zhang, J.-C. Liu and W. Bauman, On the adaptive detection of blood vessels in retinal images, *Biomedical Engineering, IEEE Transactions on*, vol. 53, pp. 341–343, 2006.

41. C. Sinthanayothin, J. F. Boyce, H. L. Cook and T. H. Williamson, Automated localisation of the optic disc, fovea, and retinal blood vessels from digital colour fundus images, *British Journal of Ophthalmology*, vol. 83, pp. 902–910, 1999.

42. L. Tusheng and Z. Yibin, Adaptive image enhancement for retinal blood vessel segmentation, *Electronics Letters*, vol. 38, pp. 1090–1091, 2002.

43. G. Yang, L. Gagnon, S. Wang and M. C. Boucher, Algorithm for detecting micros-aneurysms in low resolution color retinal images, in *Vision Interface 2001*. S.S. Beauchemin, F. Nouboud, G. Roth, Eds. Ottawa, Canada, 2001, pp. 265–271.

44. A. D. Hoover, V. Kouznetsova and M. Goldbaum, Locating blood vessels in retinal images by piecewise threshold probing of a matched filter response, *Medical Imaging, IEEE Transactions on*, vol. 19, pp. 203–210, 2000.

45. S. Chaudhuri, S. Chatterjee, N. Katz, M. Nelson and M. Goldbaum, Detection of blood vessels in retinal images using two-dimensional matched filters, *Medical Imaging, IEEE Transactions on*, vol. 8, pp. 263–269, 1989.

46. R. C. Gonzalez and R. E. Woods, *Digital Image Processing*, 3rd ed. Upper Saddle River, NJ: Prentice-Hall, 2008.

47. M. Pavel, G. Sperling, T. Riedl and A. Vanderbeek, Limits of visual communication: The effect of signal-to-noise ratio tin the intelligibility of American Sign Language, *Journal of the Optical Society of America A*, vol. 4, pp. 2355–2365, 1987.

48. G. S. Rubin and K. Siegel, Recognition of low-pass filtered forces and letters, *Investigative Ophthalmology and Visual Science (Suppl.)*, vol. 25, pp. 71–84, 1984.

49. D.-C. Chang and W.-R. Wu, Image contrast enhancement based on a histogram transformation of local standard deviation, *Medical Imaging, IEEE Transactions on*, vol. 17, pp. 518–531, 1998.

50. B. Moulden, F. Kingdom and L. F. Gatley, The standard deviation of luminance as a metric for contrast in random-dot images, *Perception*, vol. 19, pp. 79–101, 1990.

51. E. Peli, Contrast in complex images, *Journal of the Optical Society of America*, vol. 7, pp. 2032–2040, 1990.

52. J. A. Frankle and J. J. McCann, Method and apparatus for lightness imaging, U.S. Patent 4, 348,336, 1983.

53. J. McCann, Lessons learned from Mondrians applied to real images and color gamuts, in *Proceedings of the IS&T/SID Seventh Color Imaging Conference: Colour Science, Systems and Applications*, Scottsdale, Arizona, 1999, pp. 1–8.

54. E. H. Land and J. J. McCann, Lightness and retinex theory, *Journal of the Optical Society of America*, vol. 61, pp. 1–11, 1971.

55. B. Funt, F. Ciurea and J. McCann, Retinex in MATLAB™, *Journal of Electronic Imaging*, vol. 13, pp. 48–57, 2004.

56. P. Comon, Independent component analysis, A new concept? *Signal Processing*, vol. 36, p. 287, 1994.

57. A. Hyvarinen and E. Oja, Independent component analysis: Algorithms and applications, *Neural Networks*, vol. 13, p. 411, 2000.

58. M. H. A. Fadzil, H. A. Nugroho, P. A. Venkatachalam, H. Nugroho and L. Iznita Izhar, Determination of retinal pigments from fundus images using independent component analysis, in *IFMBE Proceedings: 4th Kuala Lumpur International Conference on Biomedical Engineering 2008*, Kuala Lumpur, vol. 21, N. A. A. Osman, F. Ibrahim, W. A. B. W. Abas, H. S. A. Rahman and H.-N. Ting, Eds. Berlin, Springer: 2008, pp. 555–558.

59. A. Hyvarinen, Fast and robust fixed-point algorithms for independent component analysis, *Neural Networks, IEEE Transactions on*, vol. 10, pp. 626–634, 1999.

60. E. H. Land, The retinex theory of color vision, *Scientific American*, vol. 237, pp. 108–28, 1977.

61. F. Pukelsheim, The three sigma rule, *American Statistician*, vol. 48, pp. 88–91, 1994.

62. M. Oren and S. Nayar, Seeing beyond Lambert's law in *Computer Vision — ECCV '94*, vol. 801, J.-O. Eklundh, Ed. Berlin: Springer, 1994, pp. 269–280.

63. J. H. Lambert, *Photometria sive de mensura de gratibus luminis, colorum umbrae*. Eberhard Klett: Augsburg, 1760.

64. R. Jain, R. Kasturi and B. G. Schunck, *Machine Vision*. New York: McGraw-Hill, 1995.
65. S. M. Pizer, E. P. Amburn, J. D. Austin, R. Cromartie, A. Geselowitz, T. Greer, B. H. Romeny, J. B. Zimmerman and K. Zuiderveld, Adaptive histogram equalization and its variations, *Computer Vision, Graphics, and Image Processing*, vol. 39, pp. 355–368, 1987.
66. M. Hitosugi, K. Omura, T. Yokoyama, H. Kawato, Y. Motozawa, T. Nagai and S. Tokudome, An autopsy case of fatal anaphylactic shock following fluorescein angiography, *Medicine Science and the Law*, vol. 44, pp. 264–265, 2004.

chapter six

Noise reduction of retinal image for diabetic retinopathy assessment

Ahmad Fadzil Mohamad Hani, Toufique Ahmed Soomro,
Ibrahima Faye, Nidal Kamel and Norashikin Yahya

Contents

6.1 Introduction

Many eye-related diseases such as diabetic retinopathy (DR) can be diagnosed through analysis of fundus image. Analysis and interpretation of fundus images are essential in the diagnosis and monitoring of vision-threatening complications.

Fundus images are commonly obtained through fundus fluorescein angiography (FFA) image and digital colour fundus image. In FFA, fluorescein dye is injected into the patient's blood vessel to increase the contrast level of retinal vasculature, a mesh of vessels in the retinal layer of fundus image [1]. The FFA method is invasive and can cause physiological reactions such as nausea, vomiting and dizziness. In the most pessimistic scenario, death can occur as well. It was reported by Yanmuzzi et al. [2] that there are 1:222,000 rate of deaths due to FFA, thus it is not recommended unless necessary.

In digital colour fundus imaging, a retinal image is obtained by fundus camera without injecting the contrast agent into the patient's blood vessels. Figure 6.1 shows typical FFA and digital colour fundus images.

Retinal vessels appeared brighter in the FFA image because of the higher contrast compared to the normal colour fundus image. Contrast of retinal vasculature of a colour fundus picture can however be enhanced using digital techniques. A closer analysis of the colour fundus images shows that the images are of varied and low contrast (averaging around 8 for contrast between vessels and background), with low peak signal-to-noise ratios (SNRs) of around 25 dB.

The varied contrast occurs due to uneven illumination of the curved retinal surface and configuration of the light source [3]. There are two types of varied contrast in the retinal fundus image, that is, inter-varying and intra-varying contrast, as shown in Figure 6.2.

The macular region shown in Figure 6.3 suffers from very low contrast and as a result, tiny capillaries cannot be observed clearly [4]. Generally, it is difficult to determine small vessels due to the small contrast between retinal blood vessels and background in retinal fundus pictures [5].

Furthermore, noise due to improper acquisition process of imaging modalities and imaging process methods can affect or occlude the appearance of retinal vessels in the macula region, as shown in Figure 6.4.

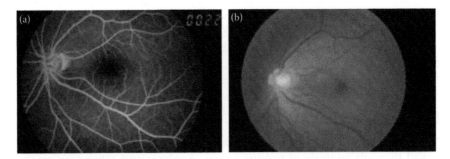

Figure 6.1 Fundus images: (a) fundus fluorescein angiogram image and (b) digital colour fundus image.

(a)

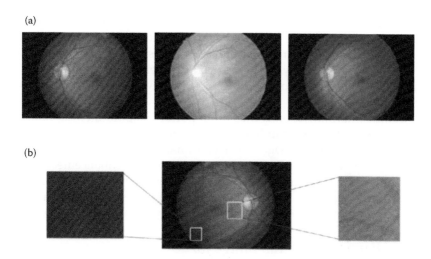

(b)

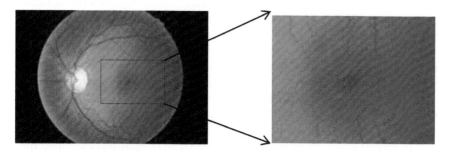

Figure 6.2 Varied contrast problem in colour fundus images: (a) inter-varying contrast and (b) intra-varying contrast.

Figure 6.3 Low contrast problem in the macula region.

(a)   (b)   (c)

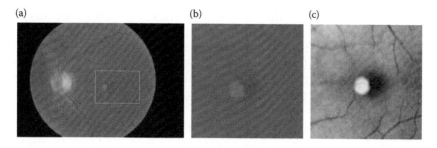

Figure 6.4 Example of noise in fundus images: (a) colour fundus image, (b) macular region and (c) green band of macula image.

Based on the above observations we can conclude that retinal fundus images require noise reduction, image correction and image enhancement. In particular, contrast normalisation is essential for many medical images to reduce varying contrast, contrast enhancement to enhance objects of interest and noise reduction to achieve better signal-to-noise (SNR) ratio quality.

Contrast normalisation is thus an important step for medical images because medical images can have varying contrast. Due to low contrast, tiny objects in medical images such as retinal blood vessels, can be very difficult to observe and process. Therefore, contrast-enhancement techniques played a vital role to enhance tiny low-contrast objects. Noise affects image quality, therefore in order to obtain a better image quality it is very important to remove noise first before any enhancements are made.

6.2 Denoising fundus image for noninvasive DR assessment

In DR assessment, the main challenge in noninvasive image enhancement is to enhance fundus images in order to determine and distinguish the object of interests such as blood vessels from other objects such as noise and artefacts. The aim is to obtain better enhanced images comparable to the image achieved by the FFA method.

Many digital image-processing techniques have been proposed for medical images including retinal images. Detection and reconstruction of retinal vasculature was achieved using image-enhancement method based on contrast limited adaptive histogram equalization (CLAHE) with good accuracy [6]. Although CLAHE gave a contrast improvement factor (CIF) of around 3, it produces noise artefacts that affected the performance of detection of retinal vasculature in fundus images. Fadzil et al. [6] developed the non-invasive image-enhancement technique named RETICA to solve the problem of varied and small contrast of coloured retinal fundus pictures.

As discussed in Chapter 5, the technique has been investigated and applied on retinal fundus model images. The performance of RETICA based on three fundus model images, as shown in Figure 6.5, confirms its ability to enhance fundus images effectively.

RETICA essentially consists of two stages: Retinex [8] for contrast normalisation and independent component analysis (ICA) [9] for contrast enhancement. RETICA accomplished a CIF of 5.38 on the fundus model images compared to CIF 5.79 achieved by FFA method on real fundus images.

The overall challenge is to implement an alternative to FFA method using non-invasive image-enhancement techniques that address the problems of noise, diverse and small contrast of fundus images. It is important to emphasise that the nature of noise in the fundus images can affect the

(a) (b) (c)

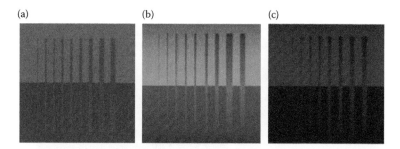

Figure 6.5 Model fundus images. (a) Small contrast model fundus image, (b) varied contrast model fundus image and (c) low and varied contrast model fundus image. (Adapted from H. A. Nugroho, Non-invasive image enhancement of colour retinal fundus image for computerised diabetic retinopathy monitoring and grading system, *PhD thesis*, Electrical and Electronics Engineering Programme, Universiti Teknologi PETRONAS, 2012.)

performance of any image-enhancement technique. The issue of recognising the characteristics of noise has been talked about by a few researchers [3,10,11]. Proposing a strategy that is reasonable for recognising the sort of noise present in a picture is very testing [12]. In most actual pictures, there is no earlier learning of the characteristics of the noise present in the picture; nevertheless, most algorithms reported for filtering (Lee, Wiener) in related literature consider the characteristics of the noise to be known. It is, however, conceivable to recognize noise referencing on adaptive Wiener filters (additive, multiplicative and additive plus multiplicative filters) and the fundus model picture; and genuine fundus pictures are used for these filters. It is known that retinal fundus pictures comprise both additive and multiplicative noise [13].

6.2.1 Image noise models

Image noise is a variation of brightness or colour information in image, and is usually an aspect of electronic noise. It can be produced by the circuitry of digital camera. In image processing, noise reduction and restoration of an image is expected to improve the qualitative inspection of an image and the performance criteria of the quantitative image analysis techniques. The main purpose of denoising the image is to restore the details of the original image as much as possible. The criteria of the noise removal problem depend on the noise type by which the image is corrupted. In the field of reducing the image noise, several types of linear and non-linear filtering techniques have been proposed.

The nature of the noise present depends on the image modality used, as shown in Figure 6.6. The noise affects the x-ray images due to which details of the image cannot be observed clearly; similarly, ultrasound

(a)   (b)

(c)

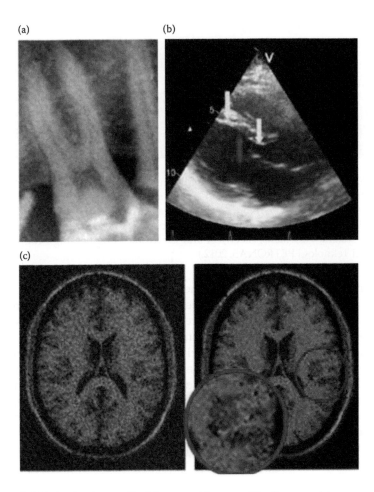

Figure 6.6 Noise in the medical images: (a) x-ray, (b) ultrasound image and (c) magnetic resonance image (MRI).

images and MRI (magnetic resonance images) are affected due to noise. But identification of these images are based on the sources of the acquisition process of the devices; like the ultrasound image that contains speckles or multiplicative noise due to the inherent characteristics of coherent imaging like ultrasound imaging.

The main source of noise in digital images occurs during image acquisition. The performance of imaging sensors is affected by a variety of factors, such as environmental conditions during image acquisition process and quality of sensing elements themselves. For example, in acquiring images with CCD camera, light levels and sensors temperature are major factors affecting the amount of noise in resultant image [3]. The basic noise models are defined below.

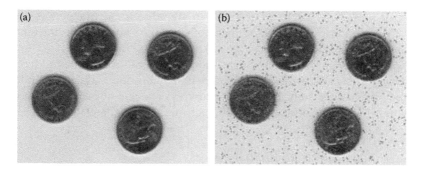

Figure 6.7 Illustration of salt and pepper noise in image. (a) Original image and (b) with added salt-and-pepper noise.

Salt-and-pepper noise is otherwise called as impulse noise, shot noise or binary noise. This debasement can be brought about by a sharp, sudden distribution in the picture and its appearance is randomly scattered white or black pixels over the image, as the example shown in Figure 6.7. Salt-and-pepper noise is modelled as [3]

$$p(z) = \begin{cases} P_a & \text{for } a = z \\ P_b & \text{for } z = b \\ 0 & \text{otherwise} \end{cases} \qquad (6.1)$$

If $p(z) > a$, intensity b will show up as light dot in the picture and a will show up as a dark dot. If either P_a and P_b is zero, the impulse (salt and pepper) noise is called unipolar. In the event that neither one of the probabilities is zero and particularly if they are around equivalent to impulse, noise values will resembles salt-and-pepper granules arbitrarily dispersed over the image.

Gaussian noise is an admired type of white noise, which is brought about by the irregular vacillation in the signals. One can watch the white noise by viewing a TV that is somewhat mistuned to a specific channel. Gaussian noise is white noise which is typically aggravated. If the picture is introduced as I and the Gaussian noise by N, it can be modelled as a noise image by just including the two, I and N. Gaussian noise is also called additive noise, the probability density function (PDF) of Gaussian noise is shown mathematically [3].

$$p(z) = \frac{1}{\sqrt{2\pi}\sigma} e^{-\frac{(z-\bar{z})}{2\sigma^2}}$$

where z represents intensity of image or signal, $\bar{z}$ is the mean value of z and σ the standard deviation of image or signal. As an example, the effect of Gaussian noise is shown in Figure 6.8.

However, Gaussian noise can be modelled by random values added to an image and speckle noise can be modelled by random values multiplied by the pixel values; hence, it is also known as speckle noise. As an example, the effect of speckle noise on the picture is highlighted in Figure 6.9.

6.2.2 Noise in retinal fundus images

It is difficult to analyse the tiny blood vessels against the surrounding background in the selected RGB (red, green and blue) macular region (Figure 6.10); the analysis is further made difficult when fundus image contains noise. The green band also contained noise. The different regions of the green band image were cropped for observation and it was seen that due to the noise, the blood vessels could not be observed.

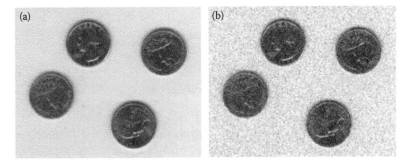

Figure 6.8 Illustration of Gaussian noise. (a) Original image and (b) with Gaussian noise.

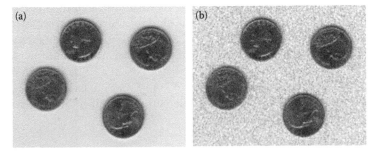

Figure 6.9 Illustration of Speckle noise. (a) Original image and (b) with Speckle noise.

(a)   (b)

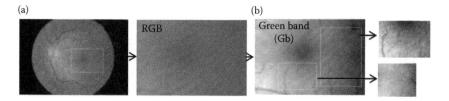

Figure 6.10 Noise in the retinal fundus images. (a) Colour fundus image and (b) macular region of fundus image.

A fundus camera has a complex optical design system and according to the principle operation of the fundus camera, it contains two illumination systems: the flash tube and photo detector (camera circuitry) [4]. Noise in the retinal fundus image may be multiplicative due to the speckle flash or iteration of the patient's eye and the flash of the fundus camera. Additive noise is also present because of the circuitry of the camera electronics because no digital image is a free additive as it is captured with cameras and camera circuitry produces noise.

However, recognition of the noise type in the retinal fundus picture enables a suitable denoising method to be selected in order to improve the retinal fundus image quality.

6.2.3   Image denoising methods

In retinal fundus imaging, image denoising problem is still a challenge for the researchers because removal of noise causes the artefacts and image blurring. Image denoising is classified into two types, that is, spatial domain filtering and transform domain filtering methods. A spatial filter is an image operation where each pixel value $I(x,y)$ is changed by a function of the intensities of pixels in a neighbourhood of (x,y). Spatial filters can be further ordered into non-linear and linear filters. A filtering method is linear when the output is a weighted sum of the input pixels such as mean filter, average filter, Wiener and Lee filter. Non-linear spatial filters cannot be calculated using just a weighted sum. Other operations (e.g. square root, log, sorting and selection) are involved in calculation of non-linear filters. Examples of non-linear filters are median filter and weighted median filters. Non-linear filters are not easy to implement as compared to linear spatial filters such as non-linear Lee filter, Roberts filter and Kirsch's template filter. Non-linear filters can smooth with less blurring edges compared to linear filters and can detect edges at all orientations simultaneously, but can be slow to compute.

Some of transform domain filtering are specifically used to remove the noise [14]. The purpose of transform domain filtering is to find a domain where signal can be more easily separated from noise. Transform domain filtering has three main techniques namely frequency transform, short frequency transform and wavelet transform and these techniques can be used for image denoising purpose. Wavelet transform is one of the most popular methods in image denoising [14].

Many researchers worked on the spatial domain and transform domain to solve the problem of removal of noise from the image. In Changyan et al.'s [15] proposed method, median filter is utilised to expel noise. Authors also centred around on comparative investigation of picture denoising methods depending on spatial filters and transform domain filters. Subjective and objective strategies are utilised for judging the efficiency of different types of spatial filters and transform filters applied to different types of noise. Folke et al. [16] proposed a de-noising procedure that is based on a blend of median and wavelets filter. Image that is tainted by two or more types of noise can be simultaneously denoised. But it is one of the drawbacks of cascaded two filters for one task (removal of noise) because it takes more time and median filters [17] gave smoothness in images and wavelet produce artefacts due to its higher frequency coefficient and details of image are lost due to smoothness of median filter [18,19].

Denoising techniques based on the subspace structure of the image have been proposed over the last decade, among them are the least squares (LS) and the minimum variance (MV) [20]. These two techniques depend on the singular value decomposition (SVD) of the original image or the eigen decomposition (ED) of the covariance in segregating the signal subspace from the noise subspace and use this information in minimising the distance between the noisy image and the signal subspace. The LS and the MV do achieve significant improvement in image denoising but at the expense of signal distortion. Recently, a novel subspace technique is suggested that deal with signal distortion and noise reduction. This technique is an extension of the time-domain constraint estimators (TDCEs) of Ephraim and Van Trees [21] and towards two-dimensional signal (image). The technique is proposed by Nidal Kamel et al. [22], and is used for retina image denoising in this research.

The signal subspace methodology was initially proposed by Ephraim and Van Trees [21] for speech improvement applications. Comprehensive research works in speech improvement had been conducted by different researchers by using time-domain constrained (TDC) estimators. The principle is based on breaking down the vector space of the noisy signal into a signal subspace. The noise expulsion is accomplished by nulling the noise subspace and controlling the noise distribution in the signal (signal + residual noise) subspace. It is observed that signal distortion and residual noise (once denoised image or signal subspace is obtained, it is also possible that it contained noise so that noise is known residual noise and its effect the details of image, it is possible also to calculate the noise residual or residual image as it is a difference between the original and denoised image [23]) cannot be minimised concurrently. Linear estimation using TDC estimator is performed on the clean picture to keep residual noise energy within the threshold while at the same time minimising the signal distortion. The strategy included decomposition of noisy pictures into two orthogonal subspaces: signal (signal + residual noise) subspace and noise subspace. The signal (signal + residual noise) subspace is prevailed by eigenvalues of clean picture and so it is termed as signal subspace.

Here, the TDC estimator is used in retinal colour fundus image to improve the SNR of image because TDC estimator can control signal distortion and reduce the noise also. TDC estimator is based on the SVD. The SVD is used to determine the signal subspace; it is defined in the subsection below. The basic standard of subspace denoising is to cancel the noise subspace and control the noise contribution in the signal subspace. Henceforth, the techniques attempt to accomplish an exchange between the amount of diminished noise and signal distortion. This can be accomplished by optimisation criteria which target to minimize signal distortion while setting a user-defined upper bound on the residual noise by means of a control parameter and this can be achieved by using TDC estimator. Table 6.1 provides the description of several denoising methods along with its strength and weakness.

6.2.4 SVD method

The SVD is one strong mathematical tool for factorising data [24]. It is a strong orthogonal matrix decomposition technique [25]. SVD becomes more regularly utilised in signal- and image-processing applications because of its conceptual and stability reasons. SVD has numerous properties that are profoundly advantageous for pictures; for example, its maximum energy packing, settling of LS issue, computing pseudo-inverse of a matrix and multivariate analysis [26,27]. A key property of SVD is its connection to the rank of a matrix and its capacity to estimate matrices of a given rank. Digital pictures are frequently represented by low rank matrices and, hence, ready to be portrayed by a sum of a generally small set of eigenvalues. This idea rises the controlling of the signal as two distinct subspaces [28,29]. SVD is constituted from two orthogonal subspaces. This property of SVD is mostly used in noise filtering to determine the signal subspace and noise subspace [30,31].

SVD depends on a hypothesis from linear algebra which says that a rectangular matrix A can be separated into the result of three matrices – an orthogonal matrix U, a diagonal matrix S and the transpose of an orthogonal matrix V and this hypothesis is shown in as

$$A_{mn} = U_{mm}S_{mn}V_{nn}^T \tag{6.2}$$

Table 6.1 Comparison between image denoising techniques

No.	Denoising method	Description	Strengths	Weaknesses
1	Mean filter	The value of each pixel is replaced by the average of all the values in the local neighbourhood	Easy to implement	Lose the details of image due to blurring in the image
2	Median filter [32]	Replace each pixel value with the median of the grey values in the local neighbourhood	Easy to implement	Lose the details of image due to blurring in the image
3	Wiener filter [33]	Wiener filter depends on statistical measurement of fundamental parameters like standard deviation, mean and window size	Local filtering is performed and it remove the noise while maintain the contrast also	Wiener filter makes the image smooth and due to its smoothness image details are gone
4	Wavelet transform [34]	Standardised localisation of the time–frequency. Wavelet transform give good image then frequency domain filtering such as spatial filtering	Removed the noise and give good information about the edges of image	Produce the artefacts. The results of wavelet transform are no longer shift-invariant
5	Least squares estimator (LSE) [18]	It minimises the length between noisy vectors and signal subspace and provides denoised picture	LSE is favourable technique in handling the level of noise	LS estimator cannot control the signal distortion that influences the subtle elements of the picture
6	The minimum variance estimator (MVE) [35]	MVE is utilised to minimize the difference as per rank of matrix	MVE is greatly improved method to handle the noise level then LSE	MVE estimator cannot control the signal distortion that influences the subtle elements of picture

where

$$U_{mm} = [u_1, u_2, \ldots, u_m], V_{nn} = [v_1, v_2, \ldots, u_n] \quad \text{and} \quad S_{mn} = \begin{bmatrix} \sigma_1 & & \\ & \sigma_2 & \\ & & \sigma_n \end{bmatrix}$$

where $U^T U = I$, $V^T V = I$; the columns of U are orthonormal eigenvectors of AA^T, the columns of V are orthonormal eigenvectors of $A^T A$ and S is a diagonal matrix containing the square roots of eigenvalues ($[\sigma_1, \sigma_2, \ldots, \sigma_n]$) from U or V in descending order [36]. For example, consider matrix A

$$A = \begin{bmatrix} 3 & 1 & 1 \\ -1 & 3 & 1 \end{bmatrix}$$

To find U we have to begin with AA^T. The transpose of A is

$$A = \begin{bmatrix} 3 & -1 \\ 1 & 3 \\ 1 & 1 \end{bmatrix}$$

$$AA^T = \begin{bmatrix} 3 & 1 & 1 \\ -1 & 3 & 1 \end{bmatrix} \begin{bmatrix} 3 & -1 \\ 1 & 3 \\ 1 & 1 \end{bmatrix} = \begin{bmatrix} 11 & 1 \\ 1 & 11 \end{bmatrix}$$

Thereafter, we have to locate the eigenvalues and interrelated eigenvectors of AA^T. We understand that eigenvectors are represented by the equation $Au = \lambda u$, where A is a square matrix of data, λ the scalar value known as eigenvalue also and v is the eigenvector and applying this to AA^T provides us

$$Au = \lambda u = \begin{bmatrix} 11 & 1 \\ 1 & 11 \end{bmatrix} \begin{bmatrix} u_1 \\ u_2 \end{bmatrix} = \lambda \begin{bmatrix} u_1 \\ u_2 \end{bmatrix}$$

This represents the system of equations

$$11u_1 + u_2 = \lambda u_1 = (11 - \lambda)u_1 + u_2 = 0 \tag{6.3}$$

$$u_1 + 11u_2 = \lambda u_2 = u_1 + (11 - \lambda)u_2 = 0 \tag{6.4}$$

In order to solve λ, we need to set the determinant of the coefficient matrix to zero,

$$\begin{vmatrix} (11-\lambda) & 1 \\ 1 & (11-\lambda) \end{vmatrix} = 0$$

It results as

$$(11-\lambda)(11-\lambda) - 1.1 = 0 \tag{6.5}$$

$$(\lambda - 10)(\lambda - 12) = 0 \tag{6.6}$$

$$\lambda = 10, \lambda = 12 \tag{6.7}$$

It gives us two eigenvalues $\lambda = 10$ and $\lambda = 12$. Inserting λ in Equations 6.3 and 6.4 gives us eigenvectors u_1 and u_2. For $\lambda = 10$ we get

$$(11-\lambda)u_1 + u_2 = 0$$

$$(11-10)u_1 + u_2 = 0$$

$$u_1 + u_2 = 0$$

$$u_1 = -u_2$$

As it is applicable for many values, we shall pick $u_1 = 1$ and $u_2 = -1$ considering they are small and less demanding to work with. Hence, we obtain the eigenvector [1, −1] interrelated to the eigenvalue $\lambda = 10$. For $\lambda = 12$ we have

$$u_1 + (11-\lambda)u_2 = 0$$

$$u_1 + (11-12)u_2 = 0$$

$$u_1 - u_2 = 0$$

$$u_1 = u_2$$

For the same reason as before, let $u_1 = 1$ and $u_2 = 1$. Currently, for $\lambda = 12$ we have the eigenvector $[1, 1]$. These eigenvectors become column vectors in a matrix ordered by the size of the interrelated eigenvalue. Explaining in another form, column one represents the eigenvector of the largest eigenvalue, column two represents the eigenvector of the next largest eigenvalue and so forth until the last column of our matrix becomes our eigenvector of the smallest eigenvalue. In the matrix below, column one is the eigenvector for $\lambda = 12$ and column two is the eigenvector for $\lambda = 10$.

$$\begin{bmatrix} 1 & 1 \\ 1 & -1 \end{bmatrix}$$

At the final stage, this matrix is converted into an orthogonal matrix by applying the Gram–Schmidt orthonormalisation method to the column vectors [37]. The following equations are used for orthogonal matrix conversion:

$$u_1 = \frac{u_1}{|u_1|} = \frac{[1,1]}{\sqrt{1^2 + 1^2}} = \frac{[1,1]}{\sqrt{2}} = \left[\frac{1}{\sqrt{2}}, \frac{1}{\sqrt{2}} \right]$$

Similarly, u_2

$$u_1 = \frac{u_2}{|u_2|} = \frac{[1,-1]}{\sqrt{1^2 + (-1^2)}} = \frac{[1,-1]}{\sqrt{2}} = \left[\frac{1}{\sqrt{2}}, \frac{-1}{\sqrt{2}} \right]$$

It gives

$$U = \begin{bmatrix} \dfrac{1}{\sqrt{2}} & \dfrac{1}{\sqrt{2}} \\ \dfrac{1}{\sqrt{2}} & -\dfrac{1}{\sqrt{2}} \end{bmatrix}$$

The calculation of V is the same. V is based on $A^T A$, therefore

$$A^T A = \begin{bmatrix} 3 & -1 \\ 1 & 3 \\ 1 & 1 \end{bmatrix} \begin{bmatrix} 3 & 1 & 1 \\ -1 & 3 & 1 \end{bmatrix} = \begin{bmatrix} 10 & 0 & 2 \\ 0 & 10 & 4 \\ 2 & 4 & 4 \end{bmatrix}$$

Find the eigenvalues of $A^T A$ by

$$Av = \lambda v = \begin{bmatrix} 10 & 0 & 2 \\ 0 & 10 & 4 \\ 2 & 4 & 2 \end{bmatrix} \begin{bmatrix} v_1 \\ v_2 \\ v_3 \end{bmatrix} = \lambda \begin{bmatrix} v_1 \\ v_2 \\ v_3 \end{bmatrix}$$

This represents the system of equations

$$10v_1 + 2v_3 = \lambda v_1$$

$$10v_2 + 4v_3 = \lambda v_2$$

$$2v_1 + 4v_2 + 2v_3 = \lambda v_3$$

These equations can be rewritten as

$$(10 - \lambda)v_1 + 2v_3 = 0 \tag{6.8}$$

$$(10 - \lambda)v_2 + 4v_3 = 0 \tag{6.9}$$

$$2v_1 + 4v_2 + (2 - \lambda)v_3 = 0 \tag{6.10}$$

This can be solved as

$$\begin{vmatrix} (10 - \lambda) & 0 & 2 \\ 0 & (10 - \lambda) & 4 \\ 2 & 4 & (2 - \lambda) \end{vmatrix} = 0$$

This will be solved as

$$(10 - \lambda) \begin{vmatrix} (10 - \lambda) & 4 \\ 4 & (2 - \lambda) \end{vmatrix} + 2 \begin{vmatrix} 0 & (10 - \lambda) \\ 2 & 4 \end{vmatrix} = 0$$

$$(10 - \lambda)[(10 - \lambda)(2 - \lambda) - 16] + 2[0 - 2(10 - \lambda)] = 0$$

$$\lambda(\lambda - 10)(\lambda - 10)$$

so $\lambda = 0$, $\lambda = 10$, $\lambda = 12$ are the eigenvalues for $A^T A$. Substituting λ back into Equation 6.3 to find corresponding eigenvectors yields for $\lambda = 12$

$$(10 - \lambda)v_1 + 2v_3 = 0$$

$$(10 - 12)v_1 + 2v_3 = 0$$

$$-2v_1 + 2v_3 = 0$$

$$v_1 = v_3$$

$$v_1 = 1, v_3 = 1$$

Substituting v_1 and v_3 in Equation 6.5.

$$2v_1 + 4v_2 + (2 - 12)v_3 = 0$$

$$2 + 4v_2 - 10 = 0$$

$$4v_2 = 8$$

$$v_2 = 2$$

Therefore for $\lambda = 12$, $V_1 = [1, 2, 1]$. For $\lambda = 10$,

$$(10 - \lambda)v_1 + 2v_3 = 0$$

$$(10 - 10)v_1 + 2v_3 = 0$$

$$v_3 = 0$$

Substituting v_3 in Equation 6.5

$$2v_1 + 4v_2 + (2 - \lambda)v_3 = 0$$

$$2v_1 + 4v_2 + (2 - \lambda) * 0 = 0$$

$$2v_1 + 4v_2 = 0$$

$$2v_1 = -4v_2$$

$$v_1 = -2v_2$$

$$v_1 = 2, v_2 = -1$$

Therefore for $\lambda = 10$, $V_2 = [2, -1, 0]$. For $\lambda = 0$ put $v_1 = 1$ in Equation 6.2

$$(10 - 0)v_1 + 2v_3$$

$$10v_1 = -2v_3$$

$$v_3 = -5$$

Substituting $v_3 = 5$ and $\lambda = 0$ in Equation 6.4

$$(10 - 0)v_2 + 4 * 5 = 0$$

$$10v_2 - 20 = 0$$

$$v_2 = 2$$

Substituting $v_3 = 5$, $v_2 = 2$ and $\lambda = 0$ in Equation 6.5

$$2v_1 + 4v_2 + (2 - \lambda)v_3 = 0$$

$$2v_1 + 4 * 2 + (2 - 0) * (-5) = 0$$

$$2v_1 = 2$$

$$v_1 = 1$$

Therefore, for $\lambda = 0$, $V_3 = [1, 2, -5]$. The order of V_1, V_2, V_3 as column vectors in a matrix according to the size of the eigenvalue to obtain

$$V = \begin{bmatrix} 1 & 2 & 1 \\ 2 & -1 & 2 \\ 1 & 0 & -5 \end{bmatrix}$$

At the final stage, this matrix is converted into an orthogonal matrix by using the Gram–Schmidt orthonormalisation method on the column vectors [37]. The following equations are used for orthogonal matrix conversion.

$$v_1 = \frac{v_1}{|v_1|} = \frac{[1,2,1]}{\sqrt{1^2 + 2^2 + 1^2}} = \frac{[1,2,1]}{\sqrt{6}} = \left[\frac{1}{\sqrt{6}}, \frac{2}{\sqrt{6}}, \frac{1}{\sqrt{6}}\right]$$

$$v_2 = \frac{v_2}{|v_2|} = \frac{[2,-1,0]}{\sqrt{2^2 + (-1^2)}} = \frac{[2,-1,0]}{\sqrt{5}} = \left[\frac{2}{\sqrt{5}}, \frac{-1}{\sqrt{5}}, 0\right]$$

$$v_3 = \frac{v_3}{|v_3|} = \frac{[1,2,-5]}{\sqrt{1^2 + 2^2 + (-5^2)}} = \frac{[1,2,-5]}{\sqrt{30}} = \left[\frac{1}{\sqrt{30}}, \frac{2}{\sqrt{30}}, \frac{-5}{\sqrt{30}}\right]$$

The V matrix is

$$V = \begin{vmatrix} \dfrac{1}{\sqrt{6}} & \dfrac{2}{\sqrt{5}} & \dfrac{1}{\sqrt{30}} \\ \dfrac{2}{\sqrt{6}} & \dfrac{-1}{\sqrt{5}} & \dfrac{2}{\sqrt{30}} \\ \dfrac{1}{\sqrt{6}} & 0 & \dfrac{-5}{\sqrt{30}} \end{vmatrix}$$

According to SVD theorem (Equation 6.2), V matrix is transpose V^T is

$$V^T = \begin{vmatrix} \dfrac{1}{\sqrt{6}} & \dfrac{2}{\sqrt{6}} & \dfrac{1}{\sqrt{6}} \\ \dfrac{2}{\sqrt{5}} & \dfrac{-1}{\sqrt{5}} & 0 \\ \dfrac{1}{\sqrt{30}} & \dfrac{2}{\sqrt{30}} & \dfrac{-5}{\sqrt{30}} \end{vmatrix}$$

In reference to S we need to take the square roots of the nonzero eigenvalues and insert the diagonal with them, inserting the largest in S_{11}, the next largest in S_{22} and so forth until the smallest value is inserted in S_{mn}. The nonzero eigenvalues of U and V are dependably the same, this explains why it does not matter which one is being used. The diagonal entries in S are the singular values of A, the columns in U are named left singular vectors and the columns in V are named right singular vectors as shown in below matrix.

$$S = \begin{bmatrix} \sqrt{12} & 0 & 0 \\ 0 & \sqrt{10} & 0 \end{bmatrix}$$

We have SVD equation

$$A_{mn} = U_{mm} S_{mn} V_{nn}^T$$

$$A_{mn} = \begin{bmatrix} \dfrac{1}{\sqrt{2}} & \dfrac{1}{\sqrt{2}} \\ \dfrac{1}{\sqrt{2}} & -\dfrac{1}{\sqrt{2}} \end{bmatrix} \begin{bmatrix} \sqrt{12} & 0 & 0 \\ 0 & \sqrt{10} & 0 \end{bmatrix} \begin{bmatrix} \dfrac{1}{\sqrt{6}} & \dfrac{2}{\sqrt{6}} & \dfrac{1}{\sqrt{6}} \\ \dfrac{2}{\sqrt{5}} & \dfrac{-1}{\sqrt{5}} & 0 \\ \dfrac{1}{\sqrt{30}} & \dfrac{2}{\sqrt{30}} & \dfrac{-5}{\sqrt{30}} \end{bmatrix}$$

$$A_{mn} = \begin{bmatrix} \dfrac{\sqrt{12}}{\sqrt{2}} & \dfrac{\sqrt{10}}{\sqrt{2}} & 0 \\ \dfrac{\sqrt{12}}{\sqrt{2}} & \dfrac{-\sqrt{10}}{\sqrt{2}} & 0 \end{bmatrix} \begin{bmatrix} \dfrac{1}{\sqrt{6}} & \dfrac{2}{\sqrt{6}} & \dfrac{1}{\sqrt{6}} \\ \dfrac{2}{\sqrt{5}} & \dfrac{-1}{\sqrt{5}} & 0 \\ \dfrac{1}{\sqrt{30}} & \dfrac{2}{\sqrt{30}} & \dfrac{-5}{\sqrt{30}} \end{bmatrix}$$

$$A_{mn} = \begin{bmatrix} 3 & 1 & 1 \\ -1 & 3 & 1 \end{bmatrix}$$

A_{mn} is the required SVD matrix. A_{mn} is also known as signal subspace and TDC estimator is defined in the following section because TDC estimator is used to keep residual noise energy within the threshold while at the same time minimising the signal distortion, and TDC estimator gives image without noise, well-contrasted image and maintain image details. It is very important to understand the signal and noise model before explaining the TDC estimator and both sections (signal and noise model and TDC estimator) are explained in the following sections.

6.2.5   *Time-domain constrained estimator*

An image signal is a short window that may be treated as wide sense stationary method, and therefore may be portrayed by a linear stochastic model of the form

$$X = H\theta \tag{6.11}$$

where $X \in \mathbb{R}^{m \times n}$ is a matrix of random specimens in whose rank is $n < m, H \in \mathbb{R}^{m \times m}$ is a model matrix and $\theta \in \mathbb{R}^{m \times n}$ is a zero mean random coefficient matrix obtained from multivariate distribution. Considering that a picture is distorted by additive independent white noise, N, and not correlated with the clean signal, the $m \times n$ matrix of noisy image Y is represented by

$$Y = X + N \tag{6.12}$$

where $X \in \mathbb{R}^{m \times n}$ is the noise matrix while $X \in \mathbb{R}^{m \times n}$ is the clean image. With the given noisy signal, it can be estimated that the clean signal, X, is as precise as possible in referencing to a few points of comparison. This is a classical issue in estimation theory. If H is the $m \times m$ filter matrix, therefore the linear estimator of the clean picture given Y is equal to

$$\hat{X} = YH \tag{6.13}$$

The noisy signals mentioned are a product of stochastic methodologies, which means that the study of subspace methods is according to correlation matrices. First, deliberate that the correlation matrix of the original picture is represented by the linear model of Equation 6.11, that is

$$R_X = E\{XX^T\} = E\{H\theta\theta^T H^T\} = HR_\theta H^T$$

where $R_\theta = E\{\theta\theta^T\}$. The rank of R_x is r and this matrix has $(m - r)$ zero eigenvalues. Alike, allow the correlation matrix of the noise vector be expressed by $R_N = E\{NN^T\}$. During the consideration of second-order statistics, it is meaningful to allow the following two assumptions:

1. The element of X and N are uncorrelated, that is, $R_{XN} = 0$, $R_{NX} = 0$.
2. The noise is white with variance ϑ_n^2 that is, $R_N = \vartheta_n^2 I$.

The second assumption is according to the point that the correlation matrix of noise is obtained beforehand and the mathematical methodology of the estimators utilizes the eigenvalue-decomposition (EVD) of covariance matrices R_Y, R_X and R_N given by

$$R_Y = R_N + R_X \tag{6.14}$$

It is understood that the noise power is consistently disseminated in the entire Euclidean space, while the image signal is confined to r dimensional subspace. In the actual practice, the precise information of the second-order statistic R_X is not accessible, but it is predicted from the noisy signal.

A novel subspace technique is suggested that handles the signal distortion and noise limitation and it is known as TDC estimator. This technique is an extension of the TDCEs of Ephraim and Van Trees [21] towards two-dimensional signal (image). Referring to the predicted signal in Equation 6.13, the error signal attained in the prediction is given by

$$\epsilon = \hat{X} - X$$

The estimated signal according to Equation 6.13 is $\hat{X} = YH$, then error signal becomes

$$\epsilon = YH - X$$

According to Equation 6.12, $Y = X + N$

$$\epsilon = (X + N)H - X$$

$$\epsilon = XH + NH - X$$

$$\epsilon = (H - I)X + HN \tag{6.15}$$

where $(H - I)X$ is signal distortion and it is represented as ϵ_X and HN is residual noise and it is represented as ϵ_X [21]. The energy of $m \times n$ matrix of signal distortion and residual noise is equivalent to Frobenius norm given as

$$\varepsilon_X^2 = \|\epsilon_X\|_2^2 = tr\{\epsilon_X \epsilon_X^T\} = tr((H - I)R_s(H - I)^T) \tag{6.16}$$

$$\varepsilon_N^2 = \|\epsilon_N\|_2^2 = tr\{\epsilon_N \epsilon_N^T\} = tr\{H(NN^T)H^T\} = tr\{HR_N H^T\} \tag{6.17}$$

where tr is matrix trace and it is defined as sum of diagonal elements of matrix.

Thus, assuming established value of R_N, a TDC estimator [21] contains the residual noise energy, within some threshold while diminishing the signal distortion energy. The ideal linear estimator may be attained by unlocking a constrained optimization issue

$$\min_H \varepsilon_X^2 \text{ subject to} \frac{1}{m} \varepsilon_N^2 \leq \sigma^2 \tag{6.18}$$

where σ^2 is a positive constant and m is the rank of matrix. The constrained minimization described in Equation 6.18 may be solved utilising the strategy of Lagrange multipliers [38]. In other words, H is a stationary feasible point if it complies to the gradient equation of Lagrangian [38],

$$\mathcal{L}(H,\lambda) = \varepsilon_s^2 + \lambda(\varepsilon_N^2 - m\sigma^2)$$

$$\mathcal{L}(H,\lambda) = tr\left\{(H-I)R_x(H-I)^T\right\} + \lambda(tr\left\{HR_nH^T\right\} - m\sigma^2) \quad (6.19)$$

where $\lambda \geq 0$ is the Lagrangian multiplier, λ is the Lagrangian multiplier

$$\lambda\left(\varepsilon_N^2 - m\sigma^2\right) = \lambda\left(tr\left\{HR_nH^T\right\} - m\sigma^2\right) = 0 \text{ for } \lambda \geq 0 \quad (6.20)$$

From $\nabla_H \mathcal{L}(H,\lambda)$ we obtained

$$\nabla_H \mathcal{L}(H,\lambda) = 2(H-I)R_x + 2\lambda HR_n = 0 \quad (6.21)$$

It gives

$$H_{TDC} = R_x(R_x + \lambda R_N)^{-1} \quad (6.22)$$

When N is white, $R_N = \vartheta_n^2 I$, where ϑ_n^2 is the noise variance, and I is the identity matrix, the optimal estimator H, can be written as

$$H_{TDC} = R_x(R_x + \lambda\vartheta_n^2 I)^{-1} \quad (6.23)$$

Also, from Equations 2.23 and 6.21 it can be shown that σ^2 should satisfy

$$\sigma^2 = \frac{1}{m}tr(R_x(R_x + \lambda R_N)^{-1}R_N(R_x + \lambda R_N)^{-1}R_x) \quad (6.24)$$

Equation 6.17 shows that if λ has different values from 0 to ∞ then it motivates the σ^2 to have different values from $(1/m)tr(R_N)$ to 0. In other words, the estimator does not add noise to the estimated signal. It is important to know that the value of λ builds upon picture and noise level. Thus, Equation 6.23 may be interpreted utilising the SVD of $R_x = U\Delta_X U^T$ to

$$H_{TDC} = U\Delta_X(\Delta_X + \lambda\vartheta_n^2 I)U^T \quad (6.25)$$

where the U is the unitary eigenvectors matrix and Δ_X is the diagonal eigenvalue matrix of R_x. TDC is successfully applied and as an example consider matrix A,

$$A = \begin{bmatrix} 3 & 1 & 1 \\ -1 & 3 & 1 \end{bmatrix}$$

Perform the SVD on the matrix and achieved SVD components are given below, where

$$U = \begin{bmatrix} \dfrac{1}{\sqrt{2}} & \dfrac{1}{\sqrt{2}} \\ \dfrac{1}{\sqrt{2}} & -\dfrac{1}{\sqrt{2}} \end{bmatrix}, V = \begin{bmatrix} \dfrac{1}{\sqrt{6}} & \dfrac{2}{\sqrt{6}} & \dfrac{1}{\sqrt{6}} \\ \dfrac{2}{\sqrt{5}} & \dfrac{-1}{\sqrt{5}} & 0 \\ \dfrac{1}{\sqrt{30}} & \dfrac{2}{\sqrt{30}} & \dfrac{-5}{\sqrt{30}} \end{bmatrix} D = \begin{bmatrix} \sqrt{12} & 0 & 0 \\ 0 & \sqrt{10} & 0 \end{bmatrix}$$

According to the Equation 6.19 $H_{TDC} = U\Delta_X\left(\Delta_X + \lambda\vartheta_n^2 I\right)U^T$ and Δ_X is diagonal value of R_x and Rx is equal to $R_x = AA^T$.

$$Rx = \begin{bmatrix} 3 & 1 & 1 \\ -1 & 3 & 1 \end{bmatrix} \begin{bmatrix} 3 & -1 \\ 1 & 3 \\ 1 & 1 \end{bmatrix} = \begin{bmatrix} 11 & 1 \\ 1 & 11 \end{bmatrix}$$

But Δ_X is the diagonal matrix of its Eigen value of Rx and its Eigen values are 12 and 10 then Δ_X becomes

$$\Delta_X = \begin{bmatrix} 12 & 0 \\ 0 & 10 \end{bmatrix}$$

The transpose of U is

$$U^T = \begin{bmatrix} \dfrac{1}{\sqrt{2}} & \dfrac{1}{\sqrt{2}} \\ \dfrac{1}{\sqrt{2}} & -\dfrac{1}{\sqrt{2}} \end{bmatrix}$$

According to Equation 6.19, to determine the TDC estimated image H_{TDC}

$$H_{TDC} = U\Delta_X(\Delta_X + \lambda\vartheta_n^2 I)U^T$$

$$H_{TDC} = \begin{bmatrix} \dfrac{1}{\sqrt{2}} & \dfrac{1}{\sqrt{2}} \\ \dfrac{1}{\sqrt{2}} & -\dfrac{1}{\sqrt{2}} \end{bmatrix} \begin{bmatrix} 12 & 0 \\ 0 & 10 \end{bmatrix} \left(\begin{bmatrix} 12 & 0 \\ 0 & 10 \end{bmatrix} + \begin{bmatrix} 1 & 0 \\ 0 & 1 \end{bmatrix} \right) \begin{bmatrix} \dfrac{1}{\sqrt{2}} & \dfrac{1}{\sqrt{2}} \\ \dfrac{1}{\sqrt{2}} & -\dfrac{1}{\sqrt{2}} \end{bmatrix}$$

Resultant H_{TDC} signal is

$$H_{TDC} = \begin{bmatrix} 133 & 23 \\ 23 & 133 \end{bmatrix}$$

When applied on the signals and images, TDCE achieved better results in terms of noise reduction (performance is evaluated by measuring SNR of images) while preserving image details as shown in Figures 6.11 and 6.12 [39].

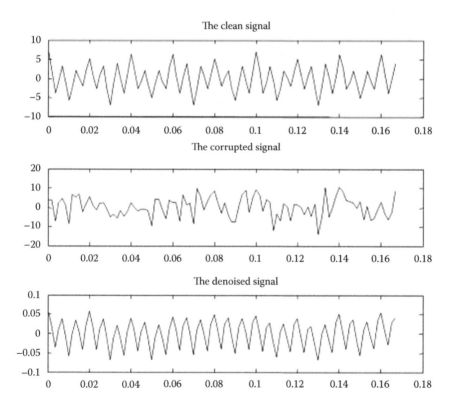

Figure 6.11 TDCE on signal. (Adapted from M. H. Ahmad Fadzil, L. I. Izhar, and H. A. Nugroho, *Computers in Biology and Medicine*, vol. 40, pp. 657–664, 2010.)

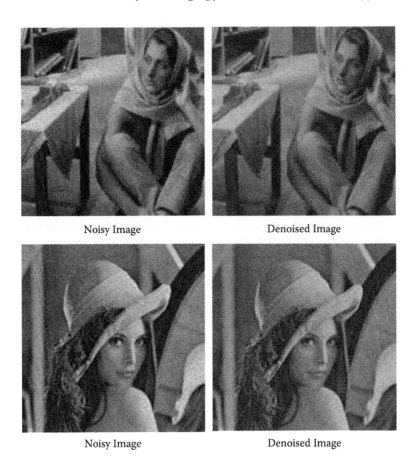

| Noisy Image | Denoised Image |

| Noisy Image | Denoised Image |

Figure 6.12 TDCE on standard test images.

6.3   *Improving RETICA*

The aim in non-invasive retinal image enhancement is to address three main problems of colour fundus image namely, diverse and small contrast, and noise in real fundus pictures. To overcome the issue of diverse and small contrast, a digital image enhancement method that combines Retinex and ICA techniques known as RETICA, is applied on real fundus images. In the preceding chapter, model fundus images were used and RETICA was effective in overcoming contrast problems. Here, the real fundus image in particular the macular region undergoes a denoising process called TDCE to improve the SNR prior to RETICA. The improvement in performance of incorporating TDCE before RETICA is investigated in terms of contrast improvement and peak SNR measurements, compared to the invasive FFA modality.

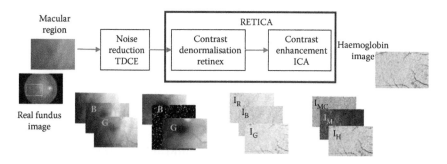

Figure 6.13 Proposed method TDCE with RETICA.

The RGB colour channels of the fundus picture are each processed through Retinex methodology to get the corresponding normalised RGB colour channels. As shown in Figure 6.13, a smaller area of the fundus picture consisting of the macular area is utilised to find out the improvement of the retinal capillaries. According to the figure, the RGB colour channels of the macular region are initially denoised by TDCE to improve the SNR. Then, in the RETICA process, the Retinex algorithm normalises the varied contrast in the colour channels followed by ICA to get the independent components (IC) that are caused by the macular, haemoglobin and melanin pigments from the colour channels. The haemoglobin picture is chosen from the three ICs as it represents an optimally contrast-enhanced retinal vasculature picture.

6.3.1   Subspace-based technique for image denoising

Various denoising techniques based on the subspace structure of the image have been proposed over the last decade, among them are the least squares estimator (LSE) and the minimum variance estimator (MVE) [40]. These two techniques depend on the SVD of the original image or the ED of the covariance, in segregating the signal subspace from the noise subspace and use this information in minimising the distance between the noisy image and the signal subspace. The LS and the MV methods can achieve significant improvement in image denoising but at the expense of signal distortion. Recently, Yahya et al. [41] proposed a novel subspace technique that takes into account both signal distortion and noise energy. This technique is an extension of the TDCEs of Ephraim and Trees [21] for two-dimensional signal (image).

6.3.2   Time-domain constraints estimator

The TDCE as mentioned by Yahya et al. [42] has been considered to minimize the signal distortion. The strategy preserves the contrast of the pictures as well as picture details while expelling noise [43]. Let $\hat{s} = Hx \in R^m$ be the linear estimator of the pure signal vector s where $H \in R^{m \times m}$. H is attained by minimising the residual signal $r = \hat{s} - s \in R^m$. Equation 6.26 shows the concept

$$r = Hx - s = H(s+n) - s = (Hs - s) + Hn = r_S + r_N \tag{6.26}$$

where the signal distortion is r_S and the noise residual is r_N. Both signal distortion and residual noise cannot be minimised concurrently. TDCE is suggested to handle the signal distortion and noise reduction. TDCE preserves the signal distortion by reducing the residual noise as the residual noise energy. This is shown below

$$\varepsilon_N^2 = \|r_N\|_2^2 = tr\{r_N r_N^T\} = tr\{H(nn^T)H^T\} = tr\{HR_n H^T\} \tag{6.27}$$

The energy of the residual noise has a threshold as shown below

$$\varepsilon_N{}^2 \leq mv^2 \text{ where } v^2 \text{ is a positive constant} \tag{6.28}$$

Equation 6.29 is utilised to minimise the energy of the signal distortion

$$\varepsilon_s{}^2 = \|e_s\|_2^2 = tr\{e_s e_s{}^T\} = tr((H - I_m)R_s(H - I_m)^T) \tag{6.29}$$

By bringing together Equations 6.28 and 6.29, it provides the TDCE,

$$\min_H \varepsilon_s^2 \text{ subject to } \varepsilon_N^2 \leq mv^2$$

The quantity of noise is cut down by lowering the threshold level, V^2, of the noise; thus, the quantity of distortion is elevated and vice versa. By utilising Kuhn-Tucker settings to minimise constraints, ideal distortion can be attained. In the event that it meets the requirement of the gradient equation of the Lagrangian, then H is a feasible point that is stationary. Alike, utlising a data matrix that contains n realisations and $X \in R^{m \times n}$, then $\hat{S} = XW \in R^{m \times n}$ where $H \in R^{n \times n}$. Utilising Equation 6.30, the residual matrix, E, is attained.

$$E = \hat{S} - S = XH - S = S(H - I_n) + NH = E_S + E_N \tag{6.30}$$

where E_S and $E_N \in R^{m \times n}$.

E_S and E_N are the signal distortion and the residual noise matrix, respectively. Equation 6.31 shows the Lagrangian formulation.

$$\mathcal{L}(H,\mu) = \varepsilon_s^2 + \mu\left(\varepsilon_N^2 - mv^2\right) \tag{6.31}$$

where, μ is the Lagrangian multiplier. With $\blacktriangledown H\ \mathcal{L}(H,\mu) = 0$, an optimum H is attained (denoised signal), as

$$H_{TDCE} = R_s(R_s + \mu R_n)^{-1} \tag{6.32}$$

6.3.3   Contrast normalisation using McCann iterative Retinex algorithm

The McCann iterative Retinex algorithm [8] is decided for contrast normalisation of fundus picture. Figure 6.14 demonstrates the flow chart of iterative Retinex [32]. Retinex algorithm is utilised on the RGB output pictures of TDCE. Each colour channel input picture is changed from linear to logarithmic form to disentangle the procedure (i.e. multiplication to addition and division to subtraction). A multi-resolution pyramid of each colour channel is made. In each progression, the distance between the pixels being compared reduces with one-shift pixel distance. The course among the pixels also adjusts clockwise at each progression. The comparison between pixels is executed at each progression to predict reflectance part utilising ratio-product-reset-average operation [8,33]. The latter comparisons between pixels are consistently done to refine the predicted reflectance at pyramid's bottom level until the distance reduces to one pixel and final product is accomplished.

The Compare Neighbour block in Figure 6.14, that is, the ratio-product-reset-average operation is the main implementation of Retinex to reduce illumination variations and thus normalise image. The operation subtracts the neighbour's log luminance (the ratio step) and then adds the result to the old product (the product step). If the result exceeds the highest value, defined by maximum, it is reset to maximum (the reset step). Finally, the new product for the pixel obtained by comparison to its neighbour is averaged with previous product (average steps).

The ratio-product-reset-average task is done by figuring the ratio between I (in specific channel) and its spatially shifted input version; and offset it by some distances formulated as Equation 6.33 and flow chart depicted in Figure 6.15.

$$\log R_{x,y}^* = \frac{\mathrm{Re\,set}\left[(\log I_{x,y} - \log I_{xs,ys}) + \log R_{xs,ys}\right] + \log R_{x,y}}{2} \tag{6.33}$$

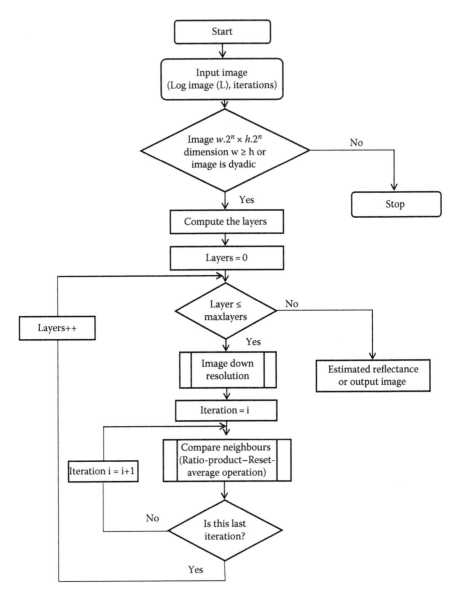

Figure 6.14 McCann Retinex algorithm.

where $[\log I(x,y) - \log L'(x,y)]$ serves as the ratio and $([\log I(x,y) - \log L'(x,y)] + \log R'(x,y))$ serves as the product in log domain. The Reset procedure is done to renew the maximum intensity value according to number of iterations. The term $\log R(x,y)^*$ is a result of averaging with $\log R'(x,y)$ and $\log R(x,y)^*$ itself is an updated output produced in each iteration that will

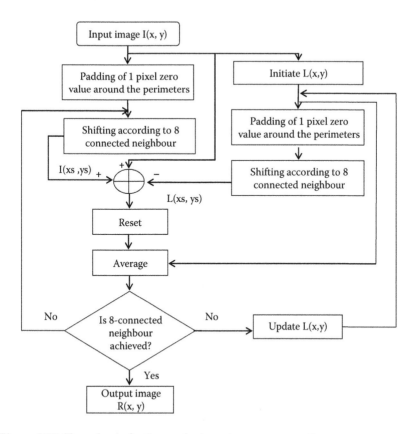

Figure 6.15 Flow chart of ratio-product-reset-average operation.

be used as an input for next iteration until the final reflectance is obtained at given last iteration.

6.3.4   Contrast enhancement using FastICA

The FastICA algorithm with the symmetrical orthogonalisation is utilised to accomplish the predicted ICs because of its exact accuracy and fast computation for high-dimensional data [44]. The output picture of the Retinex algorithm is being used as inputs to the ICA as depicted in Figure 6.16. The ICA is a methodology used to decide the original signals from the mixtures of several independent sources. For this situation, enhancement of low contrast retinal blood vessels in the digital fundus picture is done by deciding the retinal pigment make-up, namely haemoglobin I_H, melanin I_M and macular I_{MC} pigment utilising the ICA. The IC caused by the haemoglobin exhibits higher contrast for retinal blood

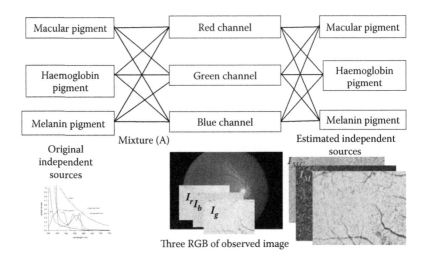

Figure 6.16 Independent component analysis.

vessels against its surrounding background (melanin and macular components), as shown in Figure 6.16.

6.3.5   *Performance of TDCE-RETICA method*

The performance of the proposed non-invasive image-enhancement TDCE-RETICA technique is based on two parameters. The first parameter is the contrast between the blood vessels against its surrounding background in the macular area of the green channel, haemoglobin and FFA pictures. The second parameter is the contrast enhancement factor of the haemoglobin image against the green channel picture; and the FFA image against the green channel picture.

Contrast determination: The absolute mean intensity difference between the retinal blood vessels and the background of the retinal image is the contrast of the retinal blood vessels and the background region. Equation 6.34 is used to determine this.

$$C_{|bv-bg|} = \left| \frac{1}{n} \left(\sum_{i=1}^{n} I_{bvi} - \sum_{i=1}^{n} I_{bgi} \right) \right| \tag{6.34}$$

Here, the contrast between the background and the retinal blood vessels $C_{|bv-bg|}$ is the contrast between the retinal blood vessels and the background. The intensities of the retinal blood vessels against its surrounding background are referred to by the terms, I_{bvi} and I_{bgi},

(a) (b)

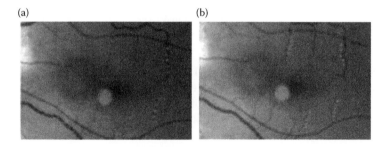

Figure 6.17 Random choice of positions of the pixels of blood vessel and background for contrast determination. (a) Green band blood vessels intensity selection and (b) green band background choice of intensity.

respectively. The number of pixels in the background of the fundus picture and the retinal blood vessels are indicated by the n variable where $n = 50$. The positions of the pixel are irregularly selected in this study, as illustrated in Figure 6.17.

Selection of data intensity for contrast measurement: In the objective of quantifying the contrast of the picture, the intensity points or pixels of the blood vessels against its surrounding background inside the macular area is chosen irregularly as shown by the blue dots in Figure 6.17. Likewise, the intensity of the retinal blood vessels against its surrounding background of macular area of green band picture, FFA picture and haemoglobin picture because of RETICA are chosen irregularly. Contrast between the blood vessels against its surrounding background of macular area of green band picture, macular area of grey scale of FFA picture and macular area of haemoglobin picture is quantified according to Equation 6.34.

Selection of haemoglobin image: The differentiation of haemoglobin-related IC from the other two ICs, which are the melanin pigments and the macular pigments, is based on the IC that has the highest contrast of blood vessels against its surrounding background [18]. Retinal blood vessels, comparing to the melanin or the macular background of the retinal fundus picture, are more visible in the haemoglobin image (Figure 6.17).

6.4 Results and analysis

The contrast between blood vessels and its surrounding background in the green band picture is utilised as the reference contrast, C_{REF}. The contrast enhancement is given by the contrast between blood vessels and its surrounding background in the haemoglobin picture, C_{HI}. The contrast ratio of C_{HI}/C_{REF} is known as the contrast improvement factor, *CIF* as shown below.

$$CIF = \frac{C_{RETICA}}{C_{REF}} \tag{6.35}$$

Peak signal-to-noise ratio (PSNR) is an engineering term for the ratio between the maximum possible power of a signal or image and the noise image power that affects the quality of image [35]. Noise in fundus picture is evaluated based on PSNR values as follows:

$$PSNR = 20\log_{10}\left(\frac{255}{\sigma}\right) \tag{6.36}$$

The term σ is the standard deviation of the picture and 255 is regarded as peak value of picture.

Signal energy is the term in the signal processing to determine the strength of signal. Signal energy of image shows how the grey levels are distributed in image or any particular channels as expressed in

$$\text{Signal energy} = \sum_{i,j}|I(i,j)|^2 \tag{6.37}$$

where $I(i,j)$ is image with intensities values.

6.4.1   Improving contrast of fundus pictures

Two fundus picture datasets are used namely, 35-Fundus dataset and FINDeRS (Fundus image for non-invasive diabetic retinopathy system) dataset. The 35-Fundus dataset contained 35 colour fundus images of various DR stages with their corresponding FFA images. Of the 35-Fundus pictures, there are 11 No_DR, 6 Mild NPDR, 6 Moderate NPDR, 4 Severe NPR and 8 PDR images. The FINDeRS dataset contains 175 colour fundus images of various DR stages, 50 No_DR, 40 Mild NPDR, 30 Moderate NPDR, 18 Severe NPDR and 37 PDR images. The achievement of the recommended methodology is assessed based on the CIF and PSNR.

Table 6.2 shows the contrast values for the green band component of the fundus pictures (C-GB), FFA images (C-FFA) and haemoglobin images (C-HI) for the 35-Fundus dataset. The CIFs for FFA (CIF-FFA) and haemoglobin images (CIF-HI) are also given for each image. The average CIFs are found to be 5.12 for FFA and 5.46 for the proposed TDCE-RETICA method.

Generally, it is observed that the application of TDCE-RETICA results in higher contrast and thus higher CIF compared to FFA images. However, as seen from Table 6.2, there are six cases where the FFA images has

Table 6.2 Contrast values and CIFs for 35-Fundus dataset

No.	Image	C-GB	C-FFA	C-HI	CIF-FFA	CIF-HI
1	No DR_1	6	33.8	34.4	5.63	5.73
2	No DR_2	6.9	38.3	39.4	5.55	5.71
3	No DR_3	5.6	28.4	31.1	5.07	5.55
4	No DR_4	6.3	31.6	35.8	5.01	5.68
5	No DR_5	6.2	33.2	35.5	5.35	5.72
6	No DR_6	11.7	53.3	60.1	4.55	5.13
7	No DR_7	6.4	34.9	35.3	5.45	5.51
8	No DR_8	9.1	47.7	48.2	5.24	5.29
9	No DR_9	8.5	34.3	47.5	4.03	5.58
10	No DR_10	7.1	40.9	36.9	5.76	5.19
11	No DR_11	8.7	35	45.5	4.02	5.22
12	Mild_1	5.2	28.7	29.9	5.51	5.75
13	Mild_2	5.3	29.2	26.9	5.50	5.07
14	Mild_3	12.9	73	68.5	5.65	5.31
15	Mild_4	12.9	50.2	67.1	3.89	5.20
16	Mild_5	5.1	26.1	29.3	5.11	5.74
17	Mild_6	10.7	54.9	58.9	5.13	5.50
18	Moderate_1	5.6	28.3	30	5.05	5.35
19	Moderate_2	5.1	27.6	26.5	5.41	5.19
20	Moderate_3	7.8	44.4	39.2	5.69	5.02
21	Moderate_4	9.3	49.5	52.8	5.32	5.67
22	Moderate_5	14.2	75.5	82.2	5.31	5.78
23	Moderate_6	9.9	42.1	53.8	4.25	5.43
24	Severe_1	6.5	34.9	36.1	5.36	5.55
25	Severe_2	5.1	29.2	31.2	5.72	6.11
26	Severe_3	10.9	54.2	54.9	4.97	5.03
27	Severe_4	11.2	59.8	59.9	5.33	5.34
28	PDR_1	5.2	26.5	29.8	5.09	5.73
29	PDR_2	5.2	27.1	29.6	5.20	5.69
30	PDR_3	3.9	14.9	21.1	3.82	5.4
31	PDR_4	6.3	32	31.8	5.07	5.04
32	PDR_5	9.5	42.8	48.7	4.50	5.12
33	PDR_6	4.6	27.2	25.6	5.91	5.56
34	PDR_7	15.8	87.3	82.2	5.52	5.20
35	PDR_8	7.4	38.5	43.4	5.20	5.86
Average		7.9	40.4	43.1	**5.12**	**5.46**

better CIF in particular, NO_DR_10, MILD_2, MILD_3, MODERATE_2, MODERATE_3 and PDR_7. For example, images of MILD_3 and PDR _7 are shown in Figure 6.18.

Figure 6.18 shows examples of haemoglobin images from green band, FFA and TDCE-RETICA for various DR stages. From Figure 6.18, it can be seen that the green band image of No_DR_6 has varied contrast (some regions are brighter and some regions are darker) and contains artefacts (specular reflection) as shown in the red circle. With TDCE-RETICA, the resultant images have uniform and higher contrast without generating artefacts (Retinex being the technique to normalise contrast). The tiny blood vessels in the macula of the green band No_DR_6 image are not clearly observable due to low contrast (yellow circle) but due to ICA in TDCE-RETICA (ICA is used to extract the blood vessels against its surrounding background) the blood vessels can be better observed in comparison to the untreated image and its corresponding FFA image. Likewise, RETICA pictures of MILD_4, MILD_6, MODERATE_5, SEVERE_3 and SEVERE_4 exhibit uniform and bigger contrast of blood vessels against its surrounding background allowing clearer observation of small capillaries comparing to FFA pictures.

MILD_3 and PDR_7 of FFA images have a slightly bigger contrast comparing to RETICA pictures. We can observe that the green band of MILD_3 contained varying and low contrast with artefacts as shown by the red circles making it difficult to analyse tiny blood vessels. However, even at a lower contrast of 68.5 for TDCE-RETICA, the tiny blood vessels are enhanced uniformly. A similar observation is obtained for the green band image of PDR_7. Clearly, TDCE-RETICA is able to enhance image contrast uniformly and to reduce artefacts.

The CIF for various DR-severity stages of the 35-Fundus dataset are shown in Figure 6.19. TDCE-RETICA performs better with an average CIF of 5.46 than FFA that has an average CIF of 5.12.

Figure 6.20 depicts the achievement of TDCE-RETICA for images from the FINDeRS dataset. The CIF varies between 4.8 and 5.22 for the various DR stages with an average CIF of 5.02.

Figure 6.21 shows the CIF by TDCE-RETICA for various DR stages of 35-Fundus and FINDeRS datasets.

Figure 6.22 shows samples of No_DR, Mild NPDR, Moderate NPDR, Severe NPDR and PDR pictures from FINDeRS dataset. Generally, the green band images of all samples suffer from varied and low contrast. After applying TDCE-RETICA, the contrast of haemoglobin images are homogeneous with a higher contrast between the blood vessels and the background.

Figure 6.22 shows several fundus images containing artefacts and the effects of applying TDCE-RETICA. In the case of the No_DR image in Figure 6.22, the green band image contains a bright spot artefact (yellow

Image	Green band	FFA picture	Haemoglobin picture
No_DR_6	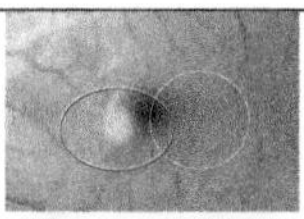 Contrast: 11.17	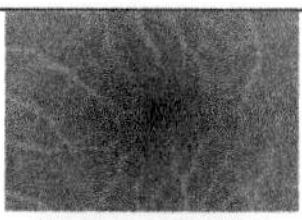 Contrast: 53.3	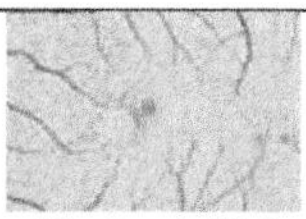 Contrast: 60.1
Mild_3	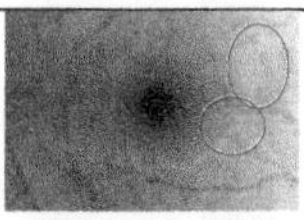 Contrast: 12.9	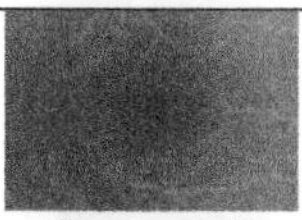 Contrast: 73	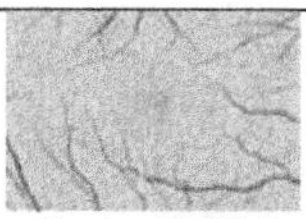 Contrast: 68.5
Mild_4	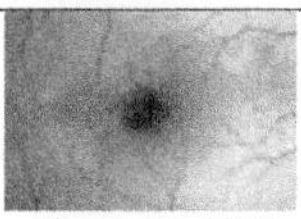 Contrast: 12.9	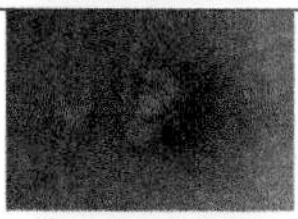 Contrast: 50.9	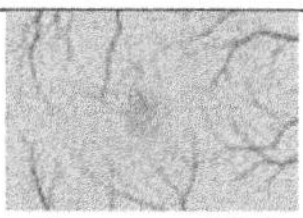 Contrast: 58.9
Mild_6	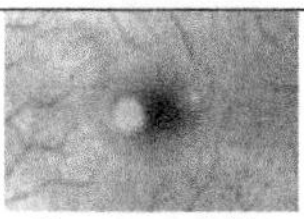 Contrast: 10.7	Contrast: 54.9	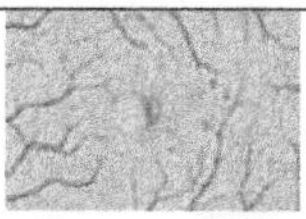 Contrast: 58.9
Moderate_5	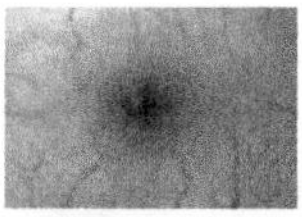 Contrast: 14.2	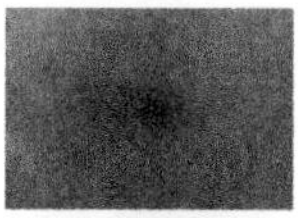 Contrast: 75.5	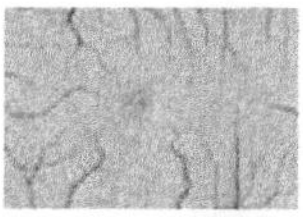 Contrast: 82.2
Severe_3	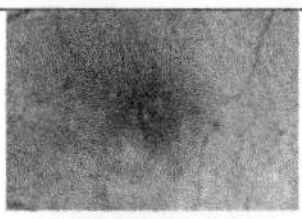 Contrast: 10.9	Contrast: 54.2	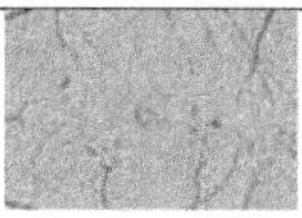 Contrast: 54.9
Severe_4	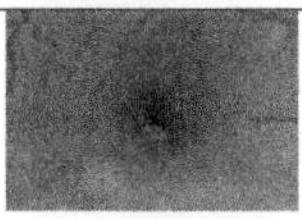 Contrast: 11.2	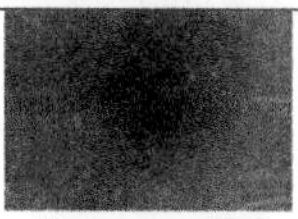 Contrast: 59.8	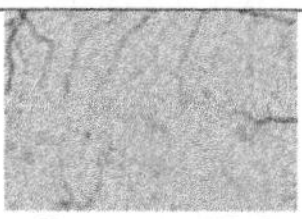 Contrast: 59.9
PDR_7	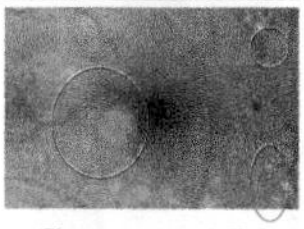 Contrast: 15.8	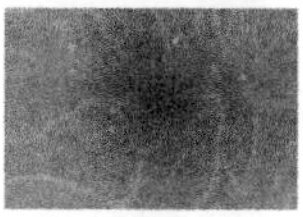 Contrast: 87.3	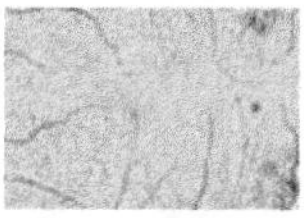 Contrast: 82.2

Figure 6.18 Comparison of selected FFA and TDCE-RETICA pictures.

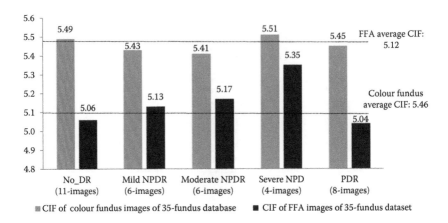

Figure 6.19 CIF of RETICA and FFA for 35-Fundus dataset.

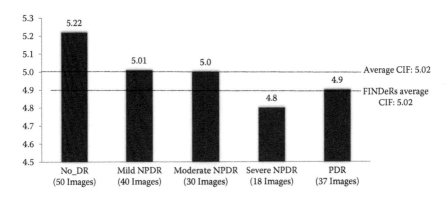

Figure 6.20 CIF of FINDeRS database.

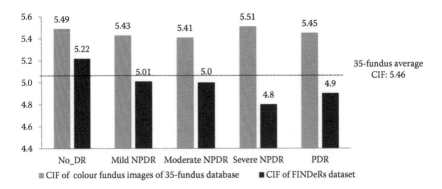

Figure 6.21 Comparison of CIF between haemoglobin (TDCE-RETICA) images from FINDeRS and 35-Fundus datasets.

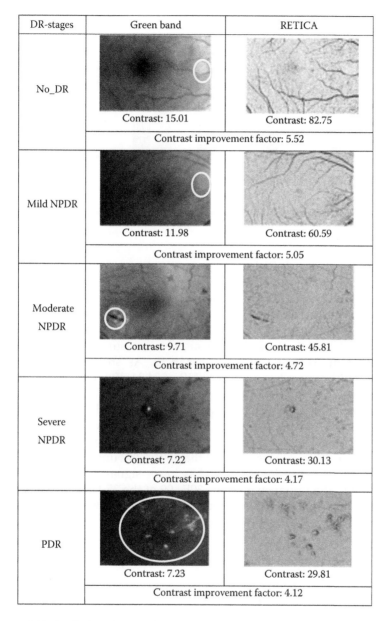

DR-stages	Green band	RETICA
No_DR	Contrast: 15.01	Contrast: 82.75
	Contrast improvement factor: 5.52	
Mild NPDR	Contrast: 11.98	Contrast: 60.59
	Contrast improvement factor: 5.05	
Moderate NPDR	Contrast: 9.71	Contrast: 45.81
	Contrast improvement factor: 4.72	
Severe NPDR	Contrast: 7.22	Contrast: 30.13
	Contrast improvement factor: 4.17	
PDR	Contrast: 7.23	Contrast: 29.81
	Contrast improvement factor: 4.12	

Figure 6.22 Analysis of green band image and RETICA image of FINDeRS dataset.

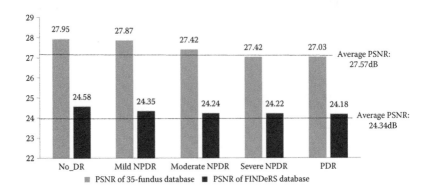

Figure 6.23 PSNR comparisons between FINDeRS database and 35-Fundus image database.

circle) but with TDCE-RETICA, a normalised image without the artefact is produced allowing better observation of tiny blood vessels. Similar results were obtained for the Mild, Moderate, Severe and PDR images. Clearly, TDCE-RETICA algorithm can normalise the image and enhance the contrast of tiny blood vessels against its surrounding background.

The PSNR of the both datasets are also measured to investigate the reason for the different CIF performances. As shown in Figure 6.23, the FINDeRS dataset has a lower PSNR of 24.34 dB while the 35-Fundus dataset has a higher PSNR of 27.57 dB.

The lower PSNR of FINDeRS database corresponds to lower CIF performance in TDCE-RETICA. The 3 dB difference shows that the noise level in FINDeRS is twice the level in the 35-Fundus database or the signal level in FINDeRS database is half of that in the 35-Fundus database. It was found that the FINDeRS database has lower signal energy of 1.42E+09 compared to the signal energy of 2.30E+09 of the 35-Fundus database as shown in Figure 6.24. This means that noise level affects the performance of RETICA.

6.4.2 Improving the SNR of the fundus image

The PSNR of fundus images in the FINDeRS dataset is improved applying the linear subspace TDCE as a denosing filter before RETICA (see Figure 6.25).

As shown in Figure 6.26, as a result of applying TDCE, the PSNR of images of FINDeRS dataset for various DR stages has been improved by nearly 3 dB.

The PSNR of improved FINDeRS dataset almost equal to the PSNR of 35-Fundus dataset as shown in Figure 6.27.

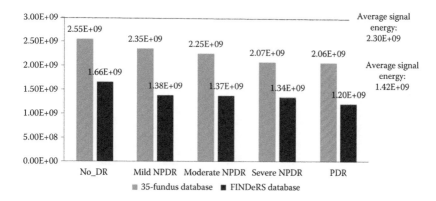

Figure 6.24 Average signal energy of fundus images for the two databases (35-Fundus and FINDeRS database) for various DR stages.

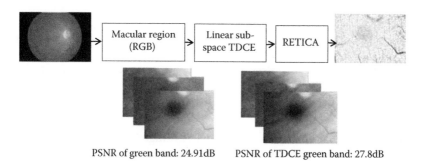

Figure 6.25 Modified RETIC.

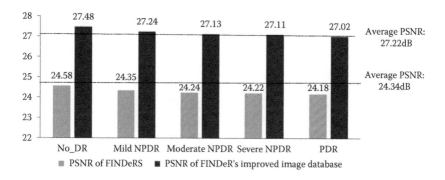

Figure 6.26 Comparison between PSNR of improved FINDeRS database and PSNR of FINDeRS database.

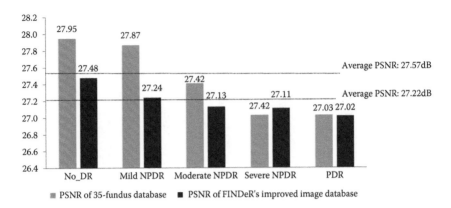

Figure 6.27 Comparison between PSNR of improved FINDeRS dataset and PSNR of 35-Fundus dataset.

It can be seen from Figure 6.28 that with improved SNR of the fundus images, the average CIF for FINDeRS dataset has been increased significantly from 5.02 to 5.56.

CIF of FINDeRS dataset is slightly higher than the CIF of 35-Fundus image dataset as shown in Figure 6.29. Note that the 35-Fundus images did not undergo the TDCE. This proves that noise levels affect the performance of RETICA.

It can be seen from Figure 6.28 that an average CIF of 0.54 of FINDeRS dataset has been achieved by improving the SNR of the FINDeRS dataset around 3dB. Figure 6.30 shows samples of enhanced images in the macular region due to RETICA method and TDCE-RETICA method. Close examination shows that the TDCE+RETICA method resulted in slightly

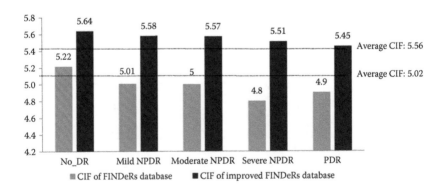

Figure 6.28 Comparison between CIF of Improved FINDeRS dataset and CIF of FINDeRS dataset.

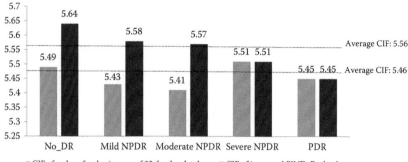

Figure 6.29 Comparison between CIF of improved FINDeRS dataset and CIF of 35-fundus dataset.

improved contrast between retinal vessels and the background allowing a better visualisation of tiny capillaries as compared to RETICA.

The TDCE-RETICA solves the three main problems of retinal fundus, that is, low contrast, varied contrast and presence of noise in the fundus image. The novelty of this technique is that the noise level has been effectively reduced by TDCE, with RETICA addressing the diverse and small contrast issue of the retinal fundus picture.

6.5 Conclusions

The small contrast between the blood vessels and the varying contrast of its surrounding background makes it visually difficult to determine the retinal vasculature accurately. In addition, fundus images are found to have both multiplicative and additive noise, and can contain artefacts. This contrast problem can be overcome by using fundus fluorescein angiography (FFA) that creates fundus images of high contrast; however, because of its invasive nature, injecting contrast agent is not a preferred method. The primary objective of this research is to solve the problems of noise, diverse and small contrast nature of colour fundus pictures and hence avoid the use of FFA.

RETICA was initially developed to deal with the diverse and small contrast of the colour fundus pictures. The performance of TDCE-RETICA with real fundus images and issue of noise are addressed in this research. Two datasets namely 35-Fundus dataset and FINDeRS dataset were processed through TDCE-RETICA. The 35-Fundus dataset contained 35 colour fundus pictures with their corresponding FFA pictures. In reference to the 35-Fundus dataset, it is observed that the application of TDCE-RETICA results in uniformly higher contrast without artefacts and thus higher CIF compared to FFA images. RETICA gave an average CIF of 5.46

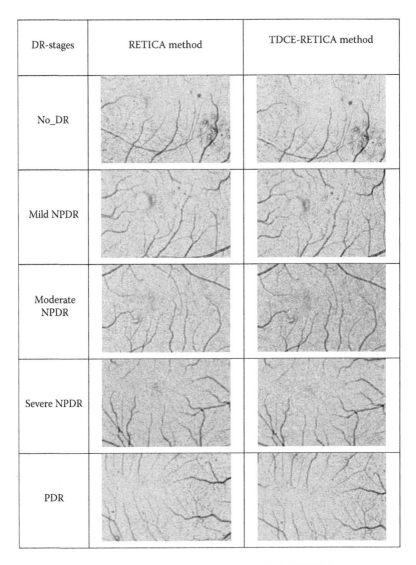

DR-stages	RETICA method	TDCE-RETICA method
No_DR		
Mild NPDR		
Moderate NPDR		
Severe NPDR		
PDR		

Figure 6.30 Comparison of RETICA image and modified RETICA image.

comparing to 5.12 for FFA images. TDCE-RETICA algorithm is successful in normalising the image contrast and in enhancing the contrast of tiny blood vessels against its surrounding background.

TDCE-RETICA gave an average CIF of 5.02 for the 175 fundus images of FINDeRS dataset. The lower CIF performance for RETICA in the case of FINDeRS dataset as compared to 35-Fundus image dataset is mainly due to higher noise level of the fundus images. Noise is found to affect

RETICA performance. The TDCE is used as denoising method to improve the noise level of fundus images of FINDeRS dataset around 3dB prior to RETICA. As a result, TDCE-RETICA gave a higher average CIF of 5.56 on improved PSNR fundus image of FINDeRS dataset as compared to 5.46 for the normal fundus images of 35-Fundus dataset. The proposed technique based on TDCE and RETICA solves the issue of noise (TDCE), small and diverse contrast (RETICA) of the fundus pictures. The modified technique TDCE+RETICA achieves comparable and better CIF and is thus a better alternative to reduce use of the invasive FFA method for eye and DR assessment using fundus camera.

RETICA with TDCE thus provides a mechanism to reduce noise and resolve low and varied contrast existing with colour fundus images that provides an efficient and non-invasive manner for retinal fundus image analysis and interpretation. It is a practical non-invasive alternative to the invasive fluorescein angiogram for retinal imaging and further analysis and interpretation for diagnosis and monitoring of vision-threatening complications.

6.6   *MATLAB codes*

Contrast calculation-based image-enhancement method for Retinal Fundus Images

```
tic
close all;
clear all;
LOAD IMAGE
pathName = 'G:\soomroo\ICT-FFA and Fundus images\D300\';
fileName =  'DFIpdr_1.jpg';
I = imread([pathName,fileName]);
Ig = double(I(:,:,2));
[m n] = size(Ig);
ratio = 0.3;
figure,imshow(I);
[x,y] = ginput(1);
x = round(x);
y = round(y);
rectOri=[(x-0.4*ratio*n) (y-0.4*ratio*m) (round(ratio*n))
(round(ratio*m))];
Ic = imcrop(I,rectOri);
[xx yy] = size(Ic(:,:,2));
Ic = Ic(1:xx-mod(xx,2),1:yy-mod(yy,2),:);
figure,imshow(Ic)
Irc = double(Ic(:,:,1));
Igc = double(Ic(:,:,2));
Ibc = double(Ic(:,:,3));
figure;imshow(Irc,[]),title('Red channel')
```

```
figure;imshow(Igc,[]),title('Green Channel')
figure;imshow(Ibc,[]),title('Blue channel')
Iteration = 7;
contrast calculation of green band
number of intensities
noI = 10;
%selection of intensity of blood vessels
imshow(Igc,[]),title('hemoglobin component image for
bloodvessels intensities');
[x2,y2] = ginput(noI);
x2 = floor(x2);
y2 = floor(y2);
for i=1:noI
   dataIntensity2(i)= Igc(y2(i),x2(i));
end
%selection of intensity of green band background
imshow(Igc,[]),title('hemoglobin component image for
background intensities');
impixelregion
[x3,y3] = ginput(noI);
x3 =floor(x3);
y3 =floor(y3);
for i=1:noI
   dataIntensity3(i)=Igc(y3(i),x3(i));
end
%mean of blood vessels intensity
z1=mean(dataIntensity2);
%mean of background intensity
u1=mean(dataIntensity3);
%determine the contrast
contrastg=abs((z1)-(u1))
% Retinex Mccann99 + swavelet
RETINEX mccann99
IrcR2 =  myretinex_mccann99(Irc, Iteration);
IgcR2 =  myretinex_mccann99(Igc, Iteration);
IbcR2 =  myretinex_mccann99(Ibc, Iteration);
figure,imshow(IrcR2,[]),title('Red Retinex ')
figure,imshow(IgcR2,[]), title('Green Retinex ')
figure,imshow(IbcR2,[]),title('Blue Retinex ')
Separation of RGB components
IR2 = double(IrcR2);
IG2 = double(IgcR2);
IB2 = double(IbcR2);
figure,imshow(IR2,[]),title('Red Retinex ')
figure,imshow(IG2,[]), title(' Green Retinex ')
figure,imshow(IB2,[]),title('Blue Retinex ')
[M2 N2] = size(IG2);
fprintf(' FastICA algorithm\n\n')
```

```
fprintf(' Number of sources = %g \n\n',M2);
fprintf(' Number of samples = %g \n\n',N2);
imgrl2 = double(IR2);
imggl2 = double(IG2);
imgbl2 = double(IB2);
Input for PCA ICA
img_in2 = [imgrl2(:) imggl2(:) imgbl2(:)]';
the next process is using the FastICA
[img_est2, A_est2, W2]=fastica(img_in2, 'approach', 'symm',
'g', 'tanh');
Rout2 = img_est2(1,:);Gout2 = img_est2(2,:);Bout2 =
img_est2(3,:);
Rescale the image intensity value from min and max log into
0 to 255
Romax2 = max(Rout2);
Romin2 = min(Rout2);
Ro2 = uint8(round((255*(Rout2 - Romin2)/(Romax2-Romin2))));
Gomax2 = max(Gout2);
Gomin2 = min(Gout2);
Go2 = uint8(round((255*(Gout2 - Gomin2)/(Gomax2-Gomin2))));
Bomax2 = max(Bout2);
Bomin2 = min(Bout2);
Bo2 = uint8(round((255*(Bout2 - Bomin2)/(Bomax2-Bomin2))));
ROim2 = reshape(Ro2,M2,N2);GOim2 = reshape(Go2,M2,N2);BOim2 =
reshape(Bo2,M2,N2);

% -----------------------------------------------------------
% -----------------------------------------------------------
Original Image
figure ; imshow(I), title('Original image');
figure ; imshow(Ig,[]), title('Green channel');

Cropped image
figure; imshow(Ic), title('Original cropped image');
figure; imshow(Igc,[]), title('Green channel');
figure; imshow(IgcR2,[]), title('Mccann99 in green');

Plot the input crop2an images and the retinca2 components
figure ; imshow(Ic(:,:,2),[]), title('Green channel');
figure ; imshow(ROim2,[]), title('RETINCA Mccann No 1');
figure ;  imshow(GOim2,[]), title('RETINCA Mccann No 2');
figure ; imshow(BOim2,[]), title('RETINCA Mccann No 3');
kur(1)=kurtosis(double(ROim2(:)));
kur(2)=kurtosis(double(GOim2(:)));
kur(3)=kurtosis(double(BOim2(:)));
% procedure to find hemoglobin image
[mkur pkur]=max(kur);
```

```
if pkur==1
    A20=ROim2;
end

if pkur==2
    A20=GOim2;
end

if pkur==3
    A20=BOim2;
end
% procedure to adjust hemoglobin image so that the intensity
of blood
vessels is lower than surrounding
A21=imcomplement(A20);

if mean2(A20)>mean2(A21)
    A1=A20;
else
    A1=A21;
end
%
A2=imcomplement(A1);
A1=double(A1);
imshow(A1,[]),title('hemoglobin component image for blood
vssels intensities ')
contrast calculation of Heamogobin image
number of intensities
noI = 10;
%selection of intensity of blood vessels
[x,y] = ginput(noI);
x = floor(x);
y = floor(y);
for i=1:noI
    dataIntensity(i)= A1(y(i),x(i));
end
%selection of intensity of background
imshow(A1,[]),title('hemoglobin component image for
background intensities');
impixelregion
[x1,y1] = ginput(noI);
x1 =floor(x1);
y1 =floor(y1);
for i=1:noI
  dataIntensity1(i)=A1(y1(i),x1(i));
end
%mean of blood vessels intensity
z=mean(dataIntensity);
%mean of background intensity
```

```
u=mean(dataIntensity1);
%determine the contrast
contrast=abs((z)-(u))
```

Denoising (Stationary Wavelet Transform)-based Image Enhancement Method Code for Retinal Images

```
tic
close all;
clear all;
LOAD IMAGE
pathName = 'G:\soomroo\Severe NPDR\';
fileName =  'SevereNPDR_UTPFINDeRSno_1.tiff';
I = imread([pathName,fileName]);
Ig = double(I(:,:,2));
[m n] = size(Ig);
ratio = 0.3;
figure,imshow(I);
[x,y] = ginput(1);
x = round(x);
y = round(y);
rectOri=[(x-0.4*ratio*n) (y-0.4*ratio*m) (round(ratio*n))
(round(ratio*m))];
Ic = imcrop(I,rectOri);
[xx yy] = size(Ic(:,:,2));
Ic = Ic(1:xx-mod(xx,2),1:yy-mod(yy,2),:);
figure,imshow(Ic)
Irc = double(Ic(:,:,1));
Igc = double(Ic(:,:,2));
Ibc = double(Ic(:,:,3));
figure;imshow(Irc,[]),title('Red channel')
figure;imshow(Igc,[]),title('Green Channel')
M=imcrop(Igc,[])
figure;imshow(M,[]),title('Blue channel')
figure;imshow(Ibc,[]),title('Blue channel')
Iteration = 7;
contrast calculation of green band
number of intensities
noI = 10;
%selection of intensity of blood vessels
imshow(Igc,[]),title('hemoglobin component image for
bloodvessels intensities');
[x2,y2] = ginput(noI);
x2 = floor(x2);
y2 = floor(y2);
for i=1:noI
    dataIntensity2(i)= Igc(y2(i),x2(i));
end
%selection of intensity of green band background
```

```
imshow(Igc,[]),title('hemoglobin component image for
background intensities');
impixelregion
[x3,y3] = ginput(noI);
x3 =floor(x3);
y3 =floor(y3);
for i=1:noI
  dataIntensity3(i)=Igc(y3(i),x3(i));
end
%mean of blood vessels intensity
z1=mean(dataIntensity2);
%mean of background intensity
u1=mean(dataIntensity3);
%determine the contrast
contrastg=abs((z1)-(u1))
% Retinex Mccann99 + swavelet
RETINEX mccann99
IrcR2 =  myretinex_mccann99(Irc, Iteration);
IgcR2 =  myretinex_mccann99(Igc, Iteration);
IbcR2 =  myretinex_mccann99(Ibc, Iteration);
figure,imshow(IrcR2,[]),title('Red Retinex ')
figure,imshow(IgcR2,[]), title('Green Retinex ')
impixelregion
figure,imshow(IbcR2,[]),title('Blue Retinex ')
XDENr = func_denoise_sw2d(IrcR2);
XDENg = func_denoise_sw2d(IgcR2);
XDENb = func_denoise_sw2d(IbcR2);
figure;imshow(XDENr,[]),title('swt red image')
figure;imshow(XDENg,[]),title('swt green image')
figure;imshow(XDENb,[]),title('swt blue image')
Separation of RGB components
IR2 = double(XDENr);
IG2 = double(XDENg);
IB2 = double(XDENb);
figure,imshow(IR2,[]),title('Red Retinex ')
figure,imshow(IG2,[]), title(' Green Retinex ')
figure,imshow(IB2,[]),title('Blue Retinex ')
[M2 N2] = size(IG2);
fprintf(' FastICA algorithm\n\n')
fprintf(' Number of sources = %g \n\n',M2);
fprintf(' Number of samples = %g \n\n',N2);
imgrl2 = double(IR2);
imggl2 = double(IG2);
imgbl2 = double(IB2);
Input for PCA ICA
img_in2 = [imgrl2(:) imggl2(:) imgbl2(:)]';
the next process is using the FastICA
[img_est2, A_est2, W2]=fastica(img_in2, 'approach', 'symm',
'g', 'tanh');
```

```
Rout2 = img_est2(1,:);Gout2 = img_est2(2,:);Bout2 =
img_est2(3,:);
Rescale the image intensity value from min and max log into
0 to 255
Romax2 = max(Rout2);
Romin2 = min(Rout2);
Ro2 = uint8(round((255*(Rout2 - Romin2)/(Romax2-Romin2))));
Gomax2 = max(Gout2);
Gomin2 = min(Gout2);
Go2 = uint8(round((255*(Gout2 - Gomin2)/(Gomax2-Gomin2))));
Bomax2 = max(Bout2);
Bomin2 = min(Bout2);
Bo2 = uint8(round((255*(Bout2 - Bomin2)/(Bomax2-Bomin2))));
ROim2 = reshape(Ro2,M2,N2);GOim2 = reshape(Go2,M2,N2);BOim2
= reshape(Bo2,M2,N2);


% --------------------------------------------------------------
% --------------------------------------------------------------
Original Image
figure ; imshow(I), title('Original image');
figure ; imshow(Ig,[]), title('Green channel');

Cropped image
figure; imshow(Ic), title('Original cropped image');
figure; imshow(Igc,[]), title('Green channel');
figure; imshow(IgcR2,[]), title('Mccann99 in green');

Plot the input crop2an images and the retinca2 components
figure ; imshow(Ic(:,:,2),[]), title('Green channel');
figure ; imshow(ROim2,[]), title('RETINCA Mccann No 1');
figure ;  imshow(GOim2,[]), title('RETINCA Mccann No 2');
figure ; imshow(BOim2,[]), title('RETINCA Mccann No 3');
kur(1)=kurtosis(double(ROim2(:)));
kur(2)=kurtosis(double(GOim2(:)));
kur(3)=kurtosis(double(BOim2(:)));
%  procedure to find hemoglobin image
[mkur pkur]=max(kur);

if pkur==1
    A20=ROim2;
end

if pkur==2
    A20=GOim2;
end

if pkur==3
```

```
      A20=BOim2;
end
% procedure to adjust hemoglobin image so that the intensity
of blood
vessels is lower than surrounding
A21=imcomplement(A20);

if mean2(A20)>mean2(A21)
    A1=A20;
else
    A1=A21;
end
%
A2=imcomplement(A1);
A1=double(A1);
imshow(A1,[]),title('hemoglobin component image for blood
vssels intensities ')
contrast calculation of Heamogobin image
number of intensities
noI = 10;
%selection of intensity of blood vessels
[x,y] = ginput(noI);
x = floor(x);
y = floor(y);
for i=1:noI
    dataIntensity(i)= A1(y(i),x(i));
end
%selection of intensity of background
imshow(A1,[]),title('hemoglobin component image for
background intensities');
impixelregion
[x1,y1] = ginput(noI);
x1 =floor(x1);
y1 =floor(y1);
for i=1:noI
   dataIntensity1(i)=A1(y1(i),x1(i));
end
%mean of blood vessels intensity
z=mean(dataIntensity);
%mean of background intensity
u=mean(dataIntensity1);
%determine the contrast
contrast=abs((z)-(u))
```

Denoising (LSE)-based Image Enhancement Method Code for Retinal Images

```
tic
close all;
```

```
clear all;
LOAD IMAGE
pathName ='C:\Users\CISIR\Desktop\subspace image\PDR\';
fileName =  '3.tiff';
I = imread([pathName,fileName]);
Ig = double(I(:,:,2));
[m n] = size(Ig);
ratio = 0.3;
figure,imshow(I);
[x,y] = ginput(1);
x = round(x);
y = round(y);
rectOri=[(x-0.4*ratio*n) (y-0.4*ratio*m) (round(ratio*n))
(round(ratio*m))];
Ic = imcrop(I,rectOri);
[xx yy] = size(Ic(:,:,2));
Ic = Ic(1:xx-mod(xx,2),1:yy-mod(yy,2),:);
figure,imshow(Ic)
Irc = double(Ic(:,:,1));
Igc = double(Ic(:,:,2));
Ibc = double(Ic(:,:,3));
figure;imshow(Irc,[]),title('Red channel')
figure;imshow(Igc,[]),title('Green Channel')
figure;imshow(Ibc,[]),title('Blue channel')
Iteration = 7;
RETINEX mccann99
IrcR2 =  myretinex_mccann99(Irc, Iteration);
IgcR2 =  myretinex_mccann99(Igc, Iteration);
IbcR2 =  myretinex_mccann99(Ibc, Iteration);
IR2 = double(IrcR2);
IG2 = double(IgcR2);
calculate PSNR of Green Retinex
R=255;
std=std2(IG2);
PSNRgretinex=20*log10(R/std);
blue retinex
IB2 = double(IbcR2);
Red channel
Rx       = IR2*IR2';
[Vx,Dx] = eig(Rx);
Vx       = fliplr(Vx);
Vs       = Vx(:,1:250);
S1       = (Vs*Vs')*IR2;
figure;imshow(IR2,[]);title('The red Retinex image')
figure;imshow(S1,[]);title('The RED denoised image')
Green Channel
Rx1      = IG2*IG2';
[Vx1,Dx1] = eig(Rx1);
```

```
Vx1       = fliplr(Vx1);
Vs1       = Vx1(:,1:250);
S2        = (Vs1*Vs1')*IG2;
figure;imshow(IG2,[]);title('The GREEN Retinex image')
figure;imshow(S2,[]);title('The GREEN denoised image')
calculate PSNR of Green subspace Retinex
R=255;
std1=std2(S2);
PSNRsubspace=20*log10(R/std1);
blue Channel
Rx2       = IB2*IB2';
[Vx2,Dx2] = eig(Rx2);
Vx2       = fliplr(Vx2);
Vs2       = Vx2(:,1:250);
S3        = (Vs2*Vs2')*IB2;
figure;imshow(IB2,[]);title('The BLUE Retinex image')
figure;imshow(S3,[]);title('The BLUE denoised image')
Separation of RGB components
Ir2 = double(S1);
Ig2 = double(S2);
Ib2 = double(S3);
figure,imshow(Ir2,[]),title('Red Retinex ')
figure,imshow(Ig2,[]), title(' Green Retinex ')
figure,imshow(Ib2,[]),title('Blue Retinex ')
[M2 N2] = size(Ig2);
fprintf(' FastICA algorithm\n\n')
fprintf(' Number of sources = %g \n\n',M2);
fprintf(' Number of samples = %g \n\n',N2);
imgrl2 = double(Ir2);
imggl2 = double(Ig2);
imgbl2 = double(Ib2);
Input for PCA ICA
img_in2 = [imgrl2(:) imggl2(:) imgbl2(:)]';
the next process is using the FastICA
[img_est2, A_est2, W2]=fastica(img_in2, 'approach', 'symm',
'g', 'tanh');
Rout2 = img_est2(1,:);Gout2 = img_est2(2,:);Bout2 =
img_est2(3,:);
Rescale the image intensity value from min and max log into
0 to 255
Romax2 = max(Rout2);
Romin2 = min(Rout2);
Ro2 = uint8(round((255*(Rout2 - Romin2)/(Romax2-Romin2))));
Gomax2 = max(Gout2);
Gomin2 = min(Gout2);
Go2 = uint8(round((255*(Gout2 - Gomin2)/(Gomax2-Gomin2))));
Bomax2 = max(Bout2);
Bomin2 = min(Bout2);
```

```
Bo2 = uint8(round(((255*(Bout2 - Bomin2)/(Bomax2-Bomin2)))));
ROim2 = reshape(Ro2,M2,N2);GOim2 = reshape(Go2,M2,N2);BOim2
= reshape(Bo2,M2,N2);

% -------------------------------------------------------------
% -------------------------------------------------------------
Original Image
figure ; imshow(I), title('Original image');
figure ; imshow(Ig,[]), title('Green channel');

Cropped image
figure; imshow(Ic), title('Original cropped image');
figure; imshow(Igc,[]), title('Green channel');
figure; imshow(IgcR2,[]), title('Mccann99 in green');

Plot the input crop2an images and the retinca2 components
figure ; imshow(Ic(:,:,2),[]), title('Green channel');
figure ; imshow(ROim2,[]), title('RETINCA Mccann No 1');
figure ;  imshow(GOim2,[]), title('RETINCA Mccann No 2');
figure ; imshow(BOim2,[]), title('RETINCA Mccann No 3');
kur(1)=kurtosis(double(ROim2(:)));
kur(2)=kurtosis(double(GOim2(:)));
kur(3)=kurtosis(double(BOim2(:)));
%  procedure to find hemoglobin image
[mkur pkur]=max(kur);

if pkur==1
    A20=ROim2;
end

if pkur==2
    A20=GOim2;
end

if pkur==3
    A20=BOim2;
end
% procedure to adjust hemoglobin image so that the intensity
of blood
vessels is lower than surrounding
A21=imcomplement(A20);

if mean2(A20)>mean2(A21)
    A1=A20;
else
    A1=A21;
end
%
```

```
A2=imcomplement(A1);
A1=double(A1);
imshow(A1,[]),title('hemoglobin component image for blood
vssels intensities ')
%contrast calculation of Heamogobin image
%number of intensities
noI = 10;
%selection of intensity of blood vessels
[x,y] = ginput(noI);
x = floor(x);
y = floor(y);
for i=1:noI
    dataIntensity(i)= A1(y(i),x(i));
end
%selection of intensity of background
imshow(A1,[]),title('hemoglobin component image for
background intensities');
impixelregion
[x1,y1] = ginput(noI);
x1 =floor(x1);
y1 =floor(y1);
for i=1:noI
    dataIntensity1(i)=A1(y1(i),x1(i));
end
%mean of blood vessels intensity
z=mean(dataIntensity);
%mean of background intensity
u=mean(dataIntensity1);
%determine the contrast
contrast=abs((z)-(u))
```

Denoising (MVE)-Based Image Enhancement Method Code for Retinal Images

```
tic
close all;
clear all;
LOAD IMAGE
pathName ='C:\Users\CISIR\Desktop\subspace image\PDR\';
fileName =  '3.tiff';
I = imread([pathName,fileName]);
Ig = double(I(:,:,2));
[m n] = size(Ig);
ratio = 0.3;
figure,imshow(I);
[x,y] = ginput(1);
x = round(x);
y = round(y);
```

```
rectOri=[(x-0.4*ratio*n) (y-0.4*ratio*m) (round(ratio*n))
(round(ratio*m))];
Ic = imcrop(I,rectOri);
[xx yy] = size(Ic(:,:,2));
Ic = Ic(1:xx-mod(xx,2),1:yy-mod(yy,2),:);
figure,imshow(Ic)
Irc = double(Ic(:,:,1));
Igc = double(Ic(:,:,2));
Ibc = double(Ic(:,:,3));
figure;imshow(Irc,[]),title('Red channel')
figure;imshow(Igc,[]),title('Green Channel')
figure;imshow(Ibc,[]),title('Blue channel')
Iteration = 7;
RETINEX mccann99
IrcR2 =  myretinex_mccann99(Irc, Iteration);
IgcR2 =  myretinex_mccann99(Igc, Iteration);
IbcR2 =  myretinex_mccann99(Ibc, Iteration);
IR2 = double(IrcR2);
IG2 = double(IgcR2);
IB2 = double(IbcR2);
calculate PSNR of Green Retinex
R=255;
std=std2(IG2);
PSNRgretinex=20*log10(R/std);
Red channel
[U,D,V] = svd(IR2);
r         = 100;
Vx        = V(:,1:r);
Dx        = D(1:r,1:r);
Dx1       = 1./diag(Dx);
DI        = diag(Dx1);
W         = Vx*(eye(r)-DI^2)*Vx';
S1        = IR2*W;
figure;imshow(IR2,[]);title('The Red Retinex image')
figure;imshow(S1,[]);title('The Red Retinex denoised
image')
green channel
[U1,D1,V1] = svd(IG2);
r1        = 100;
Vx1       = V1(:,1:r1);
Dx1       = D1(1:r1,1:r1);
Dx2       = 1./diag(Dx1);
DI1       = diag(Dx2);
W1        = Vx1*(eye(r1)-DI1^2)*Vx1';
S2        = IG2*W1;
figure;imshow(IG2,[]);title('The green  Retinex image')
figure;imshow(S2,[]);title('The green Retinex denoised
image')
```

```
calculate PSNR of Green subspace Retinex
R=255;
std1=std2(S2);
PSNRsubspace=20*log10(R/std1);
blue channel
[U2,D2,V2] = svd(IB2);
r2       = 100;
Vx2      = V2(:,1:r2);
Dx2      = D2(1:r2,1:r2);
Dx3      = 1./diag(Dx2);
DI2      = diag(Dx3);
W2       = Vx2*(eye(r2)-DI2^2)*Vx2';
S3       = IG2*W2;
figure;imshow(IB2,[]);title('The BLUE  Retinex image')
figure;imshow(S3,[]);title('The BLUE Retinex denoised
image')
Separation of RGB components
Ir2 = double(S1);
Ig2 = double(S2);
Ib2 = double(S3);
figure,imshow(Ir2,[]),title('Red Retinex ')
figure,imshow(Ig2,[]), title(' Green Retinex ')
figure,imshow(Ib2,[]),title('Blue Retinex ')
[M2 N2] = size(Ig2);
fprintf(' FastICA algorithm\n\n')
fprintf(' Number of sources = %g \n\n',M2);
fprintf(' Number of samples = %g \n\n',N2);
imgrl2 = double(Ir2);
imggl2 = double(Ig2);
imgbl2 = double(Ib2);
Input for PCA ICA
img_in2 = [imgrl2(:) imggl2(:) imgbl2(:)]';
the next process is using the FastICA
[img_est2, A_est2, W2]=fastica(img_in2, 'approach', 'symm',
'g', 'tanh');
Rout2 = img_est2(1,:);Gout2 = img_est2(2,:);Bout2 =
img_est2(3,:);
Rescale the image intensity value from min and max log into
0 to 255
Romax2 = max(Rout2);
Romin2 = min(Rout2);
Ro2 = uint8(round((255*(Rout2 - Romin2)/(Romax2-Romin2))));
Gomax2 = max(Gout2);
Gomin2 = min(Gout2);
Go2 = uint8(round((255*(Gout2 - Gomin2)/(Gomax2-Gomin2))));
Bomax2 = max(Bout2);
Bomin2 = min(Bout2);
Bo2 = uint8(round((255*(Bout2 - Bomin2)/(Bomax2-Bomin2))));
```

```
ROim2 = reshape(Ro2,M2,N2);GOim2 = reshape(Go2,M2,N2);BOim2 =
reshape(Bo2,M2,N2);

% -----------------------------------------------------------
% -----------------------------------------------------------
Original Image
figure ; imshow(I), title('Original image');
figure ; imshow(Ig,[]), title('Green channel');

Cropped image
figure; imshow(Ic), title('Original cropped image');
figure; imshow(Igc,[]), title('Green channel');
figure; imshow(IgcR2,[]), title('Mccann99 in green');

Plot the input crop2an images and the retinca2 components
figure ; imshow(Ic(:,:,2),[]), title('Green channel');
figure ; imshow(ROim2,[]), title('RETINCA Mccann No 1');
figure ;  imshow(GOim2,[]), title('RETINCA Mccann No 2');
figure ; imshow(BOim2,[]), title('RETINCA Mccann No 3');
kur(1)=kurtosis(double(ROim2(:)));
kur(2)=kurtosis(double(GOim2(:)));
kur(3)=kurtosis(double(BOim2(:)));
%  procedure to find hemoglobin image
[mkur pkur]=max(kur);

if pkur==1
    A20=ROim2;
end

if pkur==2
    A20=GOim2;
end

if pkur==3
    A20=BOim2;
end
% procedure to adjust hemoglobin image so that the intensity
of blood
vessels is lower than surrounding
A21=imcomplement(A20);

if mean2(A20)>mean2(A21)
    A1=A20;
else
    A1=A21;
end
%
A2=imcomplement(A1);
```

```
A1=double(A1);
imshow(A1,[]),title('hemoglobin component image for blood
vssels intensities ')
%contrast calculation of Heamogobin image
%number of intensities
noI = 10;
%selection of intensity of blood vessels
[x,y] = ginput(noI);
x = floor(x);
y = floor(y);
for i=1:noI
   dataIntensity(i)= A1(y(i),x(i));
end
%selection of intensity of background
imshow(A1,[]),title('hemoglobin component image for
background intensities');
impixelregion
[x1,y1] = ginput(noI);
x1 =floor(x1);
y1 =floor(y1);
for i=1:noI
  dataIntensity1(i)=A1(y1(i),x1(i));
end
%mean of blood vessels intensity
z=mean(dataIntensity);
%mean of background intensity
u=mean(dataIntensity1);
%determine the contrast
contrast=abs((z)-(u))
```

Denoising (TDCE)-Based Image Enhancement Method Code for Retinal Images

```
tic
close all;
clear all;
LOAD IMAGE
pathName = 'G:\research data\soomroo\ICT-FFA and Fundus
images\D80\';
fileName =  'DFIpdr_1.jpg';
I = imread([pathName,fileName]);
Ig = double(I(:,:,2));
[m n] = size(Ig);
ratio = 0.3;
figure,imshow(I);
[x,y] = ginput(1);
x = round(x);
y = round(y);
rectOri=[(x-0.4*ratio*n) (y-0.4*ratio*m) (round(ratio*n))
(round(ratio*m))];
```

```
Ic = imcrop(I,rectOri);
[xx yy] = size(Ic(:,:,2));
Ic = Ic(1:xx-mod(xx,2),1:yy-mod(yy,2),:);
figure,imshow(Ic)
Irc = double(Ic(:,:,1));
Igc = double(Ic(:,:,2));
Ibc = double(Ic(:,:,3));
figure;imshow(Irc,[]),title('Red channel')
figure;imshow(Igc,[]),title('Green Channel')
figure;imshow(Ibc,[]),title('Blue channel')
Iteration = 7;
R=255;
std1=std2(Igc);
PSNRgreen=20*log10(R/std);

RETINEX mccann99
IrcR2 =  myretinex_mccann99(Irc, Iteration);
IgcR2 =  myretinex_mccann99(Igc, Iteration);
IbcR2 =  myretinex_mccann99(Ibc, Iteration);
figure,imshow(IrcR2,[]),title('Red Retinex ')
figure,imshow(IgcR2,[]), title('Green Retinex ')
figure,imshow(IbcR2,[]),title('Blue Retinex ')
IR2 = double(IrcR2);
IG2 = double(IgcR2);
IB2 = double(IbcR2);
calculate PSNR of Green Retinex
R=255;
std=std2(IG2);
PSNRgretinex=20*log10(R/std);
Red Channel
[U,D,V] = svd(IR2);
r        = 300;
mu       = 1;
Vx       = V(:,1:r);
Dx       = D(1:r,1:r);
M        = 1./diag(Dx+ mu*eye(r));
M1       = diag(M);
H        = Vx*M1*Dx*Vx';
S1       = IR2*H;
figure;imshow(S1,[]);title('The red denoised image')
green channel
[U1,D1,V1] = svd(IG2);
r1       = 300;
mu1      = 1;
Vx1      = V1(:,1:r1);
Dx1      = D1(1:r1,1:r1);
M1       = 1./diag(Dx1+ mu1*eye(r1));
M2       = diag(M1);
H1        = Vx1*M2*Dx1*Vx1';
```

```
S2        = IG2*H1;
figure;imshow(S2,[]);title('The GREEN denoised image')
calculate PSNR of Green subspace Retinex
R=255;
std1=std2(S2);
PSNRsubspace=20*log10(R/std1);
Blue Channel
[U2,D2,V2] = svd(IB2);
r2        = 300;
mu2       = 1;
Vx2       = V2(:,1:r2);
Dx2       = D2(1:r2,1:r2);
M2        = 1./diag(Dx2+ mu2*eye(r2));
M3        = diag(M2);
H2         = Vx2*M3*Dx2*Vx2';
S3        = IB2*H2;
figure;imshow(S3,[]);title('The BLUE denoised image')
Separation of RGB components
Ir2 = double(S1);
Ig2 = double(S2);
Ib2 = double(S3);
figure,imshow(Ir2,[]),title('Red Retinex ')
figure,imshow(Ig2,[]), title(' Green Retinex ')
figure,imshow(Ib2,[]),title('Blue Retinex ')
[M2 N2] = size(Ig2);
fprintf(' FastICA algorithm\n\n')
fprintf(' Number of sources = %g \n\n',M2);
fprintf(' Number of samples = %g \n\n',N2);
imgrl2 = double(Ir2);
imggl2 = double(Ig2);
imgbl2 = double(Ib2);
Input for PCA ICA
img_in2 = [imgrl2(:) imggl2(:) imgbl2(:)]';
the next process is using the FastICA
[img_est2, A_est2, W2]=fastica(img_in2, 'approach', 'symm',
'g', 'tanh');
Rout2 = img_est2(1,:);Gout2 = img_est2(2,:);Bout2 =
img_est2(3,:);
Rescale the image intensity value from min and max log into
0 to 255
Romax2 = max(Rout2);
Romin2 = min(Rout2);
Ro2 = uint8(round((255*(Rout2 - Romin2)/(Romax2-Romin2))));
Gomax2 = max(Gout2);
Gomin2 = min(Gout2);
Go2 = uint8(round((255*(Gout2 - Gomin2)/(Gomax2-Gomin2))));
Bomax2 = max(Bout2);
Bomin2 = min(Bout2);
Bo2 = uint8(round((255*(Bout2 - Bomin2)/(Bomax2-Bomin2))));
```

```
ROim2 = reshape(Ro2,M2,N2);GOim2 = reshape(Go2,M2,N2);BOim2 =
reshape(Bo2,M2,N2);

% ------------------------------------------------------------
% ------------------------------------------------------------
Original Image
figure ; imshow(I), title('Original image');
figure ; imshow(Ig,[]), title('Green channel');

Cropped image
figure; imshow(Ic), title('Original cropped image');
figure; imshow(Igc,[]), title('Green channel');
figure; imshow(IgcR2,[]), title('Mccann99 in green');

Plot the input crop2an images and the retinca2 components
figure ; imshow(Ic(:,:,2),[]), title('Green channel');
figure ; imshow(ROim2,[]), title('RETINCA Mccann No 1');
figure ;  imshow(GOim2,[]), title('RETINCA Mccann No 2');
figure ; imshow(BOim2,[]), title('RETINCA Mccann No 3');
kur(1)=kurtosis(double(ROim2(:)));
kur(2)=kurtosis(double(GOim2(:)));
kur(3)=kurtosis(double(BOim2(:)));
%  procedure to find hemoglobin image
[mkur pkur]=max(kur);

if pkur==1
    A20=ROim2;
end

if pkur==2
    A20=GOim2;
end

if pkur==3
    A20=BOim2;
end
% procedure to adjust hemoglobin image so that the intensity
of blood
vessels is lower than surrounding
A21=imcomplement(A20);

if mean2(A20)>mean2(A21)
    A1=A20;
else
    A1=A21;
end
%
A2=imcomplement(A1);
A1=double(A1);
```

```
imshow(A1,[]),title('hemoglobin component image for blood
vssels intensities ')
contrast calculation of Heamogobin image
%number of intensities
noI = 10;
%selection of intensity of blood vessels
[x,y] = ginput(noI);
x = floor(x);
y = floor(y);
for i=1:noI
   dataIntensity(i)= A1(y(i),x(i));
end
%selection of intensity of background
imshow(A1,[]),title('hemoglobin component image for
background intensities');
impixelregion
[x1,y1] = ginput(noI);
x1 =floor(x1);
y1 =floor(y1);
for i=1:noI
   dataIntensity1(i)=A1(y1(i),x1(i));
end
%mean of blood vessels intensity
z=mean(dataIntensity);
%mean of background intensity
u=mean(dataIntensity1);
%determine the contrast
contrast=abs((z)-(u))
```

References

1. G. Zahlmann, B. Kochner, I. Ugi, D. Schuhmann, B. Liesenfeld, A. Wegner et al., Hybrid fuzzy image processing for situation assessment [diabetic retinopathy], *Engineering in Medicine and Biology Magazine, IEEE*, vol. 19, pp. 76–83, 2000.

2. L. A. Yannuzzi, K. T. Rohrer, L. J. Tindel, R. S. Sobel, M. A. Costanza, W. Shields et al. Fluorescein angiography complication survey, *Ophthalmology*, vol. 93, pp. 611–617, 1986.

3. C. Yixin and M. Das, An automated technique for image noise identification using a simple pattern classification approach, in *Circuits and Systems, 2007. MWSCAS 2007. 50th Midwest Symposium on*, Montreal, Canada, 2007, pp. 819–822.

4. J. Gilchrist, Computer processing of ocular photographs – A review*, *Ophthalmic and Physiological Optics*, vol. 7, pp. 379–386, 1987.

5. M. H. A. Fadzil, H. A. Nugroho, P. A. Venkatachalam, H. Nugroho, and L. I. Izhar, Determination of retinal pigments from fundus images using independent component analysis, in *4th Kuala Lumpur International Conference on Biomedical Engineering 2008*, vol. 21, N. A. Abu Osman, F. Ibrahim, W. A. B. Wan Abas, H. S. Abdul Rahman, H.-N. Ting, and R. Magjarevic, Eds. Berlin: Springer, 2008, pp. 555–558.

6. M. H. A. Fadzil, L. I. Izhar, and H. A. Nugroho, Determination of foveal avascular zone in diabetic retinopathy digital fundus images, *Computers in Biology and Medicine*, vol. 40, pp. 657–664, 2010.

7. H. A. Nugroho, Non-invasive image enhancement of colour retinal fundus image for computerised diabetic retinopathy monitoring and grading system, *PhD thesis*, Electrical and Electronics Engineering Programme, Universiti Teknologi PETRONAS, 2012.

8. B. Funt, F. Ciurea, and J. McCann, Retinex in MATLAB™, *Journal of Electronic Imaging*, vol. 13, pp. 48–57, 2004.

9. A. Hyvärinen and E. Oja, Independent component analysis: Algorithms and applications, *Neural Networks*, vol. 13, Issues 4–5, June 2000, pp. 411–430.

10. S. Kollias, Y. Boutalis, and G. Carayannis, Fast adaptive identification and restoration of images degraded by blur and noise, in *Circuits and Systems, 1988, IEEE International Symposium on*, Espoo, Finland, vol. 3. 1988, pp. 2073–2076.

11. K. Chehdi and M. Sabri, A new approach to identify the nature of the noise affecting an image, in *Acoustics, Speech, and Signal Processing, 1992. ICASSP-92, 1992 IEEE International Conference on*, San Franscisco, USA, vol. 3. 1992, pp. 285–288.

12. H. Kun, L. Xin-Cheng, L. Chun-Hua, and L. Ran, Gaussian noise removal of image on the local feature, in *Intelligent Information Technology Application, 2008, IITA '08, Second International Symposium on*, Shanghai, China 2008, pp. 867–871.

13. A. F. M. Hani, T. A. Soomro, I. Faye, N. Kamel, N. Yahya, Identification of noise in the fundus images, Control System, Computing and Engineering (ICCSCE), 2013 *IEEE International Conference on*, 2013, DOI: 10.1109/ ICCSCE.2013.6719957. 2013.

14. L. A. Yannuzzi, K. T. Rohrer, Fluorescein angiography complication survey, *Ophthalmology*, vol. 93, pp. 611–617, 1986.

15. C. Chang-yan, Ji-xian, and L. Zheng-jun, *Study on Methods of Noise Reduction in A Stripped Image*, The International Archives of the Photogrammetry, Remote Sensing and Spatial Information Sciences, Vol. XXXVII, Part B6b, 2008, pp. 213–216.

16. M. Folke, L. Cernerud, M. Ekström, and B. Hök, Critical review of non-invasive respiratory monitoring in medical care, *Medical and Biological Engineering and Computing*, vol. 41, pp. 377–383, 2003.

17. C. Yixin and M. Das, An automated technique for image noise identification using a simple pattern classification approach, in *Circuits and Systems, 2007. MWSCAS 2007. 50th Midwest Symposium on*, 2007, pp. 819–822.

18. J. F. Cardoso and A. Souloumiac, Blind beamforming for non-Gaussian signals, *Radar and Signal Processing, IEE Proceedings F*, vol. 140, pp. 362–370, 1993.

19. Christos M. Michail, Non-invasive and quantitative near-infrared haemoglobin spectrometry in the piglet brain during hypoxic stress, using a frequency-domain multidistance instrument, *Physics in Medicine & Biology*, vol. 46, p. 41, 2001.

20. P. Hansen, Signal subspace methods for speech enhancement, Ph.D Thesis, *Technical University of Denmark*, 1997.

21. Y. Ephraim and H. L. V. Trees, A signal subspace approach for speech enhancement, *IEEE Trans. Speech Audio Process.*, vol. 3, pp. 251–266, 1995.

22. Nidal Kamel. N. S. Yahya, Aamir S. Malik, Subspace-based technique for speckle noise reduction in SAR images, *Accepted for publication in IEEE Transactions on Geoscience and Remote Sensing*, 2013.

23. D. Brunet, E. Vrscay, and Z. Wang, The Use of Residuals in Image Denoising, in *Image Analysis and Recognition*. vol. 5627, M. Kamel and A. Campilho, Eds. Springer Berlin Heidelberg, 2009, pp. 1–12.

24. S. Jha and R. D. S. Yadava, Denoising by Singular Value Decomposition and Its Application to Electronic Nose Data Processing, *Sensors Journal, IEEE*, vol. 11, pp. 35–44, 2011.

25. M. Fan and A. L. Tits, Toward a structure singular value decomposition, in *Decision and Control, 1987. 26th IEEE Conference on*, 1987, pp. 1742–1743.

26. M. Moonen, P. V. Dooren, and J. Vandewalle, A singular value decomposition updating algorithm for subspace tracking, *SIAM Journal on Matrix Analysis and Applications*, vol. 13, pp. 1015–1038, 1992.

27. T. Konda and Y. Nakamura, A new algorithm for singular value decomposition and its parallelization, *Parallel Computing*, vol. 35, pp. 331–344, 2009.

28. H. Patterson, Singular value decompositions and digital image processing, *IEEE Trans. on Acoustics, Speech, and Signal Processing*, vol. ASSP-24, pp. 26–53, 1976.

29. Julie L. Kamm, SVD-Based Methods For Signal And Image Restoration. *PhD Thesis* (1998). Emory University United States.

30. B. Konstantinides and G. S. Yovanof, Noise Estimation and Filtering Using Block-Based Singular Value Decomposition, *IEEE Transactions on Image Processing*, vol. 6, pp. 479–483, 1997.

31. L. Gorodetski, V. Samoilov, and V. A. Skormin, SVD-Based Approach to Transparent Embedding Data into Digital Images, *Proceeding International Workshop on Mathematical Methods, Models and Architecture for Computer Network Security, Lecture Notes in Computer Science*, vol. 2052, Springer Verlag, 2001.

32. A. F. M. Hani, T. Ahmed Soomro, H. Nugroho, and H. A. Nugroho, Enhancement of colour fundus image and FFA image using RETICA, in *Biomedical Engineering and Sciences (IECBES), 2012 IEEE EMBS Conference on*, Langkawi, Malaysia, 2012, pp. 831–836.

33. R. Sobol, Improving the Retinex algorithm for rendering wide dynamic range photographs, *Journal of Electronic Imaging*, vol. 13, pp. 65–74, 2004.

34. D. L. Donoho, De-noising by soft-thresholding, *Information Theory, IEEE Transactions on*, vol. 41, pp. 613–627, 1995.

35. L. Jong-Sen, Digital image enhancement and noise filtering by use of local statistics, *Pattern Analysis and Machine Intelligence, IEEE Transactions on*, vol. PAMI-2, pp. 165–168, 1980.

36. K. Baker, Singular Value Decomposition Tutorial, *Proceeding International Workshop on Mathematical Methods, models and Architecture for Computer Network Security, Lecture Notes in Computer Science*, vol. 2052, Springer Verlag, 2001.

37. W. C. Mitchell and D. L. McCraith, Heuristic analysis of numerical variants of the Gram-Schmidt orthonormalization process, Stanford University 1969.

38. E. Haykin, *Adaptive Filter Theory*, NJ: Prentice-Hall, 1991.

39. N. S. Yahya, N. Kamel, and A. S. Malik, Subspace-based technique for image denoising, in *National Postgraduate Conference (NPC), 2011*, 2011, pp. 1–5.

40. P. S. K. Hansen, Signal subspace methods for speech enhancement,*PhD thesis*, Technical University of Denmark, Denmark, 1997.

41. N. S. K. N. Yahya, Aamir S. Malik, Subspace-based technique for speckle noise reduction in SAR images, *IEEE Transactions on Geoscience and Remote Sensing*, vol. 52, issue 10, October 2014.

42. N. Yahya, N. S. Kamel, and A. S. Malik, Subspace-based technique for image denoising, in *National Postgraduate Conference (NPC), 2011* , Universiti Teknologi PETRONAS, Malaysia, 2011, pp. 1–5.

43. M. Z. Yusoff and N. Kamel, A subspace approach with pre-whitening for measurements of latencies in visual evoked potentials, in *Intelligent and Advanced Systems (ICIAS), 2010 International Conference on*, Kuala Lumpur, Malaysia, 2010, pp. 1–6.

44. E. H. Land and J. J. McCann, Lightness and retinex theory, *Journal of the Optical Society of America*, vol. 61, pp. 1–11, 1971.

chapter seven

Hyperspectral image analysis for subcutaneous veins localization

Aamir Shahzad, Mohamad Naufal Mohamad Saad, Fabrice Meriaudeau and Aamir Saeed Malik

Contents

7.1 Anatomy and physiology of blood vessels

The human circulation system generally consists of three kinds of blood vessels: arteries, veins and capillaries. These blood vessels are used to transport blood that behaves like a transport medium within the body. The blood is pumped by the heart into the arteries, which carry it to all

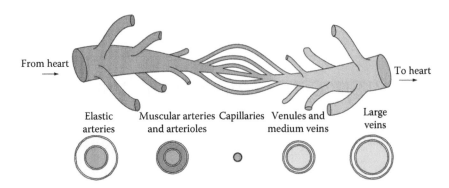

Figure 7.1 Depiction of three types of blood vessels with the direction of blood flow. (From *Anatomy and Physiology of the Cardiovascualr System*. Jones and Bartlett Publishers, 2008.)

parts of the body. Capillaries are the smaller vessels which exchange the nutrients, oxygen etc. with the tissues. Veins carry the deoxygenated blood back from the tissues to the heart. These three blood vessels are interconnected and create the closed circulation system for the body. Figure 7.1 depicts the anatomy of blood vessels at the capillaries level [1].

7.1.1 Arteries

Arteries are the high pressure blood-carrying circulatory tubes that carry oxygenated blood from the heart to the tissues of the body. The largest artery connected to the left ventricle of the heart is called aorta, which divides into smaller branches named as arterioles and capillaries at the tissue level [2]. The muscular layers of arteries are strong and are designed to bear the high pressure applied by the heart in order to make sure that the oxygenated blood and nutrients reach at the tissue level. Arteries are generally surrounded by the nerves which make the accidental artery puncture more painful [3]. Further, the high pressure of blood in arteries makes it difficult to puncture them. In situations when an artery is punctured or cut, blood spurts out with great pressure and it becomes difficult to stop it with normal procedures such as applying pressure dressing. Thus, injections in the arteries are not practiced. Furthermore, arterial injection would send concentrated dose to the extremity while venous injections return to the heart and are distributed systematically.

7.1.2 Capillaries

These are the smallest, thin-walled blood vessels that are connected to the smallest arteries and the smallest veins. The capillaries are responsible for the exchange of nutrients, oxygen, waste products and electrolytes between tissues and the blood [4]. The oxygenated blood carried by arteries reaches the tissue's level through capillaries and the de-oxygenated blood is distributed to the veins, which are responsible to carry it towards the heart. The blood flow is slower in capillaries and this provides sufficient time diffusion for the exchange of materials between blood and tissues. Capillaries have dense interconnected network called capillary bed throughout the body. An estimated length of capillaries bed is about 60,000–100,000 miles long in an average human adult [5].

7.1.3 Veins

Veins carry deoxygenated blood from tissues to the heart. The heart pumps this blood through the pulmonary artery to the lungs for the process of oxygenation. Veins are chosen for intravenous (IV) medication since the direction of the flow of blood is towards the heart from where it is pumped to every part of the body after oxygenation through the lungs. This way, medication delivered through veins can be distributed systematically in the body. The human venous system is generally divided into two types of veins: deep and subcutaneous veins.

Deep veins: The deep veins are larger in diameter and can be considered as the major pipelines residing in the deeper vicinities of the body. These veins cannot be seen with the naked eye. Different imaging modalities like MRI (magnetic resonance imaging), CT (computed tomography) and ultrasound can be used to localize these veins in case of any vascular disorder. In most of the cases there is an artery beside each of these deep veins. This pair of vein and artery usually shares the same name for identification. The larger veins maintain the flow of blood from the tissues to the heart with the help of valves. These valves are important especially when the blood flows against gravity, for example, from lower body to the heart. Furthermore, the muscles of body help the flow of blood by contraction, for example, while walking; the muscles in the leg squeeze the blood to the heart.

Subcutaneous veins: Subcutaneous or superficial veins lie near to the surface of skin. These are present in the third layer of skin called hypodermis which contains the subcutaneous tissues. The word subcutaneous means "situated under the skin." These veins communicate with deep veins through a complex network underneath the skin. The most commonly known subcutaneous veins are present in the forearm and back of the hand regions of the human body. These appear blue in colour since the absorption of the red component of visible light is much higher in deoxygenated blood as compared to the oxygenated blood in arteries [6]. These veins are used for the venous puncture procedure due to their location in the body. The pressure inside the veins is lesser than arteries which

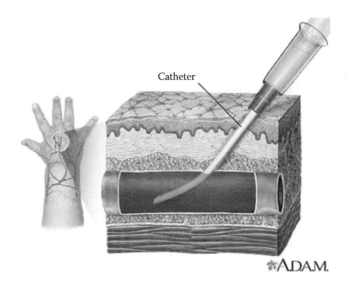

Figure. 7.2 IV catheterization process. (Reproduced from *Anatomy and Physiology of the Cardiovascualr System*. Jones and Bartlett Publishers, 2008.)

make them suitable for IV catheterization and fluid administration purposes. Figure 7.2 depicts the IV catheter insertion at the backhand site of a patient.

7.2   Problem in IV catheterization

IV catheterization is the first and most important step whenever a medical procedure involves the infusion of liquid substances directly into a vein. This process is required for anaesthesia, surgical procedure, trauma and labouring patients, and patients requiring emergency medication. Each year in the United States only, around 25 million catheters are placed in patients [7]. Studies have reported that around 80% of all hospitalized patients and several outdoor patients require catheters for the injection of medication and for blood sampling [8,9].

Trained medical personnel are required to perform the procedure of peripheral IV catheterization. Localizing and selecting a suitable vein is performed by sight and by feeling with the fingers of the targeted site of a patient's body typically at the lower arm, hand or foot. A suitable vein for holding the catheter is the vein oriented longitudinally and having a relative larger diameter than the catheter. It is a difficult and challenging task to localize such veins in patients having physiological characteristics such as darker skin tone, deep veins and the presence of scars, tattoos or hair on skin. The task of veins localization becomes very difficult in the case of infants, obese, elderly, dehydrated patients or IV drug abusers [10].

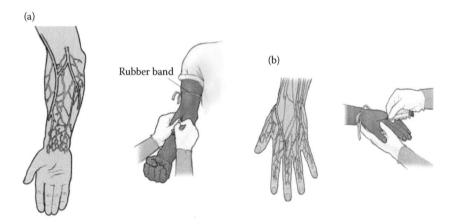

Figure 7.3 Venous access in (a) forearm and (b) backhand. Images reproduced with modification. (Reproduced from R. Bergman, Intra venous blood sampling, January 2014 [Online]. Available: http://www.anatomyatlases.org/firstaid/DrawingBlood.shtml.)

The term peripheral difficult venous access (PDVA) is used when veins are difficult to be localized. In such cases, the number of attempts due to unsuitable catheterization increases. It has been reported that the success rate of first attempt in infants is only 45% and even lesser in the infants of age less than 6 months [11]. The situation can be even worse in an emergency department for children where a large number of children are admitted with chronic medical condition. Studies have revealed that on average, 2.18 venous puncture attempts are needed for a patient who needs IV medication [12]. It was reported that the first attempt failure rate can reach up to 26% in adults and 54% in children in emergency cases [13]. Figure 7.3 illustrates the IV medication process to the subcutaneous veins of forearm and hand.

Wrong catheterization can result in serious consequences such as complex regional pain syndrome, hematoma, infiltration and extravasation [15]. In the case of hematoma, internal bleeding due to the vein rupture appears as skin bruises, as shown in Figure 7.4. Infiltration is another serious IV catheter complication. If the vein is damaged, medication can leak into the tissues, which could cause firm swelling, redness and could even be poisonous to tissues for most chemotherapy treatments. Figure 7.5 depicts the infiltration and damage of veins when needle pierces through the back wall of the vein.

Surgical interventions may be required in cases of vein damage and medication delivered to surrounding tissues due to a wrong catheterization. Multiple numbers of IV catheterization attempts cause pain, trauma and emotional distress in patients, especially in children [18,19]. A higher number of attempts also cause anxiety for the patients and to the parents

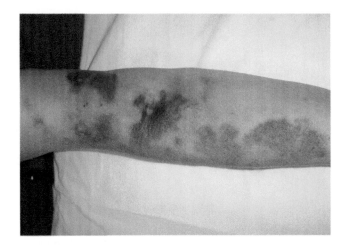

Figure 7.4 Depiction of hematoma caused by wrong catheterization. (Image reproduced from M. Haimov, *Surgery, Gynecology & Obstetrics*, vol. 141, pp. 619–625, 1975.)

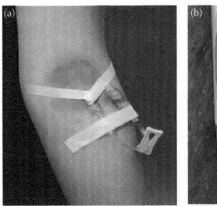
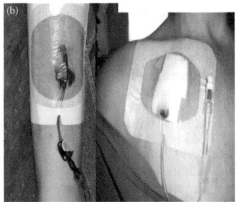

Figure 7.5 Depiction of infiltration in (a) and vein rupture in (b). (Images reproduced from Intravenous Access, Clinical Essentials, Paramedic Care, December 2014 [Online]. Available: http://what-when-how.com/paramedic-care/intravenous-access-clinical-essentials-paramedic-care-part-5/.)

in the case of a child. This also results in a lack of confidence in medical procedures and the personnel performing them [20]. In order to minimize the risk of a wrong catheterization and to reduce the number of attempts, imaging tool is proposed to aid in subcutaneous vein localization.

One of the effective solution is to use near-infrared (NIR) imaging to locate the veins. However, the PDVA problem depends on several physical characteristics of patients including skin colour and depth of subcutaneous veins. The skin tone of the patient is one of the main characteristic which contributes to the PDVA problem. People with darker skin tone are more likely to have difficult venous access due to non-visibility of veins. Patient's skin tone should therefore be considered when designing the veins localization systems. Illumination plays an important role in terms of venous imaging for different skin tone patients. This problem gives rise to the need of optimized illumination for different skin tone patients. Therefore, NIR imaging systems should have optimized illumination for all types of skin tones in order to deal with varying skin tones. Another vital point is the limited resources for wearable systems including power and space. With optimized illumination, systems can be designed for different skin tone patients while utilizing the lesser power and space. At present, there is no consensus on the band of NIR illumination to be used in order for optimal image quality for all skin tones. Various veins localization devices use different NIR illumination wavelengths and none has proven to be effective for all skin tone patients.

7.3   Imaging veins using NIR

NIR imaging work on the principle of light propagation, that is, absorption, reflection and scattering in the tissues. It has vast applications in the field of biomedical imaging, and has several advantages over the other radiological methods used for medical spectroscopy. NIR light spectrum is non-ionizing, therefore, it can be applied on patients without any harmful effects [16]. Through optical methods, skin tissues can be differentiated from veins based on their respective reflection, absorption and scattering coefficients. The non-invasive capability of this technique leads to its wide acceptance in the field of biomedical applications.

Light in the NIR spectrum (optical window) can penetrate deeper (a few millimetres) into the biological tissue because it is weakly absorbed by proteins, collagen, haemoglobin and water, as seen from Figure 7.6. In the spectral range of the optical window (750–950 nm), oxygenated haemoglobin (HbO_2), and de-oxygenated haemoglobin (Hb) are present at relatively higher concentrations and regarded as the main absorbers, even though other substances have higher absorption coefficients [17].

Hence, this optical window can be utilized for imaging subcutaneous veins that lie in the hypodermis layer of skin, at an average depth of 2–4 mm depending on the physical characteristics of a person and the location of skin analysed on the body. Persons having a high amount of body fat are more likely to have deeper veins. The vein depth is also dependent on the location on the human body; for example, the skin on the human back is much thicker as compared to the skin on the forearm.

Apart from NIR, two other techniques namely, trans-illumination and photoacoustic techniques have been proposed for vein localisation.

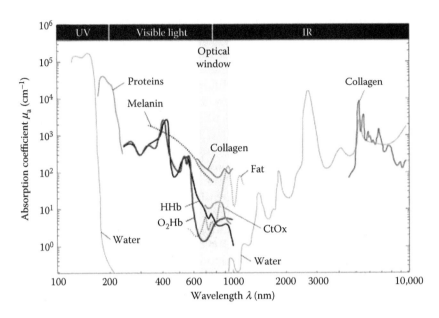

Figure 7.6 Absorption spectra for different chromophores present in human tissue. (Reproduced from F. Scholkmann et al., *NeuroImage*, vol. 85, (Part 1), pp. 6–27, 2014.)

Trans-illumination in which the body tissue is illuminated by transmitted light is relatively cost effective and mostly used for the normal cases. The tissues of the body when illuminated produce a red glow due to red blood cells absorbing other wavelengths of light. However, the trans-illumination technique is less effective in PDVA situations, especially in cases of deeper veins and darker skin tones. In photoacoustic technique, non-ionizing laser pulses are delivered into biological tissues leading to transient thermoelastic expansion and wideband (MHz) ultrasonic emission that are detected by ultrasonic transducers and then analysed to produce images associated with physiological properties, such as haemoglobin concentration and oxygen saturation. The technique is effective but the cost and portability issues limit the usage of this technique for veins localization process. Furthermore, sensitivity to environmental noise is a major drawback of this technique.

NIR imaging is found to be the most suitable technique for the process of subcutaneous veins localization compared to the trans-illumination and photoacoustic techniques, as reported in a review of imaging techniques for subcutaneous vein location [22]. It is cost effective, can be made portable and is easy to use during routine medical practices. It is also effective in situations where veins localization in patients becomes problematic. In this work, hyperspectral analysis has been performed to optimize the NIR illumination in order to get good contrast for every skin type with a lesser amount of power and space used for the illumination system.

7.3.1   Hyperspectral data acquisition

Hyperspectral and multispectral imaging are well-established spectroscopy techniques in remote sensing, satellite imaging, agriculture, physics and military. In recent years, it has gained attention in the field of biomedical imaging, especially where the standard imaging techniques fail to provide the desired outcomes [23]. Hyperspectral sensor records spectroscopic information of the entire field of view for each band and combine the collected information as a data cube, as shown in Figure 7.7, containing the image of the scene for each wavelength or band [24]. Each pixel has a specific reflectance value for a certain wavelength. The three-dimensional data cube often called hypercube is formed with two spatial and one spectral dimension [25]. With higher spectral resolution, it provides the ability to analyse data on wavelength or sub-wavelength scale. Furthermore, it also provides the ability to see beyond the visible range giving more details of the scene. Hyperspectral venous imaging allows us to look deeper in the NIR window to determine the optimal wavelength range that ensures a high contrast between skin and veins. The goal is to acquire and process hyperspectral images in the visible and NIR ranges in order to define optimized illumination for all skin tones.

The hyperspectral image acquisition system Specim® Spectral Camera PS V10E, as shown in Figure 7.8 has the ability to acquire images in the visible and NIR range, that is, 380–1055 nm wavelength range with a spectral resolution of 2.8 nm (the width of each band of the captured spectrum). Total numbers of bands are 1040, which give an average step size of 0.65 nm

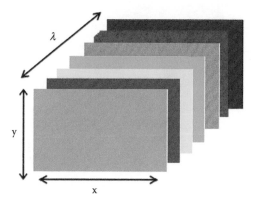

Figure 7.7 Hyperspectral image cube illustration.

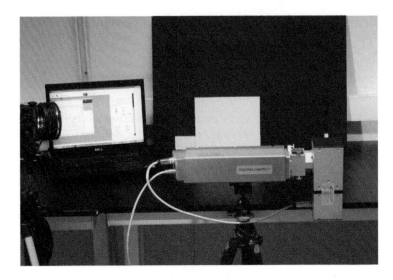

Figure 7.8 Hyperspectral image acquisition setup with Specim spectral camera.

between each central wavelength. This camera provides a high spatial and spectral resolution with an adjustable field of view to be scanned.

The images of the forearm area of each subject are acquired, as the subcutaneous veins of this region are of our interest. Projector (halogen) lamps with a constant illumination range from 350 to 2500 nm were used to illuminate the targeted region, as shown in Figure 7.9. Each acquired hyperspectral image is in the form of cube with the spatial resolution of

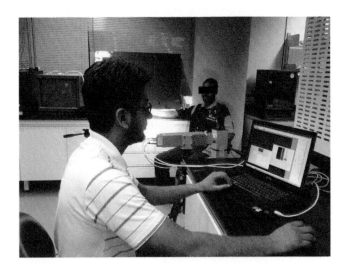

Figure 7.9 Hyperspectral data acquisition process.

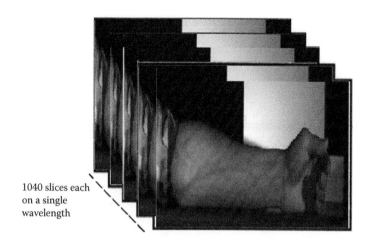

1040 slices each
on a single
wavelength

Figure 7.10 Hyperspectral cube with forearm of a subject.

450 × 1310 and 1040 spectral bands. A complete image of the scene on every single wavelength is acquired and saved in the form of hypercube, presented in Figure 7.10.

Spectral DAQ software from Specim® was used to set the camera parameters and data acquisition. The angle for the mirror scanner was set in such a way that it should scan only the forearm region of the subject, allowing the minimum data size of each hyperspectral cube for each subject. The scanning time of hyperspectral image for one subject is about 40 s. It depends on the selected scanning range of mirror scanner used with Specim VNIR image sensor. The targeted area is the forearm region of the subject, hence around 21° of scanning range (which covers the region from elbow to the tip of subject's fingers) is selected. The distance of mirror scanner is set to be about 1 m from the subject's position. The spectral images acquired are in the form of data cubes which are saved in an environment for visualizing images (ENVI) compatible formats. MATLAB is used to read the raw data (.raw) cubes using ENVI toolbox.

The data acquisition protocol is shown in Figure 7.11. The consent form is to be signed by each subject prior to the data collection steps. Subject's weight and height are measured and recorded to calculate the BMI (body

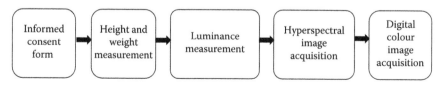

Figure 7.11 Data acquisition protocol.

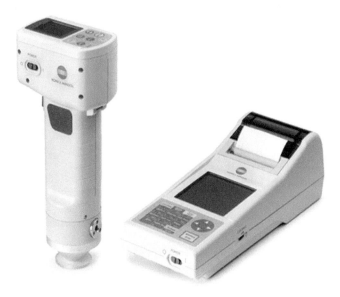

Figure 7.12 Konica Minolta chromameter.

mass index) at a later stage. Using the Konica Minolta Chromameter, the CIE *L*a*b**value is recorded at the subject's forearm region (shown in Figures 7.12 and 7.13). Measurements are taken at three different locations on the forearm to derive the average Luminance *L**value of the subject to be used in the classification of skin tone.

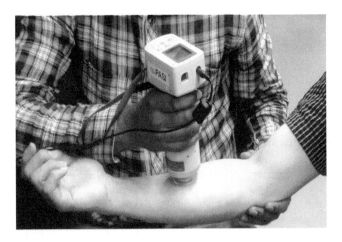

Figure 7.13 Measuring CIE *L*a*b**value from forearm of a subject with a chromameter.

The hyperspectral image of forearm of each subject is then acquired using Specim® spectral VNIR camera with the spectral range 380–1055 nm. A digital image of each subject's forearm is also taken using a Canon EOS 500D DSLR camera to record the subject's skin colour.

A total of 252 subjects were recruited as volunteers. Data were collected from two different locations. Initially, data were obtained from 80 subjects at the Universiti Teknologi PETRONAS (UTP) campus. The subjects were selected based on different nationalities and ethnicity for diversity according to four chosen skin tone classes namely fair, light brown, dark brown and dark. Next, the local community was engaged in the dataset formulation. Here, 172 subjects from UTP, community and School (Sekolah Kebangsaan Seri Selamat, Sitiawan) were recruited. In this phase, the diversity in terms of age of subjects has been achieved. The ages of the subjects vary from 2 to 72 years old. This large range of age was classified into four different groups namely, children below 12 years old, teenagers' ages ranging from 13 to 20 years old, adults with ages from 21 to 49 years old and elderly people more than 50 years old. Figure 7.14 shows the subject's distribution with respect to age groups. The image of the youngest subject is shown in Figure 7.15.

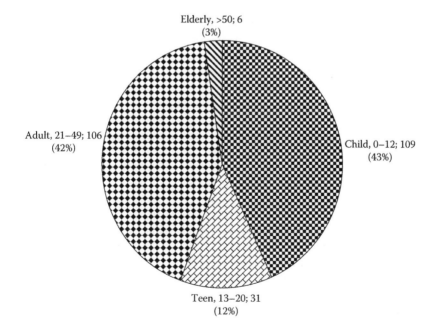

Figure 7.14 Distribution of age groups.

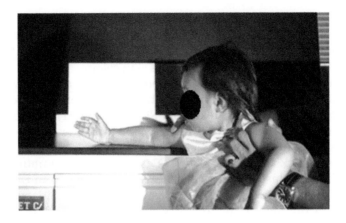

Figure 7.15 Youngest subject; a child with age of 2 years.

7.3.2 Skin tone classification

The skin tone is an important factor that affects the veins localization process. People with darker skin are more likely to have non-visibility of veins, that is, PDVA problem. In order to achieve better insight of veins viewing in subjects having different skin tones, the skin is classified into four classes as reported by Fadzil et al. [26]. The skin tone classes are fair, light brown, dark brown and dark. Luminance (CIE L^*) values of the forearm skin of subjects were obtained using a chromameter (Konica Minolta). The average value of luminance (L^*) from three different locations of the forearm of each subject is then fed into a classifier to obtain the final skin tone class.

Data can be classified using either supervised or unsupervised techniques. Unsupervised classification is often known as clustering while supervised classification is termed as discriminant analysis. In supervised classification, a training set is provided to algorithm to classify unlabelled data. While in clustering (unsupervised classification), unlabelled data are clustered into meaningful groups [27]. The objective of clustering is to separate given data objects into a certain number of categories or groups in order to provide suitable insight for further analysis [28].

Clustering algorithms can be further classified into two types. One is hard clustering algorithms such as k-means and second is fuzzy (or soft) clustering algorithms such as fuzzy c-mean (FCM) algorithm. Both k-means and FCM are widely used algorithms for clustering of data into certain number of clusters. The difference lies in the probabilities of data belonging to clusters. Since k-means is a hard clustering algorithm, data can belong to a single cluster only by making the probability of one at its cluster and zero in any other cluster. In soft clustering, a membership degree is defined as probability of data belonging to any cluster. A membership function is used to determine the membership degrees. In this way, a data point can simultaneously belong to a number of clusters, but the parent cluster is chosen on the basis of highest membership degree [26]. Since soft clustering is more natural than hard clustering, it has been chosen for the classification of skin tone. In case of data points on cluster boundaries, the method allows data belonging to more than one cluster based on membership degree.

7.3.2.1 FCM for skin tone classification

Figure 7.16 depicts the classification of skin tones into four different classes using FCM classifier. The membership function is constructed by applying Gaussian curve fitting to the dataset. The process of curve fitting is used to construct a mathematical function or curve to infer the value of function where data points are not available [29]. It is also used to visualize the data clustering results [30]. Curve fitting can be best fit or exact fit, based on the number of data points and parameters. In exact fitting (often called interpolation) curve passes through every point, but it is suitable only for small number of parameters. The best-fit curves do not pass through every possible point but the value of data point is estimated on curve keeping it close enough to exact value of data point. The residual error is made as small as possible in best-fit curves [31–33].

In this, the Gaussian curve fitting function is used to visualize the clustering results of Luminance (L^*) data values. The general Gaussian

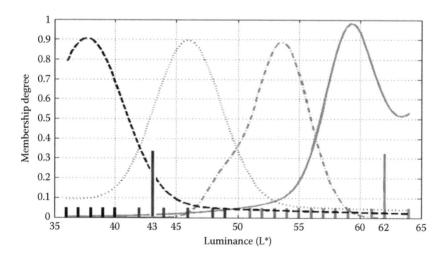

Figure 7.16 Skin tone classification using FCM into four classes: dark, dark brown, light brown and fair.

equation for four skin tone groups can be expressed in Equation 7.1. Coefficient a_i is $1/(\sigma_i(2\pi)^{1/2})$, b_i is μ_i (mean of Gaussian distribution), and c_i is $\sigma_i 2^{1/2}$ (standard deviation of the distribution).

$$T_n(L) = \sum_{i=1}^{3} a_i \exp\left(-\frac{(L-b_i)^2}{c_i^2}\right) \tag{7.1}$$

In Figure 7.16, the small bar lines on x-axis show the occurrences of the L^* value in dataset. Note that at a particular point on x-axis, multiple occurrences can be possible but those are shown by the single bar only.

For demonstration purpose, Tables 7.1 and 7.2 depicts the output for two random values of L^* which are fed to the algorithm. The cluster is decided on the basis of the highest membership degree of provided data point. Two values of L^* fed to the algorithm are '43' and '62'. Tables 7.1 and 7.2 depict the results of clustering, respectively.

Figure 7.17 shows typical digital colour image (zoomed) of four different skin tones. These are taken from subjects of four different skin classes (i.e. fair, light brown, dark brown and dark). In Figure 7.18, the pie chart of the data set showing the number of subjects for each skin class is given. According to the skin tone classification, 78 subjects were with fair skin, 107 with light brown, 51 with dark brown and 16 were with dark skin tone out of a total of 252 subjects in the hyperspectral dataset.

Table 7.1 Clustering results for luminance (L^*) value provided ($L^* = 43$)

Skin tone	Centroid (c_k)	Luminance (L^*)	Membership degree (u_{ij})	Decision on skin tone
Fair	58.9278	43	0.0162	X
Light brown	53.5736	43	0.2310	X
Dark brown	46.3221	43	0.5234	✓
Dark	37.8644	43	0.2296	X

Table 7.2 Clustering results for luminance (L^*) value provided ($L^* = 62$)

Skin tone	Centroid (c_k)	Luminance (L^*)	Membership degree (u_{ij})	Decision on skin tone
Fair	58.9278	62	0.5995	✓
Light brown	53.5736	62	0.1860	X
Dark brown	46.3221	62	0.1432	X
Dark	37.8644	62	0.0253	X

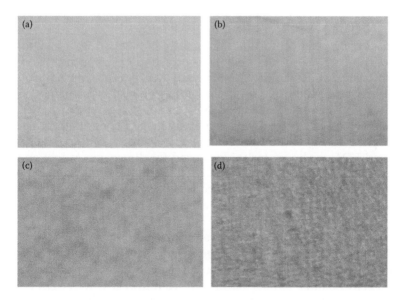

Figure 7.17 Digital (zoomed) image of four skin classes: (a) fair, (b) light brown, (c) dark brown and (d) dark skin. Images acquired with Canon EOS 500D indoor fluorescent lighting.

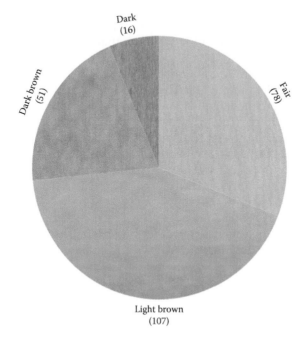

Figure 7.18 Ratio of subjects with different skin tones in the dataset of 252 subjects.

7.3.3 Hyperspectral data analysis

The goal of hyperspectral data analysis is to have an insight into the relationship between venous image contrast and the spectral bands of illumination used to acquire these images. In order to achieve the objective of optimum illumination for subcutaneous veins localization, the hyperspectral data obtained from NIR imaging of the forearm of subjects are processed with dimension reduction techniques namely, *principal component analysis* (PCA) and *linear discriminant analysis* (LDA). Both PCA and LDA are linear techniques used for dimension reduction and classification. By applying PCA and LDA, the dimensions (wavelengths) of hyperspectral data cube are reduced and classified into veins and skin tissues based on contrast, in which veins have higher contrast than skin tissues.

Hyperspectral dataset are pre-processed before applying PCA and LDA. The raw data are converted to '.mat' files with dimension $x*y*1040$, where 'x' and 'y' represent the image spatial dimensions with 1040 spectral bands. Ninety bands (50 from lowest wavelength bands and 40 from highest wavelength bands) out of 1040 bands are discarded due to high noise content. The hyperspectral cubes now have reduced dimensions of $x*y*950$. A mean image is created by taking mean of the bands from 750 to 950 nm (NIR optical window). The veins localization method is used to detect veins pixels from the mean image. A matrix of veins pixels named IV is created for each subject for the analysis. The dimensions for IV are $10 \times 10 \times 950$, that is, 10-by-10 pixel by 950 bands.

For experimentation, data cubes of eight subjects from each skin class are selected to make IVs. These IVs are then combined to make one large matrix named against skin type, for example, IV_f for fair skin, IV_d for dark skin, etc. The dimensions for IV_x are $80 \times 10 \times 950$. In a similar manner, a large matrix for skin tissue pixels are created and named as IT_x. Skin tissue pixels are the non-veins pixels in the hyperspectral image. Both IV_x and IT_x for each skin type are then concatenated to create IVT_x. The data matrix IVT_x was normalized to their mean values. In order to maximize the separation between both veins and skin pixels, PCA and LDA are applied on these large matrices separately. Table 7.3 illustrates the formulation of data matrix for implementation of PCA. The data matrix IVT_x was normalized with the formula given by

$$X_{norm} = \frac{X - \mu}{\sigma},\qquad(7.2)$$

where 'μ' is the mean and 'σ' is the standard deviation of data matrix.

Table 7.3 Illustration of creating of data matrix for implementation of PCA

Skin type	IV_Subj-1	...	IV_Subj-8	...	IT_Subj-1	...	IT_Subj-8	IVT_x
Fair	$10 \times 10 \times 950$	...	$10 \times 10 \times 950$	...	$10 \times 10 \times 950$	...	$10 \times 10 \times 950$	$IVT_f = 160 \times 10 \times 950$
Light brown	$10 \times 10 \times 950$	...	$10 \times 10 \times 950$	...	$10 \times 10 \times 950$	...	$10 \times 10 \times 950$	$IVT_{lb} = 160 \times 10 \times 950$
Dark brown	$10 \times 10 \times 950$	...	$10 \times 10 \times 950$	...	$10 \times 10 \times 950$	...	$10 \times 10 \times 950$	$IVT_{db} = 160 \times 10 \times 950$
Dark	$10 \times 10 \times 950$	...	$10 \times 10 \times 950$	...	$10 \times 10 \times 950$	...	$10 \times 10 \times 950$	$IVT_d = 160 \times 10 \times 950$

7.3.4 Principal component analysis

PCA is a well-known linear, unsupervised dimensionality reduction technique [34]. It projects a high-dimensional space to a lower dimensional space in order to reduce the data size while preserving the quality of the reconstruction by controlling the quantity of data loss [35]. It is widely used to reduce the number of features by removing irrelevant, noisy, redundant and less important features from a large feature matrix [36]. The stepwise method to apply PCA on a data set is given below:

1. Normalizing the dataset.
2. Finding covariance matrix.
3. Finding singular vectors and singular values of covariance matrix with singular value decomposition (SVD) method.
4. Sort the singular values and corresponding vectors.
5. The 'k' singular vectors corresponding to 'k' highest singular values are the principle components of the dataset.
6. Project the image data on first 'k' principle components.
7. Reconstruct the data to the original format by reshaping.

The data matrix is normalized for each skin tone. This normalized matrix is then fed into PCA algorithm which returns the principal components (PCs). The singular vectors and singular values of the covariance matrix are calculated by SVD.

$$X = U \times S \times V',\qquad(7.3)$$

where S is a diagonal matrix containing singular values of data matrix as its diagonal entries in descending order. U and V are orthogonal matrices containing the pair of singular vectors where $Vt\ V = I$ and $Ut\ U = I$. In the matrix U, first singular vector corresponding to the highest singular value is the first principal component (PC) of the data. Second singular vector is the second PC and so on. The initial few PCs possess highest energy [34,35,37].

7.3.4.1 PCA on hyperspectral data

In this work, the PCA is applied on the data from four skin tone classes. The data are pre-processed and arranged in the form of hyperspectral matrices named IVT_x according to their respective skin tone class. The PCs are calculated for all four skin classes with their respective data matrices IVT_x. Once PCs have been calculated, the image data are projected to the respective first, second and third component in order to visualize the separation between veins, and skin tissue pixels. The first three PCs are chosen since the energy contained in the first three components is more than 90% on average for all skin classes. Hence, the image is reconstructed by projecting image data on these first three components.

Figure 7.19a depicts the projection of image data of a subject from fair skin class to the first three PCs calculated from the respective IVT_f data matrix. Three PCs are depicted in Figure 7.19b, first in blue, second in red and third in green colour plot. Similarly, Figure 7.20 depicts the projection of image data of a subject from light brown skin class to the first three PCs calculated from IVT_{lb} data matrix. Figure 7.21 depicts the projection of image data of a subject from dark brown skin class to the first three PCs calculated from IVT_{db} data matrix. Figure 7.22 depicts the projection of image data of a subject from dark skin class to the first three PCs calculated from IVT_d data matrix.

The image data of different subjects from all four skin classes are projected on the first three PCs obtained from PCA. From the resultant images it can be seen that the veins and skin tissues contrast is enhanced in case of projection on the second PC. On closer examination of the second PC plot, it can be seen that the higher values lie in the NIR window, that is, 750–950 nm. In Reference 38, it has been stated that the contrast between veins and skin tissue is higher due to the deeper penetration of

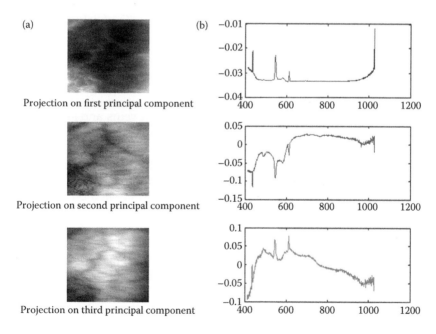

(a)

Projection on first principal component

Projection on second principal component

Projection on third principal component

(b)

Figure 7.19 (a) Projection of image data of a subject belonging to fair skin on first three PCs of fair skin tone. (b) First three PCs of fair skin tone with wavelength (nm) on x-axis.

(a)

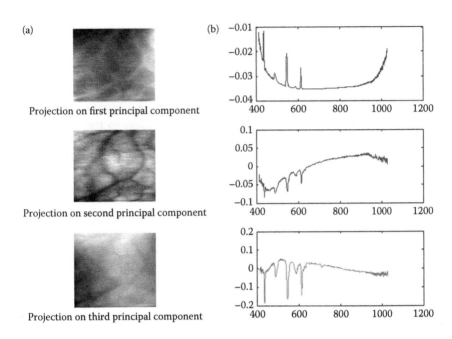

Projection on first principal component

Projection on second principal component

Projection on third principal component

Figure 7.20 (a) Projection of image data of a subject belonging to light brown skin on first three PCs of light brown skin tone. (b) First three PCs of light brown skin tone with wavelength (nm) on x-axis.

light in the NIR window. Figures 7.23 through 7.26 show the comparison of the contrast between original NIR images to reconstructed images with second PCs for the subjects of different skin tone classes. It can be seen through the histogram plots; the contrast between veins and skin pixels for the reconstructed image is higher in comparison to the corresponding original NIR image for each skin tone class.

In this section, it is established that skin/veins contrast is higher in the images captured with the NIR illumination range. In Section 7.3.4.2, the NIR range is further studied through the PCA applied on four sub-bands within NIR range.

7.3.4.2   PCA on four NIR sub-bands

In order to get optimized wavelength range for better skin contrast in venous image, PCA is applied on four different sub-bands within the NIR window of hyperspectral data. The wavelengths range of first, second, third and fourth sub-band are 750–800 nm, 800–850 nm, 850–900 nm and 900–950 nm, respectively. PCA is applied on these four sub-bands and the image data are projected on the corresponding first PC to reconstruct the image for display. This is because first PC contains the maximum energy

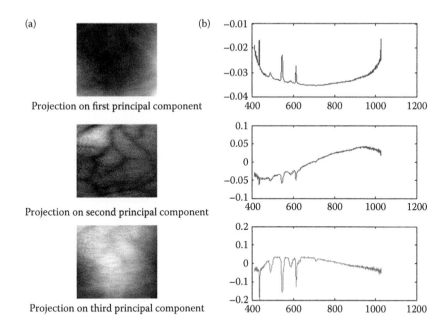

Figure 7.21 (a) Projection of image data of a subject belonging to dark brown skin on first three PCs of dark brown skin tone. (b) First three PCs of dark brown skin tone with wavelength (nm) on x-axis.

and projecting image data on that will contain maximum information out of image. In order to have quantitative measure of image quality, the structure similarity (SSIM) [39] index is computed for each reconstructed image. It is the measure to compute the similarity between two images on the basis of three components, that is, change in luminance 'L', contrast 'C' and structure 'S' in image.

The following equation gives the SSIM between two images x and y.

$$\text{SSIM}(x,y) = \left[L(x,y)\right]^{\alpha} \cdot \left[C(x,y)\right]^{\beta} \cdot S\left[x,y\right]^{\gamma} \tag{7.4}$$

where α, β and γ are the scale factors to adjust the importance of three parameters in the equation.

In this case, the comparisons of four reconstructed images are made with the reference image created by taking mean on the entire NIR window. The mean image created from the NIR range is supposed to have best quality in terms of higher peak signal-to-noise ratio (PSNR) due to highly random nature of noise. By taking average of the image slices in this range, noise is significantly reduced.

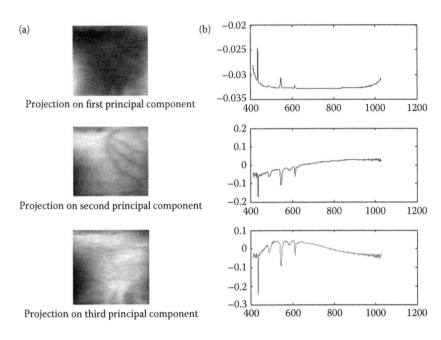

Figure 7.22 (a) Projection of image data of a subject belonging to dark skin on first three PCs of dark skin tone. (b) First three PCs of dark skin tone with wavelength (nm) on x-axis.

Figures 7.27 through 7.30 depict the reconstructed image from the application PCA on four sub-bands defined earlier. The SSIM values are given on top of each image. The image reconstruction is performed on the hyperspectral images on all four skin class subjects. It was found that the reconstructed image from the PCA on 800–850 nm sub-band has better image quality (SSIM value is higher) as compared to other sub-bands. The results of image quality in all fair, light brown, dark brown and dark skin tone classes are shown in Figures 7.27 through 7.30, respectively.

These results of PCA implementation on four different sub-bands show that the projected image on the PC computed from PCA on 800–850 nm sub-band has highest image quality among all. It is therefore suggested that the illumination band in the range of 800–850 nm is the optimal band for NIR imaging system for all skin tone class subjects. Further analysis of hyperspectral data is performed with LDA detailed in the following section.

7.3.5   Linear discriminant analysis

LDA is used to reduce dimensionality of multidimensional dataset. LDA maximizes the between-class separation and minimizes the within-class

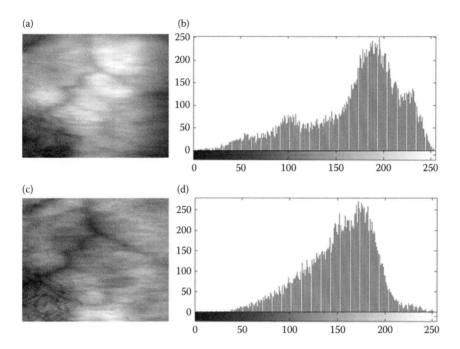

Figure 7.23 Comparison of original NIR image to the reconstructed image with second PC for a subject of fair skin tone class. (a, b) NIR image and its histogram and (c, d) reconstructed image and its histogram.

scatter [37,38]. It preserves the class discriminatory information as much as possible. Hence it can be used in applications like face recognition and feature extraction [40,41]. Two-class LDA is implemented on the hyperspectral dataset. Here, veins and tissues make a two-class problem and the separation of these classes is intended. LDA maximizes an objective function, which is the ratio of between-class scatter to the within-class scatter. The Fisher linear LDA considers maximizing the objective function given as [42]

$$J(w) = \frac{w^T S_B w}{w^T S_w w},\tag{7.5}$$

where 'S_B' is the between-class scatter, 'S_w' is within-class scatter and 'w' is the projection vector. Scatter of a class is the covariance and is defined as

$$S_i = \sum_{j=1}^{N} (x_j - \mu_i)(x_j - \mu_i)^T \tag{7.6}$$

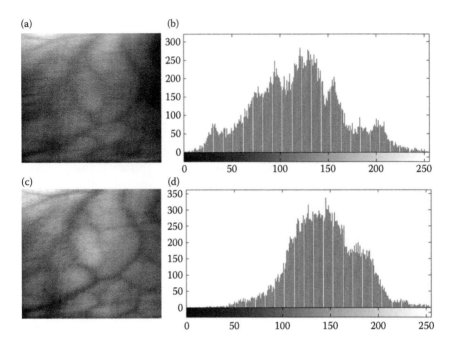

Figure 7.24 Comparison of original NIR image to the reconstructed image with second PC for a subject of light brown skin tone class. (a, b) NIR image and its histogram and (c, d) reconstructed image and its histogram.

where 'N' is the number of samples in a class and 'μ_i' is the mean of the class defined as

$$\mu_i = \frac{1}{N}\sum_{j=1}^{N}x_j \tag{7.7}$$

and, 'S_w' can be defined as

$$S_w = \sum_{i=1}^{c}S_i \tag{7.8}$$

where c is the number of classes

$$S_B = \sum_{i=1}^{c}(\mu_i - \mu)(\mu_i - \mu)^T \tag{7.9}$$

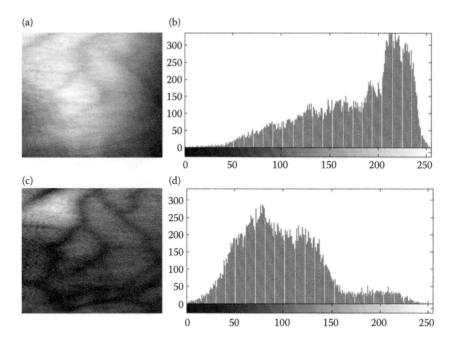

Figure 7.25 Comparison of original NIR image to the reconstructed image with second PC for a subject of dark brown skin tone class. (a, b) NIR image and its histogram and (c, d) reconstructed image and its histogram.

where μ is the total mean of the entire data and is given as

$$\mu = 1/c \sum_{i=1}^{c} \mu_i \qquad (7.10)$$

After determining 'S_B' and 'S_W', we solve to maximize the $J(w)$ value. To find the maximum value, Equation 7.5 is differentiated and equated with zero.

$$\frac{d}{dW} J(w) = \frac{d}{dW}\left(\frac{w^T S_B w}{w^T S_w w}\right) = 0 \qquad (7.11)$$

$$(w^T S_w w)\frac{d}{dW}(w^T S_B w) - (w^T S_B w)\frac{d}{dW}(w^T S_w w) = 0$$

$$(w^T S_w w)(2 S_B w) - (w^T S_B w)(2 S_w w) = 0$$

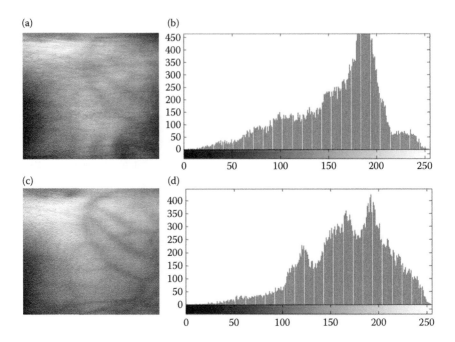

Figure 7.26 Comparison of original NIR image to the reconstructed image with second PC for a subject of dark skin tone class. (a, b) NIR image and its histogram and (c, d) reconstructed image and its histogram.

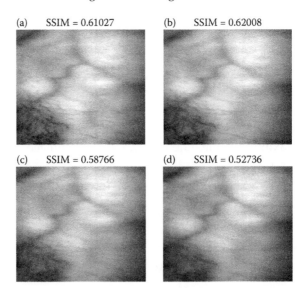

Figure 7.27 Fair Skin: reconstructed images from first PC from PCA on four sub-bands: (a) 750–800 nm, (b) 800–850 nm, (c) 850–900 nm and (d) 900–950 nm.

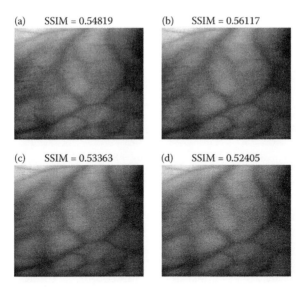

Figure 7.28 Light brown skin: reconstructed images from first PC from PCA on four sub-bands: (a) 750–800 nm, (b) 800–850 nm, (c) 850–900 nm and (d) 900–950 nm.

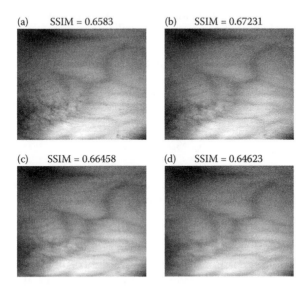

Figure 7.29 Dark brown skin: reconstructed images from first PC from PCA on four sub-bands: (a) 750–800 nm, (b) 800–850 nm, (c) 850–900 nm and (d) 900–950 nm.

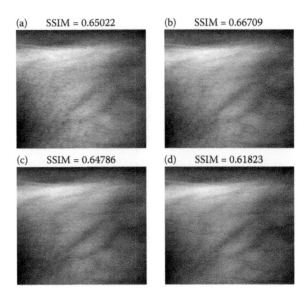

Figure 7.30 Dark skin: reconstructed images from first PC from PCA on four sub-bands: (a) 750–800 nm, (b) 800–850 nm, (c) 850–900 nm and (d) 900–950 nm.

Dividing by $2w^T S_w w$:

$$\left(\frac{w^T S_w w}{2w^T S_w w}\right)(2S_B w) - \left(\frac{w^T S_B w}{2w^T S_w w}\right)(2S_w w) = 0$$

$$S_B w - J(w) S_w w = 0$$

$$S_w^{-1} S_B w - J(w) w = 0$$

$$S_w^{-1} S_B w = J(w) w \tag{7.12}$$

Equation 7.12 can be solved as an eigenvalue problem, which means we can find the eigenvectors and eigenvalues.

7.3.5.1 *LDA on hyperspectral data*

The main purpose of applying LDA on two-class hyperspectral data matrices is to obtain the spectrum band where the contrast between these two classes is enhanced making it easier to distinguish between skin and veins visually. The contrast between both skin and veins tissues can be enhanced if the variance between both classes is maximized and variance within the classes is minimized. In this work, LDA was applied as a two-class problem on the data matrix containing veins and skin tissues samples, that is, the IVT_x matrices. In order to feed into LDA, both veins and skin classes are separated into two matrices, that is, IV_x and IT_x, respectively. The data are normalized with respect to the mean (Equation 7.3). The total within-class scatter 'S_w' is the sum of scatter parameters of all classes given in Equation 7.8. The between-class scatter 'S_B' is obtained using Equation 7.9. Eigenvectors and eigenvalues are computed for the two-class data matrices for all skin tone clusters. The image data of each subject is projected on the corresponding first three eigenvectors that are computed from the LDA algorithm. The resultant images are displayed in Figures 7.31 through 7.34, each depicting one case from each skin tone cluster.

Figure 7.31 depicts the projection of image data of a fair skin class subject on the first three eigenvectors using the fair skin data matrix, that is, IVT_f. Similarly, Figures 7.32 through 7.34 depict the projection of image data of light brown, dark brown and dark skin subjects on their corresponding three eigenvectors, respectively.

Unfortunately, the peaks in the plots of the eigenvectors do have steep rise (or fall) in the entire NIR range. In the case of dark brown skin shown

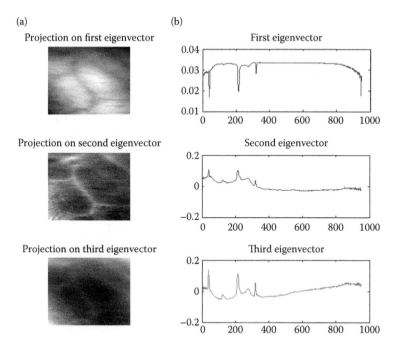

Figure 7.31 (a) Projection of a fair skin subject's image data on first three eigenvectors of LDA on fair skin data matrix. (b) First three eigenvectors with wavelength (nm) on the x-axis.

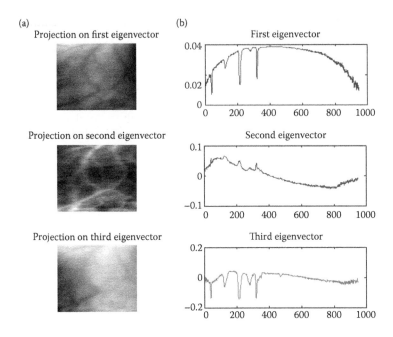

Figure 7.32 (a) Projection of a light brown skin subject's image data on first three eigenvectors of LDA on light brown skin data matrix. (b) First three eigenvectors with wavelength (nm) on the x-axis.

in Figure 7.33, the second eigenvector has relatively sharp rise and its peak lies in the NIR range around 850 nm. Similar to analysis of PCA on four bands in section 7.3.4.2. LDA is implemented on four NIR sub-bands in order to get the optimized wavelengths within NIR window. Results of implementation of LDA on four sub-bands are discussed in the following section.

7.3.5.2   LDA on four NIR sub-bands

In order to validate the results of PCA on four NIR sub-bands to get an optimized range of illumination, LDA is applied on predefined four sub-bands. The wavelength ranges of these sub-bands are 750–800, 800–850, 850–900 and 900–950 nm as the first, second, third and fourth sub-bands, respectively. Figures 7.35 through 7.38 depict the results of LDA implementation on the four sub-bands for the four different skin tone classes, that is, fair, light brown, dark brown and dark, respectively. The quantitative measure of image quality (SSIM) is given for each of the reconstructed image. It can be observed that the SSIM value is highest in the 800–850 nm band for all cases.

From these results, it can be seen that the quality of image projected on the first eigenvector from the LDA on the band of 800–850 nm is highest as

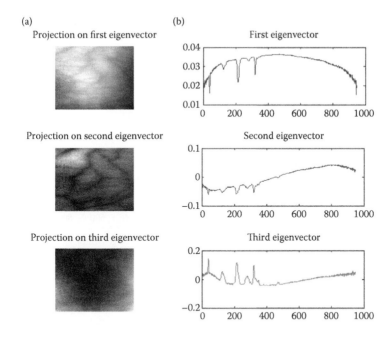

Figure 7.33 (a) Projection of a dark brown skin subject's image data on first three eigenvectors of LDA on dark brown skin data matrix. (b) First three eigenvectors with wavelength (nm) on the x-axis.

compared to the images in other three NIR sub-bands. These results are consistent for all skin tones.

7.4   Objective image quality assessment results and analysis

The goal of optimization of illumination wavelength can be achieved only if there exists a sub-band within NIR range on which the contrast is maximum between veins and skin tissues. From the analysis of hyperspectral image data using PCA and LDA discussed in sections 7.3.4 and 7.3.5 respectively, it is clear that the illumination in NIR range will produce higher venous contrast, particularly in the 800–850 nm wavelength range. To further validate these findings, hyperspectral image quality assessment based on the image quality parameters such as mean square error (MSE), PSNR and universal image quality index (Q) is performed on the hyperspectral image data of all four skin tone classes.

This section discusses the outcome of the objective analysis done on hyperspectral images for optimum illumination selection for four different skin tones. Optimum illumination is crucial for better image

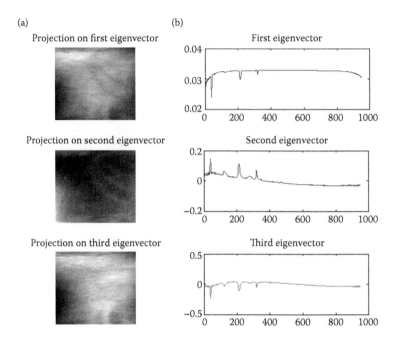

Figure 7.34 (a) Projection of a dark skin subject's image data on first three eigenvectors computed from LDA applied on dark skin data matrix. (b) First three eigenvectors with wavelength (nm) on the x-axis.

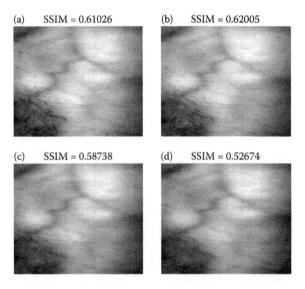

Figure 7.35 Fair skin: reconstructed images from LDA on four sub-bands: (a) 750–800 nm, (b) 800–850 nm, (c) 850–900 nm and (d) 900–950 nm.

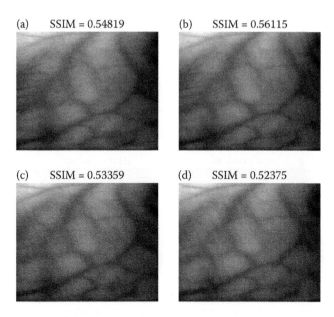

Figure 7.36 Light brown skin: reconstructed images from LDA on four sub-bands: (a) 750–800 nm, (b) 800–850 nm, (c) 850–900 nm and (d) 900–950 nm.

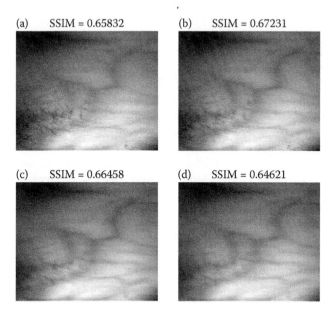

Figure 7.37 Dark brown skin: reconstructed images from LDA on four sub-bands: (a) 750–800 nm, (b) 800–850 nm, (c) 850–900 nm and (d) 900–950 nm.

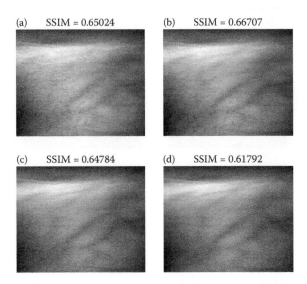

Figure 7.38 Dark skin: reconstructed images from LDA on four sub-bands: (a) 750–800 nm, (b) 800–850 nm, (c) 850–900 nm and (d) 900–950 nm.

quality and enhanced contrast between skin and veins, keeping in view the limited power and space on wearable imaging systems. To optimize the illumination for different classes of skin tone, hyperspectral image quality analysis is performed on the venous images of different subjects. This optimum illumination range is considered to achieve the best contrast while designing the wearable prototype system for veins localization.

The low absorption window, also known as the NIR window in electromagnetic spectrum is the range of wavelengths within NIR region, for which light can penetrate deeper inside skin tissues. This is due to the low absorption spectra of haemoglobin, oxy-haemoglobin and water which are main absorbers of radiations in skin. The span of window is approximately from 750 to 950 nm. Different NIR imaging devices use different wavelengths or range of wavelengths from this low absorption window to illuminate the target site for venipuncture procedure [43–46]. To define an optimum range for illumination, NIR window is divided into four sub-bands and mean images are formed from the hyperspectral slices. These images are analysed with objective quality measures to define the best wavelength range where the image quality is highest when compared to the mean reference image.

The ultimate users of images are human beings. The most trustworthy way of quality assessment of images is subjective analysis. It is based on the human visual system (HVS). The mean opinion score (MOS) is measured by human viewers. However, this measure is expensive and time consuming [47]. Furthermore, the MOS is severely affected by the image viewing conditions. The objective image quality assessment is chosen due to the following reasons:

1. Human subjects were unable to distinguish between the image quality of all sub-mean images since they look quite similar.
2. Contrast between veins and skin tissues cannot be determined fairly based on the HVS.
3. The acquired NIR images are fed to veins detection algorithm which provide an objective assessment observation.

Objective quality measurement is important for machine vision applications. Mathematical measures are used to measure and compare the image quality with respect to reference images. The factors like MSE, PSNR and universal image quality index (Q) are widely used to calculate the quality of images with a reference image which is considered the best image of the scene [48]. In this work, these three factors are chosen to find out the best range of wavelengths that will ensure good quality NIR venous images.

The images are converted into one-dimensional vectors before calculating the MSE. For simplicity of notation, we named reference image I_m as 'x' and the sub-mean image for which we want to calculate MSE, PSNR and Q as 'y'.

The following equations define the MSE and PSNR, respectively,

$$MSE = \frac{1}{N}\sum_{i=1}^{N}(x_i - y_i)^2 \tag{7.13}$$

$$PSNR = 10\log_{10}\frac{L^2}{MSE} \tag{7.14}$$

where 'N' is the total number of pixels in both images and L is 255 in these 8-bit grey-scale images. Furthermore, 'x_i' and 'y_i' are the ith pixels in image x and y, respectively [49].

The universal image quality index (Q) [48,50] is a measure that is independent of viewing conditions. It is called universal since the method to measure the quality of an image is independent of image nature, viewing conditions and the observers. The range of Q is [−1, 1], where the best value is 1 which is resultant of the comparing reference image to itself. The following equation defines the universal quality factor:

$$Q = \frac{\sigma_{xy}}{\sigma_x\sigma_y} \times \frac{2\bar{x}\,\bar{y}}{(\bar{x})^2 + (\bar{y})^2} \times \frac{2\sigma_x\sigma_y}{\sigma_x^2 + \sigma_y^2} \tag{7.15}$$

where

$$\bar{x} = \frac{1}{N}\sum_{i=1}^{N} x_i, \quad \bar{y} = \frac{1}{N}\sum_{i=1}^{N} y_i$$

$$\sigma_x^2 = \frac{1}{N-1}\sum_{i=1}^{N}(x_i - \bar{x})^2, \quad \sigma_y^2 = \frac{1}{N-1}\sum_{i=1}^{N}(y_i - \bar{y})^2$$

$$\sigma_{xy} = \frac{1}{N-1}\sum_{i=1}^{N}(x_i - \bar{x})(y_i - \bar{y})$$

There are three components of Q: the first component $'\sigma_{xy}/(\sigma_x\sigma_y)'$ is the coefficient of correlation between images, the reference image and the one whose quality factor is being measured. The second component $2\bar{x}\bar{y}/((\bar{x})^2 + (\bar{y})^2)$ is to measure the relation of luminance of both images. The third component $(2\sigma_x\sigma_y)/(\sigma_x^2 + \sigma_y^2)$ is the measurement of the similarity of contrast between two images.

To define an optimum range for illumination, NIR window is divided into four sub-bands and mean images are formed from the hyperspectral slices in these sub-bands. These images are analysed using the objective image quality measures. These are, MSE, PSNR and universal image quality index (Q) to define best wavelength range where the image quality is highest when compared to the mean reference image.

A mean NIR image (I_m) is created for each subject, by taking mean of the bands from 750 to 950 nm. This spans the whole NIR low absorption window. These mean NIR images serve as reference images since the contrast of these images is higher than the mean images obtained in other spectral regions. Moreover, the noise present in each band (of 2 nm), is minimum in the mean image due to the highly random nature of noise. Four sub-mean images are created by taking mean of the bands in the following ranges:

I_m = mean ($I(x, y,$ 750:950)
Image-1 = mean (I ($x, y,$ 750:800)
Image-2 = mean (I ($x, y,$ 800:850)
Image-3 = mean (I ($x, y,$ 850:900)
Image-4 = mean (I ($x, y,$ 900:950)

From the hyperspectral dataset, 12 subjects from each skin class were selected randomly. With the data from selected subjects, mean

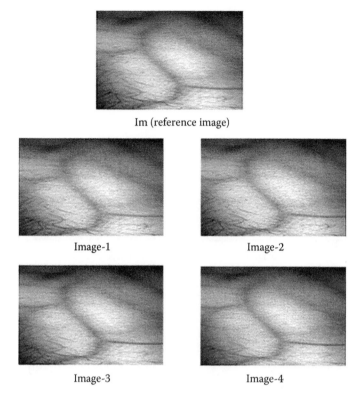

Im (reference image)

Image-1   Image-2

Image-3   Image-4

Figure 7.39 The reference image 'I_m' and four sub-mean images for fair skin subject.

reference image named as 'I_m' and four sub-mean images, named 'Image1–4', were created for the subjects of all four classes. Figures 7.39 through 7.42 depict reference images 'I_m' and four sub-mean images for a random subject among each skin class. These sub-mean images are then analysed with the reference of corresponding mean reference image 'I_m'.

In Figure 7.43, the mean value of MSE calculated for four sub-mean images for all 12 subjects of each class is plotted. In this plot, it can be observed that the MSE for the sub-mean image (Image-2), which was formed by taking mean in the range of 800–850 nm bands, has the lowest value of MSE for all skin classes. The fourth image (Image-4) which was formed by taking mean in the range of 900–950 nm bands has the highest MSE for all skin classes. Similarly, the PSNR value of Image-2 is highest for all skin classes. This suggests that the image formed with the wavelengths bands ranging from 800 to 850 nm has higher quality as compared to the other three sub-mean images. The mean PSNR value for all

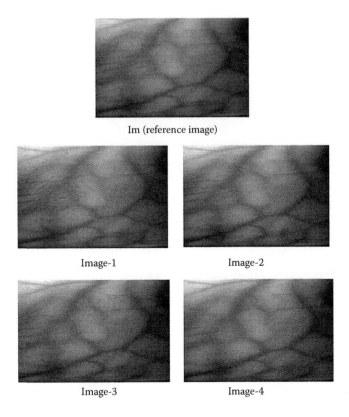

Im (reference image)

Image-1   Image-2

Image-3   Image-4

Figure 7.40 The reference image 'I_m' and four sub-mean images for light brown skin subject.

subjects of four sub-mean images for all 12 subjects of each class is plotted in Figure 7.44.

The quality analysis of sub-mean images is further performed with the help of universal image quality index (Q). It is an objective quality measure that is independent of viewing conditions. The results from the Q factor analysis are plotted in Figure 7.45. In this plot, the value of Q factor is highest for Image-2 as compared to the other three images in case of light brown, dark brown and dark skin tones. This indicates that the Image-2 has best quality as compared to the other three images. In case of fair skin, the Q factor is high for both Image-1 and Image-2 with a minor difference. In this case, the Q value for Image-1 is slightly higher than Image-2, but the difference is small, which does not lead to any conclusive remarks. Nevertheless, for the darker (than fair) skin tone classes, the Image-2 has best quality among all four sub-mean images. Furthermore, the overall results are consistent with the MSE and PSNR results, which indicate that the quality of Image-2 is highest among all four sub-mean images of NIR range.

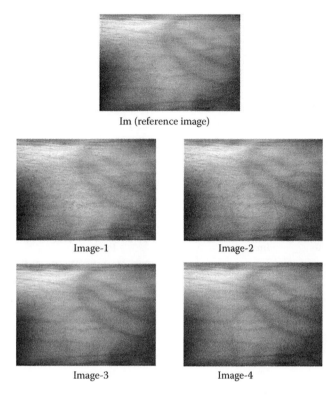

Im (reference image)

Image-1   Image-2

Image-3   Image-4

Figure 7.41 The reference image 'I_m' and four sub-mean images for dark brown skin subject.

Through this work, it is determined that the image (Image-2) which was created by taking mean of bands in the range 800–850 nm from hyperspectral data has the best quality among the other sub-mean images in NIR window. The parameters like MSE, PSNR and universal image quality (Q) was calculated. Keeping in mind the image acquisition setup explained in Section 1.3, it is concluded that the best-quality image is obtained in the spectral range of 800–850 nm. These findings serve the basis for defining optimized illumination for the prototype NIR system for subcutaneous veins localization. For this system, our choice was the LEDs with a central wavelength lying within 800–850 nm range.

7.5   Conclusion

IV catheterization is the first and probably the most important step in the majority of medical treatments especially for hospitalized patients. This is required to deliver immediate medication/nutrients to the patients,

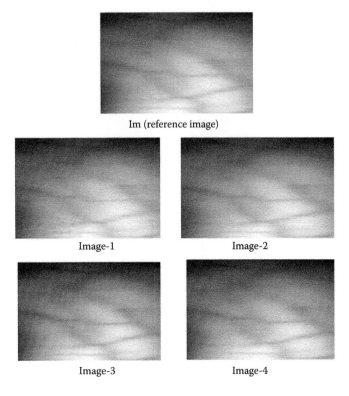

Figure 7.42 The reference image 'I_m' and four sub-mean images for dark skin subject.

anaesthesia and to draw blood for blood donation and laboratory examination purposes. Subcutaneous veins are used for IV catheterization and are localized either by sight and/or by feeling with the fingers by touching the targeted site of a patient's body. It is a difficult and challenging task to localize suitable vein in patients having the physiological characteristics like dark skin tone, deep veins and the presence of scars, tattoos or hair on skin. The error in suitable vein localization may lead to several complications including severe pain, hematoma, infiltration, veins rupture and multiple attempts. To overcome the problem of difficult venous access, several techniques can be used. NIR imaging is considered to be the most suitable among the techniques in terms of usability, cost and efficiency. This chapter focuses on the optimization of NIR illumination in order to overcome the difficulty of veins localization for different skin tone subjects. To achieve this objective, a hyperspectral data analysis is performed. Hyperspectral venous image data were acquired from 252 subjects. These data were later analysed with PCA and LDA. The hyperspectral

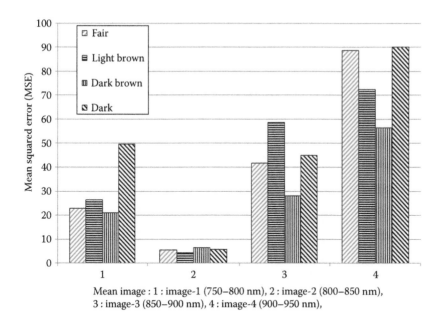

Figure 7.43 MSE plot for four sub-mean images of four skin classes.

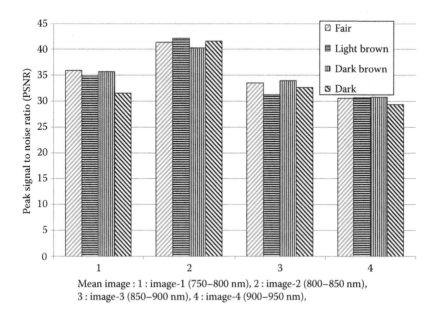

Figure 7.44 PSNR plot for four sub-mean images of four skin classes.

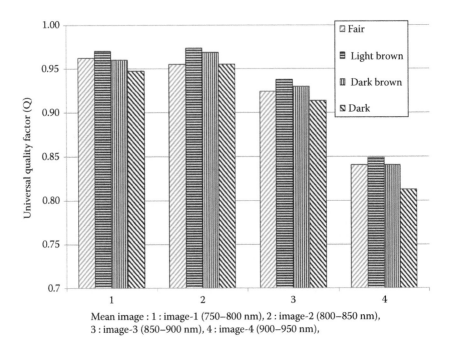

Mean image : 1 : image-1 (750–800 nm), 2 : image-2 (800–850 nm),
3 : image-3 (850–900 nm), 4 : image-4 (900–950 nm),

Figure 7.45 Q factor plot for four sub-mean images of four skin classes.

image quality assessment was performed with the parameters like MSE, PSNR and universal image quality index to define an optimized range of illumination wavelengths. It was concluded that the wavelength range of 800–850 nm is the optimum range for illumination in NIR imaging for all skin tone subjects. This conclusion was drawn from the assessment on the hyperspectral venous images of four different skin classes.

7.6   MATLAB code: PCA on 4 bands

```
clear all ; close all; clc
%   dataset_fair=[];
%   load('dataset_fair.mat');
load('wavelengths');
w = wavelengths(50:999);
w1 = w(535:610);
w2 = w(611:687);
w3 = w(688:761);
w4 = w(762:836);

load('file_name');
x=file_name;
```

```
x1=x(:,:,535:610);
[r1,c1,d1]=size(x1);


x2=x(:,:,611:687);
[r2,c2,d2]=size(x2);


x3=x(:,:,688:761);
[r3,c3,d3]=size(x3);


x4=x(:,:,762:836);
[r4,c4,d4]=size(x4);


X1=reshape(x1,(size(x1,1)*size(x1,2)),size(x1,3));
X2=reshape(x2,(size(x2,1)*size(x2,2)),size(x2,3));
X3=reshape(x3,(size(x3,1)*size(x3,2)),size(x3,3));
X4=reshape(x4,(size(x4,1)*size(x4,2)),size(x4,3));


[X_norm1, mu1, sigma1]  =  featureNormalize(X1);
[X_norm2, mu2, sigma2]  =  featureNormalize(X2);
[X_norm3, mu3, sigma3]  =  featureNormalize(X3);
[X_norm4, mu4, sigma4]  =  featureNormalize(X4);


[U1,  S1]  =  pca(X_norm1);
[U2,  S2]  =  pca(X_norm2);
[U3,  S3]  =  pca(X_norm3);
[U4,  S4]  =  pca(X_norm4);


Z1  =  projectData(X1, U1, 1);
Z2  =  projectData(X2, U2, 1);
Z3  =  projectData(X3, U3, 1);
Z4  =  projectData(X4, U4, 1);


Y1=reshape(Z1,r1,c1,1);  % reshaping data to original image form
Y2=reshape(Z2,r2,c2,1);
Y3=reshape(Z3,r3,c3,1);
Y4=reshape(Z4,r4,c4,1);


imwrite(mat2gray(-(Y1)),'I1.png');
imwrite(mat2gray(-(Y2)),'I2.png');
imwrite(mat2gray(-(Y3)),'I3.png');
imwrite(mat2gray(-(Y4)),'I4.png');
I1=imread('I1.png');
I2=imread('I2.png');
I3=imread('I3.png');
I4=imread('I4.png');
format compact;
```

```
I=mean(x(:,:,535:836),3);
[mssim1,ssimmap]=ssim(I,I1);
[mssim2,ssimmap]=ssim(I,I2);
[mssim3,ssimmap]=ssim(I,I3);
[mssim4,ssimmap]=ssim(I,I4);

name_ui=sprintf('%d',mssim1)
mssim1
mssim2
mssim3
mssim4

figure(1);
subplot(221);imshow(I1);title(['SSIM = ' num2str(mssim1)]);
subplot(222);imshow(I2);title(['SSIM = ' num2str(mssim2)]);
subplot(223);imshow(I3);title(['SSIM = ' num2str(mssim3)]);
subplot(224);imshow(I4);title(['SSIM = ' num2str(mssim4)]);
```

FUNCTION FEATURE NORMALIZE:

```
function [X_norm, mu, sigma] = featureNormalize(X)
%FEATURENORMALIZE Normalizes the features in X
% FEATURENORMALIZE(X) returns a normalized version of X where
% the mean value of each feature is 0 and the standard deviation
% is 1. This is often a good preprocessing step to do when
% working with learning algorithms.
mu = mean(X);
X_norm = bsxfun(@minus, X, mu);
sigma = std(X_norm);
X_norm = bsxfun(@rdivide, X_norm, sigma);
end
```

FUNCTION PCA:

```
function [U, S] = pca(X)
%PCA Run principal component analysis on the dataset X
% [U, S, X] = pca(X) computes eigenvectors of the
  covariance matrix of X
% Returns the eigenvectors U, the eigenvalues (on diagonal) in S
% Useful values
[m, n] = size(X);
% You need to return the following variables correctly.
U = zeros(n);
S = zeros(n);
% Instructions: You should first compute the covariance
  matrix. Then, you
%         should use the "svd" function to compute the
          eigenvectors
%         and eigenvalues of the covariance matrix.
```

```
% Note: When computing the covariance matrix, remember to
   divide by m (the
%    number of examples).
sigma=(X'*X)/size(X,1); %finding covariance
[U,S,V]=svd(sigma);
end
```

FUNCTION PROJECT DATA:

```
function Z = projectData(X, U, K)
% PROJECTDATA Computes the reduced data representation when
   projecting only
% on to the top k eigenvectors
% Z = projectData(X, U, K) computes the projection of
% the normalized inputs X into the reduced dimensional space
   spanned by
% the first K columns of U. It returns the projected
   examples in Z.
% You need to return the following variables correctly.
Z = zeros(size(X, 1), K);
% Instructions: Compute the projection of the data using
   only the top K
%      eigenvectors in U (first K columns).
%      For the i-th example X(i,:), the projection on to the
       k-th
%      eigenvector is given as follows:
%         x = X(i, :)';
%         projection_k = x' * U(:, k);
Ureduce=U(:,1:K);
Z=X*Ureduce;
end
```

References

1. *Anatomy and Physiology of the Cardiovascualr System*, Jones and Bartlett Publishers, 2008.
2. M. D. Ezekowitz, *Peripharal Vascular Disease, Heart Book*, Yale University School of Medicine, London, UK: Academic Press, 1992.
3. P. Hignell, Peripheral Intravenous Initiation, Self Learning Module. *FH Vascular Access Regional Shared Work Team*, New Jersey: Wiley Online Library, 2012.
4. A. Noordergraaf, *Circulatory System Dynamics*, vol. 1: Elsevier, 2012.
5. W. Aird, Spatial and temporal dynamics of the endothelium, *J Thromb Haemost*, vol. 3, pp. 1392–1406, 2005.
6. A. Kienle, L. Lilge, I. A. Vitkin, M. S. Patterson, B. C. Wilson, R. Hibst et al., Why do veins appear blue? A new look at an old question, *Appl Opt*, vol. 35, p. 1151, 1996.
7. N. E. Soifer, S. Borzak B. R. Edlin and R. A. Weinstein, Prevention of peripheral venous catheter complications with an intravenous therapy team: A randomized controlled trial, *Arch Intern Med*, vol. 158, pp. 473–477, 1998.

8. A. F. Jacobson and E. H. Winslow, Variables influencing intravenous catheter insertion difficulty and failure: An analysis of 339 intravenous catheter insertions, *Heart & Lung: The Journal of Acute and Critical Care*, vol. 34, pp. 345–359, 2005.

9. A. Rivera, K. Strauss, A. van Zundert and E. Mortier, Matching the peripheral intravenous catheter to the individual patient, *Acta Anæsthesiologica Belgica*, vol. 58, p. 19, 2006.

10. D. Mbamalu and A. Banerjee, Methods of obtaining peripheral venous access in difficult situations, *Postgrad Med J*, vol. 75, pp. 459–462, 1999.

11. D. Rauch, D. Dowd, D. Eldridge, S. Mace, G. Schears and K. Yen, Peripheral difficult venous access in children, *Clinical Pediatrics*, vol. 48, pp. 895–901, 2009.

12. A. J. Barton, G. Danek, P. Johns and M. Coons, Improving patient outcomes through CQI: Vascular access planning, *J Nurs Care Qual*, vol. 13, pp. 77–85, 1998.

13. A. Sabri, J. Szalas, K. S. Holmes, L. Labib and T. Mussivand, Failed attempts and improvement strategies in peripheral intravenous catheterization, *Bio-Med Mater Eng*, vol. 23, pp. 93–108, 2013.

14. R. Bergman, Intra venous blood sampling, January 2014. *[Online] Available:* http://www.anatomyatlases.org/firstaid/DrawingBlood.shtml

15. L. Hadaway, Infiltration and extravasation, *AJN The American Journal of Nursing*, vol. 107, pp. 64–72, 2007.

16. M. Haimov, Vascular access for hemodialysis, *Surgery, Gynecology & Obstetrics*, vol. 141, pp. 619–625, 1975.

17. Intravenous Access, Clinical Essentials, Paramedic Care, *December 2014, [Online]. Available:* http://what-when-how.com/paramedic-care/intravenous-access-clinical-essentials-paramedic-care-part-5/

18. E. A. Cummings, G. J. Reid, G. A. Finley, P. J. McGrath and J. A. Ritchie, Prevalence and source of pain in pediatric inpatients, *Pain*, vol. 68, pp. 25–31, 1996.

19. K. A. Burling and P. J. Collipp, Emotional responses of hospitalized children results of a pulse-monitor study, *Clinical Pediatrics*, vol. 8, pp. 641–646, 1969.

20. J. Pector, Vascular access problems, *Support Care Cancer*, vol. 6, pp. 20–22, 1997.

21. F. Scholkmann, S. Kleiser, A. J. Metz, R. Zimmermann, J. M. Pavia, U. Wolf and M. Wolf, A review on continuous wave functional near-infrared spectroscopy and imaging instrumentation and methodology, *Neuroimage*, vol 85, (Part 1), pp. 6–27, 2014.

22. A. Shahzad, N. M. Saad, N. Walter, A. S. Malik and F. Meriaudeau. A review on subcutaneous veins localization using imaging techniques. *Current Medical Imaging Reviews* 10 (2), 125–133, 2014.

23. J. Freeman, F. Downs, L. Marcucci, E. N. Lewis, B. Blume and J. Rish, Multispectral and hyperspectral imaging: Applications for medical and surgical diagnostics, in Engineering in Medicine and Biology Society, 1997. *Proceedings of the 19th Annual International Conference of the IEEE*, Chicago, IL: IEEE Engineering in Medicine and Biology Society, 1997, vol. 2, pp. 700–701.

24. C.-I. Chang, *Hyperspectral Data Exploitation: Theory and Applications.* New Jersey: John Wiley & Sons, Inc., 2007.

25. G. Lu and B. Fei, Medical hyperspectral imaging: A review, *J Biomed Opt*, vol. 19, pp. 010901–010901, 2014.

26. A. F. M. Hani, E. Prakasa, H. Nugroho and V. S. Asirvadam, Implementation of fuzzy c-means clustering for psoriasis assessment on lesion erythema, in *Industrial Electronics and Applications (ISIEA), 2012 IEEE Symposium on*, New York: ACM, 2012, pp. 331–335.

27. A. K. Jain, M. N. Murty and P. J. Flynn, Data clustering: A review, *ACM Computing Surveys (CSUR)*, vol. 31, pp. 264–323, 1999.

28. R. Xu and D. C. Wunsch, Clustering algorithms in biomedical research: A review, *Biomedical Engineering, IEEE Reviews in*, vol. 3, pp. 120–154, 2010.

29. S. S. Halli and K. V. Rao, *Advanced Techniques of Population Analysis*. New York: Springer, 1992.

30. J. R. Hauser, *Numerical Methods for Nonlinear Engineering Models*. New York: Springer, 2009.

31. S. Arlinghaus, *Practical Handbook of Curve Fitting*. London: CRC Press, 1994.

32. H. Akima, A new method of interpolation and smooth curve fitting based on local procedures, *Journal of the ACM (JACM)*, vol. 17, pp. 589–602, 1970.

33. H. Motulsky and A. Christopoulos, *Fitting Models to Biological Data Using Linear and Nonlinear Regression: A Practical Guide to Curve Fitting*. Oxford, UK: Oxford University Press, 2004.

34. I. Jolliffe, *Principal Component Analysis*. New Jersey: Wiley Online Library, 2005.

35. H. Hotelling, Analysis of a complex of statistical variables into principal components, *Journal of Educational Psychology*, vol. 24, p. 417, 1933.

36. S. Yan, D. Xu, B. Zhang, H.-J. Zhang, Q. Yang and S. Lin, Graph embedding and extensions: A general framework for dimensionality reduction, *Pattern Analysis and Machine Intelligence, IEEE Transactions on*, vol. 29, pp. 40–51, 2007.

37. A. R. Webb, *Statistical Pattern Recognition*. Chichester, Hoboken, NJ: John Wiley & Sons, 2003.

38. V. Zharov, S. Ferguson, J. Eidt, P. Howard, L. Fink and M. Waner, Infrared imaging of subcutaneous veins, *Lasers Surg Med* 34(1), pp. 56–61, 2004.

39. Z. Wang, A. C. Bovik, H. R. Sheikh and E. P. Simoncelli, Image quality assessment: From error visibility to structural similarity, *Image Processing, IEEE Transactions on*, vol. 13, pp. 600–612, 2004.

40. M. Li and B. Yuan, 2D-LDA: A statistical linear discriminant analysis for image matrix, *Pattern Recognit Lett*, vol. 26, pp. 527–532, 2005.

41. K. Fukunaga, *Introduction to Statistical Pattern Recognition*. Amsterdam, Netherlands: Academic Press, 1990.

42. M. Welling, *Fisher Linear Discriminant Analysis*, vol. 3. Department of Computer Science, University of Toronto, Amsterdam, Netherlands: Elsevier, 2005.

43. V. P. Zharov, S. Ferguson, J. F. Eidt, P. C. Howard, L. M. Fink and M. Waner, Infrared imaging of subcutaneous veins, *Lasers Surg Med*, vol. 34, pp. 56–61, 2004.

44. H. D. Zeman, G. Lovhoiden, C. Vrancken, J. Snodgrass and J. A. DeLong, Projection of subsurface structure onto an object's surface, Google Patents, 2011.

45. L. Wang, G. Leedham and S.-Y. Cho, Infrared imaging of hand vein patterns for biometric purposes, *IET Comput Vis*, vol. 1, pp. 113–122, 2007.

46. Veebot, Robotic phlebotomist, November 2013. *[Online]. Available:* http://www.veebot.com/overview.html

47. Z. Wang and A. Bovik, *Modern Image Quality Assessment (Synthesis Lectures on Image, Video, and Multimedia Processing)*. San Rafael, CA: *Morgan Claypool*, 2006.
48. Z. Wang and A. C. Bovik, A universal image quality index, *Signal Processing Letters, IEEE*, vol. 9, pp. 81–84, 2002.
49. Z. Wang and A. C. Bovik, Mean squared error: Love it or leave it? A new look at signal fidelity measures, *Signal Processing Magazine, IEEE*, vol. 26, pp. 98–117, 2009.
50. Z. Wang, A. C. Bovik and L. Lu, Why is image quality assessment so difficult?, in *Acoustics, Speech, and Signal Processing (ICASSP), 2002 IEEE International Conference on*, IEEE, 2002, pp. IV-3313–IV-3316.

Index

Printed and bound by CPI Group (UK) Ltd, Croydon, CR0 4YY

01/11/2024

01782619-0014